D1731251

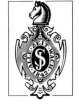

Current Concepts
of External Fixation
# of Fractures

Edited by Hans K. Uhthoff

Associate Editor Elvira Stahl

With 227 Figures

Springer-Verlag
Berlin Heidelberg New York 1982

Editor:
Hans K. Uhthoff, MD, FRCS (C)
Prof. and Head, Division of Orthopaedics
Faculty of Medicine of the University of Ottawa, Canada

Associate Editor:
Elvira Stahl, BA, FAAAS, FAMWA
2021 Atwater, Suite 1610
Montréal, Qué. H3H 2P2, Canada

ISBN 3-540-11314-2 Springer Verlag Berlin Heidelberg New York
ISBN 0-387-11314-2 Springer Verlag New York Heidelberg Berlin

Library of Congress Cataloging in Publication Data
Main entry under title: Current concepts of external fixation of fractures. Bibliogra-
phy: p. Includes index. 1. Fracture fixation. I. Uhthoff, Hans K., 1925–. II. Stahl,
Elvira. III. Title: External fixation of fractures. [DNLM: 1. Fracture fixation –
Methods – Congresses. WE 185 C975 1981]
RD101.C89 617'.15 82-5442
ISBN 0-387-11314-2 (U.S.) AACR2

Printing and bookbinding: Konrad Triltsch, Graphischer Betrieb,
D-8700 Würzburg

2124/3130-543210

Preface

External fixation is now being used widely to maintain fractures, osteotomies, and arthrodeses in a desired position during consolidation.

Whereas external fixation has been readily accepted in European countries, its use has weathered a rather stormy course in North America, especially in the treatment of fractures. Only recently has external fixation found its rightful place on this continent as well.

Many different models are on the market today, and the practitioner is faced with a difficult decision in selecting a model. Should he buy a system where the fracture has to be reduced first, or should he work with a device permitting a reduction after insertion of the pins? To enable surgeons to study the different systems, to discuss their advantages and disadvantages, and to permit them to put their hands on these devices and inspect them personally, the Division of Orthopedic Surgery, University of Ottawa organized an applied basic science course in May 1981, External Fixation of Fractures. During this course, all major systems were presented to the participants. As happened during the course "Internal Fixation of Fractures" held two years ago, the rigidity of internal fixation was frequently and intensively debated. Whereas the rigidity of internal fixation cannot be altered during the course of healing, the rigidity of external fixation can be changed. In fact, with progression of union, rods of increasing elasticity can be used.

The indications for external fixation are now firmly established, the successful treatment of infected fractures and pseudarthroses meriting special attention.

In view of the active interest shown in this subject, we are not only publishing here all the studies presented in Ottawa last May, but also papers describing the operative techniques of the various systems.

I am most grateful to all the contributors whose cooperation has made an early publication of this book possible. I should also like to thank Dr. Heinz Götze, of the Springer-Verlag, for his support and assistance.

My sincerest thanks to Mrs. Elvira Stahl. Without her devotion and untiring work this book could not have been produced.

Hans K. Uhthoff
University of Ottawa
Ottawa, Canada

Contents

X

External Fixation:
Biomechanical Considerations and Analysis of Components

R. Kleining

In recent years external fixation has undergone an impressive renaissance.
The great number of publications shows clearly, however, that problems of
stability have not yet been completely solved.

First of all, we must distinguish external fixation under a condition of
bone support from that of no bone support. The latter can be termed bridging
external fixation. The ability of a particular system to impart stability
is truly put to the test when interfragmentary compression cannot be obtained.

The only clinically relevant variables for ability to stabilize are the displacements of the fragment ends under load. We measure these displacements
in a three-dimensional system (Fig. 1) and rate the fixator according to
their magnitude - the greater the displacements, the less rigid the system.

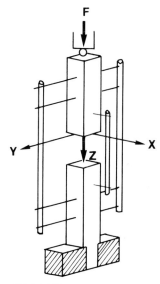

**AXIALLY LOADED
BONE MODEL**

Fig. 1. Axially-loaded bone model; x, y and z
are directions of displacements; F = applied
force.

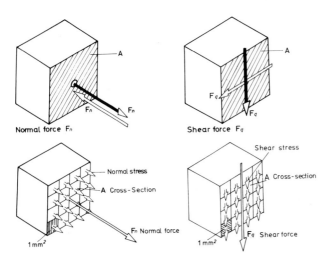

Fig. 2. Schematic representation of compressive, tensile and shear stresses in the cross section.

It is well known that of the five kinds of stresses (Fig. 2, 3) shear stresses do the greatest harm to the process of bone consolidation. Tensile stresses promote the formation of fibrous tissue, and compression per se seems not to influence bone healing. Of course, interfragmentary compression brings stability and allows bone union to result from the normal remodelling process of all living bone. To date, we have no objective and clinically relevant basis to determine exactly how much rigidity is necessary or even desired.

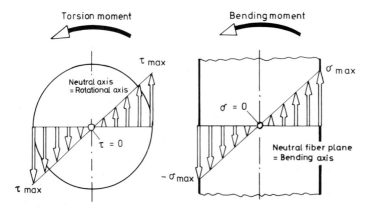

Fig. 3. Schematic representation of bending and torsion stresses in the cross section.

I would go so far as to say that external fixation is not directed at the bones themselves but at the condition of the soft tissues and at the risk or presence of infection. Every new development must fulfill three requirements:

1. The endangered area, bone and soft tissue, must be spared additional surgical trauma and the presence of foreign material.

2. An adequate immobilization must be achieved to lower the risk of infection in open fractures or to allow resolution of established infection in fractures or nonunions.

3. The application of the system must be simple.

Each analysis of rigidity must include the various responsible factors. Instabilities are always the result of deformation of all the elements under load. Stiffness is defined as the product of elastic modulus and moment of inertia divided by the length of the element. For calculations of rigidity the relationship between stress and strain is essential. By pulling on a rubber band we increase the stress and observe at the same time an elongation which we call the strain. Strain is the change in length (Δl) divided by the original or resting length (Fig. 4).

One can also say that each material has a specific relationship between stress and strain. In practice, the elastic region of the stress-strain curve is important. In this region, the curve is linear because the relationship between stress and strain is constant. The moment of inertia is a purely geometric value, that is to say, it is the result of dimensions only and has nothing to do with the kind of material used to construct the

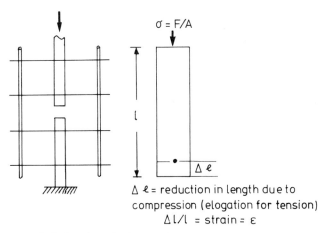

$\sigma = F/A$

$\Delta \ell$ = reduction in length due to compression (elogation for tension)
$\Delta l / l$ = strain = ε

Axially-loaded specimen

Fig. 4. Formulae for the most important mechanical relationships (axis designations are consistent with Fig. 1). δ = stress; F = force.

element. To determine a moment of inertia, one first identifies a neutral axis about which the element will be bent or twisted. The moment of inertia is the sum of the products of each bit of cross-sectional area multiplied by the square of its distance from the neutral axis.

The moment of inertia divided by the distance from the neutral axis to the most distant fiber is the moment of resistance. This moment of resistance is normally used in respect to both axes (x and y) which lie in the cross section. The moment of resistance is, like the moment of inertia, a purely geometric value which depends on the profile of the element.

An example can clarify this:

Your flat program can be easily bent. Rolled into a tube, the same cross-sectional area has a much greater resistance to bending. Knowledge of these concepts (Table I) is important for two reasons:

1. Potential weak points in fixators can be avoided through modification of the element profiles.

2. Bone defects at points of anchorage can be controlled both in size and position to maintain adequate bone strength.

Table I.

$$\sigma = \frac{F}{A} \quad \text{or} \quad \sigma = \frac{M}{W}$$

$$\frac{\sigma}{\varepsilon} = E = \text{const.}$$

$$I_y = \Sigma x^2 \, \Delta A$$

$$W_y = \frac{I_y}{e_y}$$

$$\text{STIFFNESS} = \frac{E \cdot I}{l}$$

For investigations into the properties of existing assemblies or for research on new external fixators, the various instability factors must be kept in mind. We may list the following (Table II):

Table II.

INSTABILITY FACTORS

1. BONE
2. NAILS, SCREWS
3. BINDING CLAMPS
4. CONNECTING BARS

1. Bone

The connection between nail or screw and bone must avoid two pitfalls. Pins
or screws which are too thin may, under load, cut through the bone, especially in the metaphysis. Pins or screws which are too big create a material
defect which may lead to fracture. This is the effect of loss of moment of
inertia or resistance. Clinical experience shows us that a diameter of 5 mm
(for the tibia) approaches the critical limit of size. We cannot increase
stability of the whole system by using pins which make greater defects in
the bone.

2. Pins and screws

In all common assemblies, pins or screws are deformed mainly be bending.
According to mechanical rules, the smallest deformations are seen as the
result of compression or tension. To minimize deformation to the smallest
theoretically obtainable, one would have to build a framework where joints
within the pins would transmit only tension or compression while eliminating the bending moments. Unfortunately, such a pin would be impractical.
An alternative method to increase pin stiffness is to prestress the pins
one to another within a single fragment. This is practicable and our
previous investigations showed a decrease of fragment displacement in the
long axis under load. Obviously, the longer the distance from one point
of support to the other, the less stiff the pin; the frame should be as
narrow as possible.

3. Binding clamps

Binding clamps should eliminate all modes of displacement, linear and
rotational. In a three-dimensional system that means control of 6° of
freedom: three linear and three rotational.

Both the AO and the Hoffmann fixators use friction to hold pins to binding
clamps. The Hoffmann clamps give (for a given torque on the set screw of
the binding clamp itself) more control of the pins than do the AO binding
clamps.

4. Connecting bars

It is clear that long connecting bars will more easily deflect sidewards under axial load than will short ones and that thin ones will bend more easily than the thick. Also, the profile of the connecting bar affects its stiffness. The AO traded its threaded bar for a tube to gain the advantage of a more efficient section.

In conclusion, efforts to improve the state of external fixation must be pursued with regard for biomechanical principles, limitations of materials on the one hand and biologic behavior on the other.

External fixation does not represent a concept in competition with internal fixation and traditional closed methods of treatment, but rather a modality for certain high risk and difficult clinical situations.

Biomechanical Studies of External Fixation: Clinical Application of Animal Studies

J. Hellinger and G. Mayer

The stabilization of a damaged or diseased joint segment with few metallic implants is a definite advantage of external fixation compared with methods using nails, screws, or plates.

Apart from clinical empirical reports, the problems of the mechanical strength of the external pressure osteosyntheses were rarely considered within the realm of basic research. Moreover, to date, no conclusive studies have been undertaken on the biomechanical aspects and dynamics of healing of fractures treated with compression-distraction apparatuses for compressive fragment fixation.

For this reason we investigated the stability characteristics of pressure osteosyntheses with different external compression-distraction sets both in biomechanical model tests and in animal experiments. The following compression-distraction apparatuses were available for the biomechanical model tests:

- the external fixator of the Swiss AO group
- the compression-distraction apparatus according to Hellinger-Hoffmann
- the compression-distraction apparatus according to Ilisarov
- the external fixator according to Hoffmann (double frame mounting according to Vidal)
- the compression-distraction apparatus according to Wagner
- the clamp fixator according to Hoffmann-Vidal.

A total of 13 different mounting forms were set up and tested with these basic models, giving us over 10,000 experimental results.

Sixty-seven isolated tibiae from cadavers, osteotomized in the middle of the diaphyses, were used as fracture models.

The strength of the bone-frame unit is dependent on:

1) the prestressing of the apparatus. It results from the tensile forces in the external rods produced by means of the torques at the threaded spindles.

2) the stiffness of the external rods and on the transfixing pins used for the load transmission on the bone

3) the elastic deformation of the bone

4) the amount of tension at the bone-pin interface, the critical values of which must not exceed the absolute axial pressure weight bearing capacity of bone whose lower limits are between 50 N/mm^2 and 150 N/mm^2.

The generated pressure is maintained by the elastic deformation of the bone fragments to be joined and the external mounting systems. Thus, the stability of the osteosynthesis against bending is secured and torsion is prevented by means of frictional powers through the interfragmental compression. Exact biomechanical stability testing is not possible without knowledge of the amount of pressure present in the osteotomy gap (Fig. 1).

The direct load measurements performed with strain gauges in the osteotomy gap revealed that the maximal values of deformation of the mountings differed widely from one set to another with an initial decrease in pressure due to the viscoelasticity of the bone.

The bending in sagittal and frontal planes was measured with wire strain gauges, whereas the torsional displacement of the bone fragments under rotational load was measured by means of arms with dial indicators of a high resolution.

Because of different resistance moments in the sagittal and frontal planes, different bending stability values were obtained for both load directions.

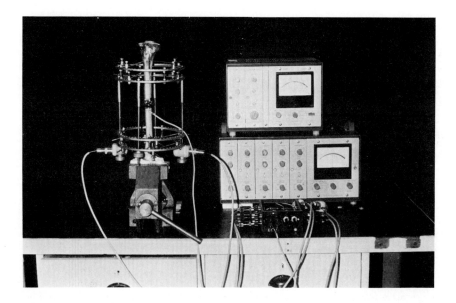

Fig. 1. Example of set-up for measurement in case of combined direct and indirect interfragmentary pressure by means of a double ring device and axial pressure load.

For a clear and efficient optical comparison, the resulting biomechanical characteristics were presented in the form of graphs for the double-sided and one-sided compression-distraction apparatuses.

The wide area occupied by the pin-fixed sets provides the basis for their efficiency. In the Hoffmann-Vidal double frame construction, optimal initial compressive values are obtained while bending at the pin level.

The advantages of the external fixator of the AO group and the wire-fixed compression-distraction apparatuses are in the production of high stability-securing tension loads, whereas the double frame construction distinguishes itself by high initial compression values. The same stability characteristics against bending and torsion load can be found in the wire-fixed apparatuses.

The triangular mountings of the external fixator surpassed all the other apparatuses. Therefore, a sufficient stability is secured with this setup, also in the presence of low prestressing forces.

Animal experiments with compression-distraction apparatuses performed in 27 sheep revealed stable osteosyntheses with roentgenologically demonstrable healing by primary intention. Moreover, interfragmentary compression was maintained for a long time. It dropped gradually within eight weeks from 40 to 50% of its initial value. About 20% of the total pressure losses result from the viscoelastic deformation of the bone, reaching its peak during the first postoperative days.

Strikingly, great pressure losses in the initial phase are due to the visco-elastic behavior of bone, to the technique of application of the apparatus, and to pressure deformation in the area of the osteotomy. Furthermore, initial loss of reduction as a result of full weight bearing immediately after the operation is also responsible for these losses.

The remaining portion of the pressure reduction must be attributed to the ossification in the area of the osteotomy since the newly-formed bone has a lower elastic pressure deformation. Greater losses of pressure at later stages are probably due to notching effects.

Roentgenologically, the typical signs of healing by primary intention were found where stability could be maintained.

Contrary to stable fixation, unstable fixation showed significantly quicker and greater pressure losses dependent on the range of instability of the compression-distraction apparatuses. Nevertheless, apart from minimal instability, the pressure contact remained stable for eight weeks as the diagram reveals. Only in the presence of gross positional changes did the interfragmental pressure drop relatively quickly to the zero-value. In such cases, fracture consolidation occurred by second intention, roentgeno-logically evident by the formation of a typical temporary callus (Fig. 2, 3, 4).

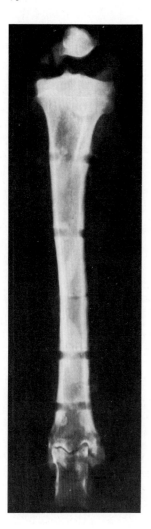

Fig. 2. Roentgenogram of sheep tibiae with primary bone healing of osteotomy by means of the Hoffmann-Vidal device, showing biomechanical stability.

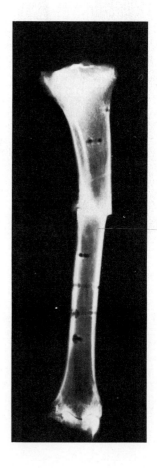

Fig. 3. Roentgenogram of sheep tibiae with mixed primary and secondary bone healing by means of the double ring device in a case of limited loss of biomechanical stability. Character- istics of fracture healing comparable to clinical results obtained by Burny. Histologically no soft tissue elements were seen in osteotomy gap.

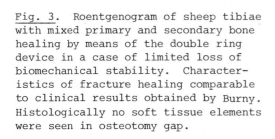

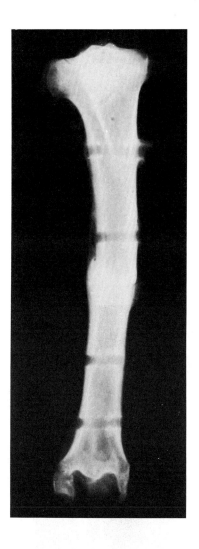

Fig. 4. Roentgenogram of sheep tibiae with secondary bone healing by means of AO-frame-fixator in the case of loss of biomechanical stability.

Histomorphologic investigations revealed that bone healing by first inten-tion had occurred under absolutely stable conditions of fixation in four osteotomies. Healing proceeded, according to the pattern of gap healing, by filling the fracture gap first with fibrous bone and later by depositing lamellar bones parallel to the longitudinal axis. Histologic sections regularly revealed that the interfragmentary filling with newly-formed fibrous and lamellar bone was dependent on the size of the fracture gap. Since osteotomies were performed with oscillating saws, broad gaps occurred causing a delay of osseous bridging. Richly vascularized loose connective tissue was found in incompletely ossified gaps which persisted until the end of the experiments. Narrow fracture gaps whose width were less than 500 µg were the only exception. Despite the existing high interfragmentary compression, no bone resorption of the cortices occurred at either end.

On the other hand, resorptive areas and more periosteal and endosteal callus formation were always observed in insignificantly or initially unstable osteosyntheses. The identification of resorptive processes was therefore a histologic criterion of instability.

Long-term results revealed that under stable conditions loss of interfragmentary compression was minimal, identical to results obtained with internal fixation. Furthermore, the curve characteristic for compression forces and their loss were nearly identical.

Based on these experimental investigations, we have successfully accomplished external fixation procedures in 213 patients up to the present time. The following two case histories demonstrate our clinical experiences with external fixation.

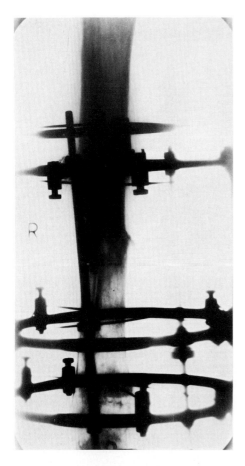

Fig. 5. Roentgenogram of the right tibia with Küntscher nail and oligotrophic pseudarthrosis.

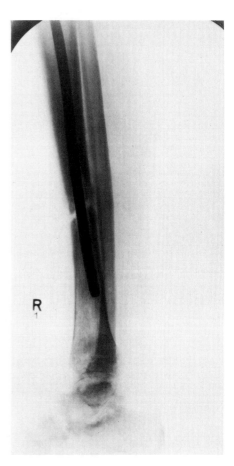

Fig. 6. Consolidation by gap healing.

A 46-year old man suffered from a missile fracture in the left tibia with a mixed infection and an oligotrophic pseudarthrosis. After the application of a wire-fixed compression-distraction apparatus, the pseudarthrosis healed by first intention through gap healing despite severe initial trauma. We attribute the healing to the double ring mounting which gave high stability (Fig. 5, 6).

A 39-year-old woman had a ski accident. The plating was delayed and was inadequate, causing a septic nonunion. After an autogenous cancellous bone graft, irrigation suction drainage, electrical stimulation in the presence of an external fixator according to Hoffmann-Vidal, a quick, callus-free consolidation of the infected pseudarthrosis occurred with a nonirritant settling of the spongiosa. Also, in this case, the healing was secured by the high stability of the double-frame mounting.

A Classification of External Fixators

F. Behrens

Every year since 1974, two to three new external fixators have appeared
on the market. While most of these fixators have similar components,
the absence of a universally applicable classification has prevented a
critical comparison of the advantages and limitations of these devices.
In the proposed classification, the basic structure of the fixators and
the ease of adjustability are used as principal criteria of distinction.

Structurally, we differentiate between pin fixators and ring fixators.

Pin Fixators

Rigid bone-holding pins, in the form of half pins or transfixion pins,
and one or more longitudinal rods form the principal structural components of these frames (Fig. 1).

The type of articulation used to connect pins and rods determines the
frame adjustability and separates simple pin fixators from modular pin
fixators.

Simple pin fixators

Each bone-holding pin is directly and independently connected to a longitudinal rod (Fig. 2).

Advantages

   i. Within the plane of pin insertion, each pin can be placed at the
       most desirable angle to the bone.

   ii. The distance between two pins in a bony fragment can be freely chosen.
       This permits considerable variability in frame geometry and rigidity.

Disadvantages

   i. The fracture fragments must be reduced before the fixator is applied.
       The ability to make subsequent adjustments depends on the design of
       the articulations. Adjustments are generally only possible in four
       or less - out of a possible six - dimensions.

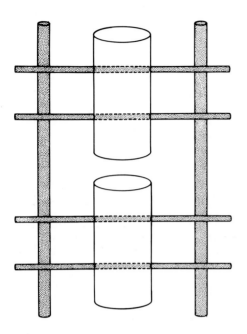

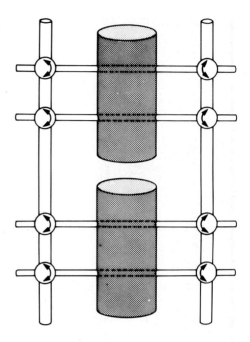

Fig. 1. Pin fixator. Bone-holding pins and longitudinal rod form the principal parts of the structure.

Fig. 2. Simple pin fixator. Each bone-holding pin is connected to a longitudinal rod over an independent clamp.

Examples of simple fixators

Denham, Murry, Oxford, Sukhtian-Hughes, Roger Anderson, Wagner leg lengthening device, ASIF "tubular" (Fig. 3).

Modular pin fixators

All bone-holding pins inserted into a bony fragment are held by one clamp which, over a universal joint, is connected to a longitudinal rod (Fig. 4).

Advantages

i. Loosening of the universal joints permits adjustments in alignment in six dimensions (translation: 3; rotation: 3).

Disadvantages

i. To provide the universal clamps with a firm grip, the bone-holding pins of each bony fragment must be inserted in the same plane and, for most modular fixators, parallel to each other. These requirements may prevent optimal pin placement and preclude the variability in frame geometry and frame rigidity possible with single pin fixators.

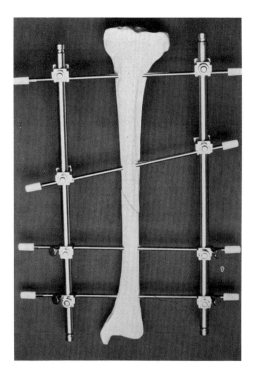

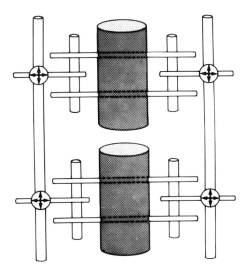

Fig. 4. Modular pin fixator. Universal joints connect pins and longitudinal rods.

Fig. 3. ASIF "tubular" fixator mounted as a bilateral frame.

Examples of modular fixators

Hoffmann (Fig. 5), ICLH, Kronner 4-bar frame.

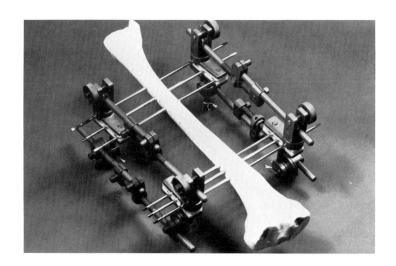

Fig. 5. Hoffmann fixator mounted as a bilateral frame.

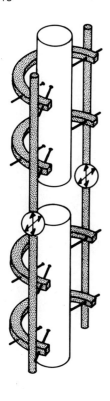

Fig. 6. Ring fixator. Circular elements and longitudinal rods form the principal parts of the frame structure.

Ring Fixators

The principal structural components of these frames (Fig. 6) are circular (rings, part-rings) elements and longitudinal rods. The bone-holding pins are not a part of the frame structure. They have the sole purpose of connecting the bony fragments to the circular elements.

Advantages

   i.   Alignment adjustments in six dimensions.

  ii.   As the bone-holding pins are not necessary parts of the frame structure they can be replaced by Kirschner wires under tension (Volkov-Oganesian, Ilisarov).

iii.   Bone-holding pins can be inserted along a circumference of 360° without complicating the frame design.

Disadvantages

i. These frames take up considerable space and limit wound access.

Examples of ring fixators

Volkov-Oganesian, Ilisarov, Ace-Fischer, Kronner circular frame.

Acknowledgments

Supported by Grant #8263 from the Medical Education and Research Foundation of St. Paul-Ramsey Medical Center, St. Paul, Minnesota.

How Stable Should External Fixation Be?

V. Mooney and B. Claudi

The simple answer on how stable should external fixation be is, "more at first". Unquestionably, initial rigid fixation has the most positive influence on the first efforts of both hard and soft tissue healing. The two questions that must be resolved, however, are how long should this rigid fixation be maintained? What are the principles necessary to achieve and maintain rigid fixation? Actually, in practice, the most critical question is - in the living, functioning human how do we maintain rigid stabilization of the fracture for as long as necessary to achieve the desired result?

The history of external fixation revolves around stability. Unfortunately, this history, at least in America, started off on a note of deceptive simplicity. "An Automatic Method of Treatment for Fractures of the Tibia and Fibula" was the title of Roger Anderson's system for fracture fixation introduced in 1934 (Anderson, 1934). It looked so easy and made so much sense that it appeared as if anyone could handle this method. Certainly, in the care of animal fractures, it offered significant advantages over open surgery and is still being used today as a viable method for fracture care in a half-pin system known as K-splints (Stader, 1937). The enthusiasm was short-lived due to the rapid development of instability even in the case of simple fractures using the Anderson device. The chronic drainage from the pins which developed as they loosened was labeled as Seattle serum - Anderson's home city. The Surgeon General ordered all Roger Anderson fixation devices to be thrown out in 1943 because of the wave of disasters related to their care. It should be pointed out that the clinicians at that time considered this system as so foolproof that they often encouraged their patients treated with external fixation to proceed to the sports field the following day and to return to active physical activity, including soccer (Nickel, 1943). Even Hoffmann's original design, although initially successful, had such a high complication rate that the innovator could not advocate its use (Hoffmann, 1938). Since this conference is being held largely to commemorate the success of external fixation in its varied clinical applications, something must have changed. Has our understanding of the principles improved since the original innovations four decades ago?

First, the indications for external fixation have greatly narrowed except in veterinary medicine (Brinker, 1975). The ideal application seems to be in settings where closed reduction and external support, or open reduction and internal fixation, are ill-advised. Thus, severely comminuted open fractures seem to be the ideal location except the initial care in pelvic fractures.

With that background, let us look at the requirements for an external fixation system. How important is stability? There is no question that motion is an adverse advent for osteogenic cells. This point has been most dramatically displayed to us with our experience of a bone graft substitute material made of sea coral. In reviewing hundreds of slides, we have not found one instance where cartilage formed before bone as the cells built up bone upon this stable lattice structure. On the other hand, in all settings showing relative motion between the coral material and surrounding soft tissues or bone, a cartilage interface develops which only later reorganizes to become solid bone. Not that this cartilage is necessarily bad. It is certainly nature's way of offering preliminary stability around fractured skeletal tissue. Millions of closed fractures treated with external support have healed by way of the stabilization and stiffness of callus cartilage. Nonetheless, in the environment wherein external fixation is most applicable, the open, potentially infected fracture, cartilage formation (implying absent blood supply) must be kept to a minimum. Moreover, the formation of fibrous tissue, which is of even lesser stiffness, must be kept to a minimum if a stable union is to result without infection. At this point, total stability is necessary, at least initially, to offer the greatest opportunity for fracture union. This is especially true in contaminated and infected settings.

On the other hand, it is quite clear from multiple experimental studies and from clinical experience, that complete stability, or stress shielding, is an adverse condition for functional healing of fractures. Whether the experimental model is a comparison of rigid versus flexible plates (Bradley et al, 1979), rigid versus flexible rods (Wang et al, 1981), or compression fixation versus oscillating movements at the fracture site (Panjabi et al, 1979), all fractures with a limited amount of stress heal faster or even more efficiently than those fractures which are maintained with total stability. Thus, although we search for complete skeletal stability initially, the advantages are rapidly diluted so that at some time during the healing phase a reduced fixation stability is advisable. There is yet no specific evidence to point to the exact amount of stability which would be ideal for most efficient fracture repair. One would assume, however, that ultimately the stability offered by the fixation system should be similar to that offered by the normal skeletal system at the site where external fixation is being used. Thus, for instance, in the case of a tibia fracture one would expect the system to absorb the amount of torque necessary to break a tibia. This amount of stiffness, of course, is far less than the amount of standard external fixation systems when applied or tested *in vitro*.

When we turn to the clinical problem, however, the problem is far more complex. In a small study wherein we compared the efficacy of the Murray fixation system with the Roger Anderson device, in Grade III tibial fractures (Lundeen et al, 1980), in spite of an average time of approximately six weeks for external fixation of the Murray system, approximately 40% of the fractures lost some position after transfer to brace or cast. (The Roger Anderson system which could be kept in external fixation only for an average of about four weeks had a slightly worse record.) Is this failure due to inherent qualities of the system or due to poor understanding of the application of the system?

In an attempt to find the answer as to the stability of various systems, we did a small series of comparisons between the Hoffmann, Roger Anderson, and Murray systems. In a transfixing pin system, they were all comparable in strength (Fig. 1); but in a single frame system ($\frac{1}{2}$ pin frame) there was some variability from one system to the other, depending on the mode of force application. (In this method of testing, the criterion of stability was the percentage of stiffness retained within the test bone after cutting it compared with the stiffness demonstrated before cutting.) Based on this small study and the test conditions, it seems that testing the systems themselves may not offer the greatest opportunity for comparing their clinical usefulness. All were about of the same strength, and the direction of force was as critical; nonetheless, in all the studies, the Murray system was as strong or stronger than the others tested.

A more sophisticated study by Chao (Chao and An, 1979) also attempted to classify the various systems as to their rate of stiffness. From this study it was clear that of greater significance in the stability was the thickness of the pin attached to the bone and distance of the side bar from the bone; of least consideration was the strength of the bar itself. Finally, as might be expected, the force which could be least resisted was that which was perpendicular to the alignment of the side bar. Thus, in a standard mediolateral configuration of external fixation for the tibia, AP loading was the least stable. Of course, triangulation of the fixation would allow considerably more stability in that forces are best resisted in fixation parallel to force.

Interestingly, to date no published study has investigated the problem of the chronic pin/bone interface and the various factors which can loosen this

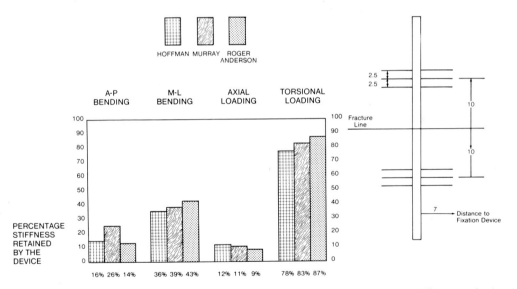

Fig. 1. Standard double frame. This graph demonstrates the efficacy of the various types of external fixation devices to resist four different methods of loading. All were comparable in their strength and all were variable in ability to withstand different types of loading. Torsional loading was best resisted by the double frame (transfixing pin system).

interface. The laboratory studies have done mechanical testing, trying to establish the most rigid system; but the clinical model is one in which multiple small forces are placed at the pin bone junction over a long period within a setting with variable potential for repair. The pin bone junction and its potential for instability probably is the ultimate key to the stability of the entire system.

What then can we take from the laboratory and clinical experience to offer guidelines as to the design of a system which will provide the highest degree of initial stability – recognizing that lesser degrees would be appropriate once preliminary union has developed. We propose three principles which offer the greatest potential for a stable system: 1) the search for inherent skeletal stability; 2) assurance of pin/bone stability; 3) distribution of stress concentration as broadly as possible.

The search for skeletal stability is probably the most important factor. As has been well demonstrated for many years by the AO system, the absence of inherent skeletal stability (uncontrolled comminution of the shaft opposite plate fixation) places such demand on the plate and screws that breakage or loosening will result. Thus, whenever possible, the fixation of fracture fragments by lag screw technique or other methods is necessary. In addition, the external fixation system ideally should be adjustable so that initial skeletal stability can be maintained in spite of some bony necrosis and resorption at the fracture ends.

Without initial skeletal stability, demands on an external fixation system may be as high as ten times that of the system when skeletal stability is present (see axial loading, Fig. 2).

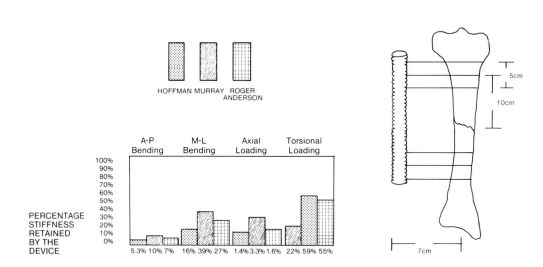

Fig. 2. Standard half pin frame. This system of a single frame is not as strong as the double frame system. In most circumstances, it is about half as strong, whereas the epoxy system was the strongest method of fixation. All of these used Steinmann pins of identical diameter - 3.2 mm.

What can be done to assure stability of the pin bone interface? First of all, the bone should be viable interfacing with the pins. Thus, failure of the pin bone interface would be encouraged by necrotic bone due to heat from drilling of cortical bone. For thick cortical bone, predrilling with a slightly smaller bit is necessary. Pin tip design is very important as is bone chip removal (Green and Matthews, 1981).

It is well known that bone tolerates compression better than any other force (Matter et al, 1975). How can compression and not tension and shear be created at the pin bone interface? Preloading of the pins places more of the force in compression than in tension. By this manner it would seem important to diminish as much as possible the pull-out force and to place the maximum in a compression loading mode. Preloading the pins before fixing to the final external system offers this opportunity.

The element which is probably most under the control of the clinician in designing an appropriate external fixation device is the distribution of mechanical forces. A principle which the engineers applied to the construction of bridges, airplanes, etc., is that stress concentration is an adverse factor. The wider distribution of stress and force along a beam, the more stable the system will be. When this principle is applied to the problem of external fixation of human fractures, it seems realistic to expect that the concentration of the stabilizing force at a single point in the proximal and distal fragment is probably not as wise as distributing the force as much as possible over the entire shaft. Thus, a wide separation of skeletal fixation in the proximal and distal fragments allows a greater distribution of the stress through the bone itself and, indeed, on to the external beam. In the metaphysis this must be modified to a wide anterior/posterior displacement; thus, the force necessary to control the other pin in a two-pin control system is diminished by the length of the lever arm of the intervening bone.

Probably the least significant element in the design of external fixation systems is the external beam which connects the pins. The strength of this beam naturally is considerably greater than that of the pin(s) and, therefore, variations in design or connections are several dimensions less significant than in the pin design itself. On this basis, therefore, improving the rigidity or method of connection to the external beam, although important, is less important compared with the other elements in the design of a system to achieve greatest stability. Finally, one must appreciate that the forces to be resisted by an external fixation system are multidimensional. Any single or two-dimensional control system has far less potential to resist all forces than a three-dimensional system. Triangulation, therefore, offers a greater opportunity for ultimate stability in a system which cannot develop inherent stability due to absence of skeletal tissue.

In summary, in an ideal system the stability of the system must be initially firmer than the bone. At a later stage in the healing process, mechanical stress allowing micromotion can be displayed to the healing bone. Our present knowledge, however, does not permit us to predict exactly when this stage has been reached.

The method by which we achieve this stability has three significant elements. The most efficient method is to achieve initial skeletal stability so that bone to bone contact is available in as many dimensions as possible at the

26

fracture area. The second method is persistent pin bone stability with
the forces applied to the bone consistently greater in compression than
in tension. Thus, preloading the pins is an important element of persistent stability at the pin bone interface. Finally, distribution of forces
as broadly as possible across the skeletal system as well as into the
external fixation system is an idealized goal of the engineering design.
Therefore, wide separation of pins rather than clustering of pins has a
theoretic advantage of broadly distributing the forces. In that same concept of broad distribution of forces, one must assume that a two-dimensional
system will be weaker than a three-dimensional system, and the adjunct of
multidimensional stabilization is necessary when ultimate stability is to
be achieved.

References

1. Anderson, R.: An automatic method for treatment for fractures of the
    tibia and fibula. Surg. Gynec. Obst. 58, 639, 1934.

2. Bradley, G.W., McKenna, G.B., Dunn, H.K., Daniels, A.U., and Statton,
    W.O.: Effects of flexural rigidity of plates on bone healing. J. Bone
    Jt. Surg. 61A, 866, 1979.

3. Brinker, W.O. and Flo, G.L.: Principles and application of external
    skeletal fixation. Vet.Clin. Nth. Am. 2, 197, 1975.

4. Chao, E.Y.S., and An, K.: Stress and rigidity analysis of external fix-
    ation devices. In, External Fixation: The Current State of the Art.
    Eds., A.F. Brooker and C.C. Edwards. The Williams and Wilkins Co.,
    Baltimore, 1979.

5. Green, C.A., and Matthews, L.S.: The thermal effects of skeletal fix-
    ation pin placement in human bone. Proc. Orth. Res. Soc., Las Vegas,
    1981, p. 103.

6. Hoffmann, R.: Rotules à os pour la réduction dirigée, non sanglante,
    des fractures. In, Cong. Franç. do Chir. 1938. pp 601-610.

7. Lundeen, M.A., Jones, R.E., and Mooney, V.: External fixation of com-
    plex open tibial fractures, Murray Universal External Fixation versus
    Roger Anderson device. Presented at Amer. Acad. Orth. Surg. Conv.,
    Atlanta, Ga., 1980.

8. Matter, P., Brennwald, J., and Perren, S.M.: The effect of static com-
    pression and tension on internal remodelling of cortical bone. Helv.
    Chir. Acta., Suppl. 12. Schabe & Co., Verlag, Basel/Stuttgart,1975.

9. Nickel, V.: Personal communication.

10. Panjabi, M.M., White, A.A. (III), and Wolf, J.W. (Jr.): A biomechanical
    comparison of the effects of constant and cyclic compression on fracture
    healing in rabbit long bones. Acta Orth. Scand. 50, 653, 1979.

11. Stader, O.: A preliminary announcement of a new method of treatment of
    fractures. Nth. Am. Vet. 18, 37, 1937.

12. Wang, G., Dunstan, J.C., Reger, S.I., Hubbard, S., Dillich, J. and
    Stamp, W.G.: Experimental femoral fracture immobilized by rigid and
    flexible rods (a rabbit model). Clin. Orthop. Rel. Res. 154, 286, 1981.

The Timing of External Fixation

Ch. C. Edwards

Is external fixation best applied immediately following injury or after
a period in traction? When, if ever, in the course of fracture healing,
should a fixator be replaced with a cast or orthosis? To what extent will
early replacement with a cast speed fracture healing and reduce pin tract
problems? Now that the use of external fixation has become widespread in
the treatment of open fractures, questions concerning the optimum timing
for its application and duration emerge with increasing frequency. Whereas
we do not have the data to answer many of these questions conclusively,
laboratory studies and extensive clinical experience with external fixation
at the University of Maryland and other trauma centers can give us some
general guidelines. In this paper I will explore the optimum timing for
external fixation as to its application and its duration.

The Application of External Fixation

Immediate applications

External fixation probably makes its greatest contribution in the first hours
and days after injury. Clinicians have long observed that both traumatized
and infected soft tissues heal better in a rigid environment (Clancy and
Hansen, 1978; Karlstrom and Olerud, 1975; Meyer et al, 1975). This may be
because the oxygen consumption requirements for injured soft tissues are
reduced when their position is rigidly fixed and also because the immobilized
tissues receive more consistant blood flow. Hence, rapid fixation of injured
segments may allow more of the ischemic soft tissues to survive than when
fixation is delayed.

Furthermore, immediate external fixation provides good wound access for
dressing changes and serial debridements. Regardless of whether surgeons
favor primary internal or external fixation for open fractures, there is substantial evidence that limb salvage is improved and complications are sub-
stantially lessened by open wound management techniques. Primary closure of
open fractures increases tissue pressure and ischemia, blocks drainage of
contaminated and necrotic material and creates an anaerobic environment con-
ducive to gas gangrene. External fixation facilitates open wound treatment.
There is sufficient wound access and patient mobilization for serial wound
debridements in the operating room every few days.

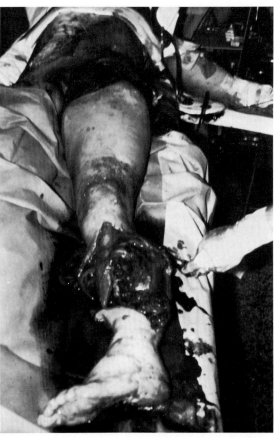

Fig. 1. Immediate application of external fixation: a) Polytrauma victim with an open tibial fracture, open pelvic dislocation, and lacerations of the liver and spleen. b) Immediate application of a quadrilateral (Vidal) Hoffmann fixator to the tibia and trapazoidal (Slätis) Hoffmann fixator to the pelvis provided 4 important advantages: 1) rigid fixation of the injured leg and pelvic tissues with prompt reduction of pelvic hemorrhage; 2) good access for future serial debridement of the tibial and pelvic wounds; 3) elevation of the injured leg, and 4) maximum mobilization to facilitate patient transportation, wound care, and respiratory management.

a

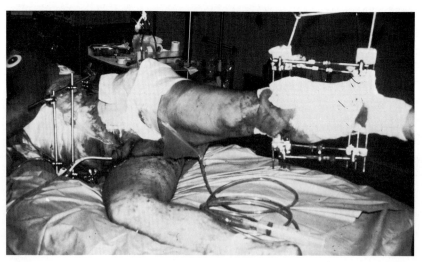

b

External fixation also facilitates elevation of the injured extremity. The fixator can be tied to an overhead bed frame to elevate the extremity and keep wound dressings away from bed sheets or other contaminated surfaces. Limb elevation is most important during the first three days following injury when soft tissue contusion, lymphatic and venous disruption all contribute to the extravasation of fluid into the injured soft tissues. Although typical compartment syndromes generally do not occur in association with large open wounds, the injured soft tissues, nevertheless, may undergo some degree of ischemic necrosis. The accumulating extracellular fluid blocks blood flow through remaining capillaries causing further soft tissue death. Open wound treatment and moderate elevation of the injured limb both serve to reduce the accumulation of edema and resultant ischemia (Fig. 1).

Moreover, immediate external fixation permits maximum mobilization for multiply-injured patients during the critical hours and days immediately following injury. Such patients require frequent turning in bed and upright posture to maximize their pulmonary ventilation-to-perfusion ratio and promote drainage of secretions; this is essential in the polytraumatized patient who remains intubated. Such patients also must be moved from their beds for diagnostic studies and surgical treatments for associated injuries.

Based on the four considerations described above, there appears to be little or no advantage to place a severely injured extremity in traction prior to the application of an external fixator. Application of external fixation at the time of debridement immediately on the patient's arrival yields maximum benefit. The importance of soft tissue stability, wound access, elevation, and patient mobilization is far greater during the first hours and days following injury than at any other time during the course of treatment. Accordingly, immediate application of external fixation is indicated for open fractures with major soft tissue injury and closed fractures requiring fasciotomies for compartment syndromes.

Delayed application of external fixation

On the other hand, there is good reason to delay the application of external fixation in the treatment of septic conditions and deformities requiring limb lengthening. In patients with cellulitis associated with previous pin tract infections or septic nonunions, it is best to initiate treatment with drainage, antibiotics and skeletal traction until the soft tissue infection resolves. Placement of external pins through infected tissues will result in pin tract infections with early pin loosening and possible osteomyelitis. In the treatment of septic nonunions, we generally favor application of the external frame after resolution of cellulitis and at the time of extensive surgical debridement of all infected and necrotic tissues.

When treating malunions or foreshortened nonunions, the first step consists of osteoclasis or debridement of interposed fibrous tissue and fasciotomies to make subsequent lengthening easier. An external fixator can then be applied to serve first as a lengthening device and then as a fixation or even compression device after the desired position of the bone has been achieved.

Duration of External Fixation

Temporary uses for external fixation

Soft tissue injury

One of the prime indications for external fixation is in the treatment of extensive injury crossing major joints. For example, where open distal femoral or proximal tibial fractures are complicated by avulsion of soft tissues from the popliteal space, standard femoral and tibial frames can be connected to fix the position of the knee (Fig. 2a). This frame configuration facilitates both treatment of the popliteal wounds and subsequent soft tissue reconstruction.

On the other hand, whenever a synovial joint is held in a fixed position for several weeks, cartilage degeneration and permanent stiffness can result. Articular cartilage is nourished by nutrients diffusing from the synovial fluid. Optimum diffusion of nutrients occurs when there is intermittent loading of the articular cartilage and movement of the synovial fluid over the articular surface (Edwards and Chrisman, 1979). Particularly when joint surfaces are fixed in compression, nutrition is impaired causing cartilage necrosis (Crelin and Southwick, 1960). The necrotic cartilage is often replaced by fibrocartilage which may form thick bands connecting both sides of the joint. Simultaneously, motionless synovium can fibrose, resulting in adhesions between the capsule and periarticular bone as well. This process quickly causes significant loss of motion in the elbow and knee and less noticeably in the hip and foot joints.

To minimize articular cartilage damage and resultant joint stiffness, external fixators should be used to limit joint motion only as a temporary measure. Once debridements of the wound are completed and edema has subsided, the components fixing the position of the joint should be loosened daily, permitting a few degrees of passive joint motion. When soft tissue coverage has been obtained, the rods connecting, for example, a femoral and tibial Hoffmann frame, can be replaced with hinges (Fig. 2b). We have found that standard polycentric knee hinges designed for cast braces can be attached

---

Fig. 2. Treatment of fractures complicated by soft tissue injury crossing the knee: a) A rod (arrow) attached by couplings is used to temporarily immobilize severely injured soft tissues crossing the joint. The rod is attached to standard femoral and tibial frames used in this case to treat open femoral and tibial fractures. The foot is held in a neutral position with an orthoplast splint attached to the tibial frame with adjustable (velcro) elastic straps. b) After early healing of soft tissues crossing the knee, the fixed rod is replaced with hinges to permit controlled knee motion. Standard castbrace polycentric hinges are attached to the Hoffmann frame with spare pin-clamps (arrow). c) When skin, ligaments, and bone no longer require hinge protection, the hinges are removed. An exerciser is then erected with pulleys attached to the tibial frame (arrow) to facilitate the return of knee motion and quadriceps strength.

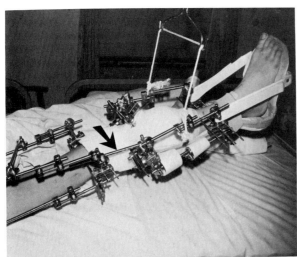

a

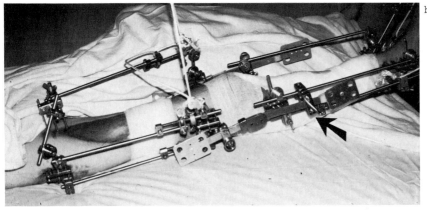

b

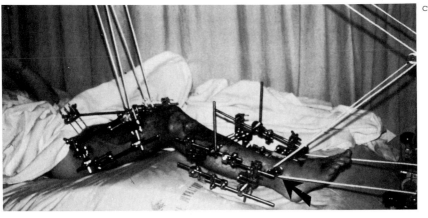

c

directly to Hoffmann frames. The flat metal pieces on either side of the hinge are sandwiched between the two sides of a standard Hoffmann pin clamp. The clamp rods can then be attached to the femoral and tibial frames with couplings. The hinges serve to provide some stability for periarticular fractures and ligamentous injuries while permitting as much flexion and extension as the soft tissues will tolerate.

Once bone and soft tissue healing has progressed to the point that no external joint articulation is necessary, hinges can be removed. When treating knee injuries, an exerciser can be constructed between the fixator and overhead frame with traction pulleys to help restore knee joint motion and quadriceps muscle strength (Fig. 2c). When using external fixation primarily to treat soft tissue injuries, it is best to remove the fixator when soft tissue coverage is mature and to protect any underlying stable fractures with a cast or brace. This will maximize physiologic loading of the fracture and minimize pin tract problems to some extent.

When pins-in-plaster or plaster alone will suffice

Another temporary role for external fixation is in the treatment of closed or Grade I fractures where reduction cannot be maintained by lesser means. Occasionally, satisfactory length or reduction may be difficult to maintain in fractures that are several days old. In certain oblique or comminuted closed tibial fractures, it may be impossible to maintain adequate length of position by simple plaster casting. In such cases, a fixator can be used to obtain and hold the fracture reduction. Once swelling subsides, plaster can be wrapped around the injured limb incorporating the external fixation pins. The fixation frame can then be removed. When there are no major wounds to treat, the pins-in-plaster method offers some advantages: It interferes less with normal gait than a tibial fixation frame. It is associated with less pin tract problems since the plaster reduces motion at the pin-skin interface and prevents contamination as well. Moreover, the hydraulic effect of the circular cast (Latta et al, 1980) can supplement the fracture stability provided by the pins.

Potentially stable open fractures and arthrodeses

The most common indication for the external fixator is in the treatment of open tibial fractures. A simple tibial fracture is frequently complicated by a major soft tissue wound. Once delayed closure or grafting of the wound is accomplished, it is difficult to justify treatment with an external fixation apparatus. Substantial clinical experience suggests that basically stable tibial (Nicoll, 1964), humeral (Reudi et al, 1974) and distal femoral fractures (Sarmiento, 1972) will heal as well in the cast as with any internal or external fixation system. Accordingly, we generally advocate converting to a cast when skin is mature and callus formation is evident.

Likewise, external fixation is ideally used only during the first several weeks following elective arthrodeses for weight-bearing joints. External fixation provides an excellent method to obtain precise alignment and rigid fixation, particularly for arthrodeses of the knee or ankle. Once bone positions are fixed by early callus, however, speed of fusion, patient convenience, and freedom from pin tract difficulties are probably all enhanced by conversion to a weight-bearing cast.

The one exception to this suggested conversion to weight-bearing casting is when extensive split thickness skin grafting has been performed on the affected limb. We have found that even split grafts that have matured for several weeks tolerate the shearing forces under a cast very poorly. Hence, in cases of extensive skin grafting, it is probably best to use the external fixator as a definitive method of treatment, even in the case of potentially stable fractures or arthrodeses.

A definitive use for external fixation: The unstable fracture

For purposes of this discussion, a fracture is classified as unstable if the degree of bone or soft tissue disruption is such without weight bearing the fragments would collapse into an unacceptable position unless they were stabilized by either internal or external fixation. Fractures may be unstable due to bone loss, extensive comminution, or extensive soft tissue disruption. Sarmiento and associates (1975) have shown that the muscular envelope and interosseous membrane play a major role in stabilizing the position of tibial fracture fragments.

In some high energy fractures the interosseous membrane of the tibia and the surrounding muscle sheath may be extensively disrupted. This soft tissue disruption will leave the bones unsupported mechanically, and will also impair the speed and volume of callus formation. In cases with extensive soft tissue injury combined with either bone loss or extensive comminution, our experience suggests that replacement of the fixator with a cast following the appearance of moderate callus usually leads to unacceptable fracture angulation and sometimes to breakdown of grafted skin as well. When a significant amount of bone must be reconstituted from healing callus or bone graft, a bone plasticity remains for some time. Hence, when treating unstable fractures with extensive soft tissue injury, it is probably best to use the fixator as a definitive means of treatment.

Borderline Judgements

The temporary use of external fixation appears most favorable in the treatment of stable fractures, and the definitive use of external fixation may be advantageous in the treatment of unstable fractures. The optimum period for external fixation is difficult to judge between these extremes. When, if ever, should casting be substituted for external fixation in the following situations: open fractures with mild comminution or a large butterfly fragment, very oblique fractures with moderate soft tissue injury, open injuries with less than circumferential bone loss, unstable fractures following extensive callus formation from successful bone grafting procedures, or potentially stable fractures with several square inches of overlying thickness skin graft? We do not have sufficient data to provide definitive answers for each of these circumstances. Nevertheless, a judgement must be made regarding the duration

of external fixation for each borderline case. To decide the optimum duration for external fixation, we must balance the following four factors based
on the characteristics of each patient's injuries:

Physiologic loading

Physiologic loading is maximized by temporary external fixation of open fractures followed by early conversion to weight-bearing cast fixation. Both
laboratory data and our clinical experience suggest that physiologic loading
speeds bone formation and promotes fracture healing. In 1892, Wolff observed
that the application of load promotes bone formation. In 1962, Bassett
showed that compaction encourages bone formation from undifferentiated
mesenchymal cells in tissue culture. Sarmiento reported that femoral fracture healing progressed more rapidly in rats allowed to walk than in those
immobilized with a cast (Sarmiento et al, 1977). More recently, White and
associates (1981), using an external fixation test device, demonstrated more
rapid initial fracture healing in rabbits whose tibial fractures were kept
compressed, but more rapid development of fracture callus strength thereafter
in rabbits whose fractures were cyclicly loaded.

Rigid fixation, on the other hand, may facilitate soft tissue healing, but
does not appear to promote bone formation or speed fracture healing after
the first few weeks. Uhthoff documented increased porosity in dog femora
unloaded by the application of rigid compression plates (Uhthoff and Dubuc,
1971). Woo, Bradley and others showed equal fracture healing rates and
greater strength in healed bones treated with less rigid plates (Bradley et
al, 1977; Woo et al, 1978).

Clinically, it is also well known that the amount of peripheral callus cor-
relates inversely with the rigidity of fixation. Rigid compression plate
fixation results in minimal peripheral callus whereas flexible intramedullary pin fixation or cast fixation is often associated with extensive
peripheral callus.

The degree to which external frames shield bone from physiologic loading is
determined by fracture configuration, frame design, and the stiffness of the
frame components. The most commonly-used external fixator today is probably
the quadrilateral Vidal configuration of the Hoffmann fixator for the tibia.
Biomechanical studies (Adrey, 1970) show the Vidal frame to be a rather rigid
appliance.

Although double frame external fixators probably reduce physiologic loading
to some extent, their overall impact on fracture healing is not clear. In
the treatment of severe open fractures it is likely that the importance of
good access and stability for injured soft tissues in the early phase of
treatment counterbalances the disadvantage of unloading the bone later in
the course of treatment. To our knowledge, no studies to date have shown
comparable injuries healing more slowly with external fixation than with
other modalities. Indeed, in our initial studies of grade III tibial fractures treated with the rigid Vidal frame, the mean healing times were as
short as any heretofore reported series treating comparable injuries with
other methods (Edwards et al, 1979; Edwards and Jaworski, 1979).

The importance of physiologic loading appears to vary with different bones. For instance, the humerus seems to heal as rapidly when stabilized with a unilateral external fixator as when treated in a cast. A tibial fracture without open wounds or extensive soft tissue damage may heal more slowly and certainly with less callus in a fixator than in a cast. In our experience, the femur heals much slower and with less callus when stablized with Hoffmann external fixation than when treated by intramedullary nailing or casting. This may be related to the greater physiologic loads normally experienced by the femur as compared with smaller or nonweight-bearing bones.

Angulation

Whereas early fixator removal and cast application promotes physiologic loading, it also increases the chances of fracture angulation. As discussed above, the rigid fixation and load shielding imparted by modern fixators inhibit peripheral callus formation. Likewise, the muscle and vascular injury usually associated with open fractures impairs callus formation as well. Resistance to bending is proportional to the third power of the radius of any structure. Hence, the less peripheral callus, the greater the chance of fracture angulation. Unstable open fractures treated with rigid external fixation are, accordingly, very subject to angulation when converted to cast fixation early in the course of callus maturation. Our preliminary results following unstable fractures converted to cast fixation shortly after the radiographic appearance of contiguous callus show an unacceptable degree of angulation in almost half of the cases (Fig. 3). In choosing between temporary versus definitive treatment with external fixation, the orthopedist must weigh the relative benefits of physiologic loading versus the risk of angulation based on the fracture pattern, degree of tissue injury, and extent of callus formation.

Pin tract problems

We commonly hear the admonition: remove external fixators to prevent pin tract problems. This raises the question to what extent pin tract problems are a function of time. To answer this question, we must consider the factors predisposing to pin tract infection.

Inadequate pin-bone contact

Muscle pull and weight bearing cause a certain amount of stress between the fixators and the fractured bone. Failure at the pin-bone interface or loosening is a function of the force per unit area. The force per unit area can be reduced by increasing the total pin-bone contact area, distributing the pins to best resist bending forces or moments, and by achieving direct contact of the fracture fragments so as to transmit some of the load through the bone and thereby relieve the pin-bone interface.

Hence, faulty placement of the pins predisposes them to loosening. The most common error is failure to achieve bicortical pin contact. For example, we find that pins placed through the anterotibial spine loosen far more frequently than pins passing through the intramedullary canal of the tibia to engage both cortices. Likewise, nonparallel pins squeezed together in a

36

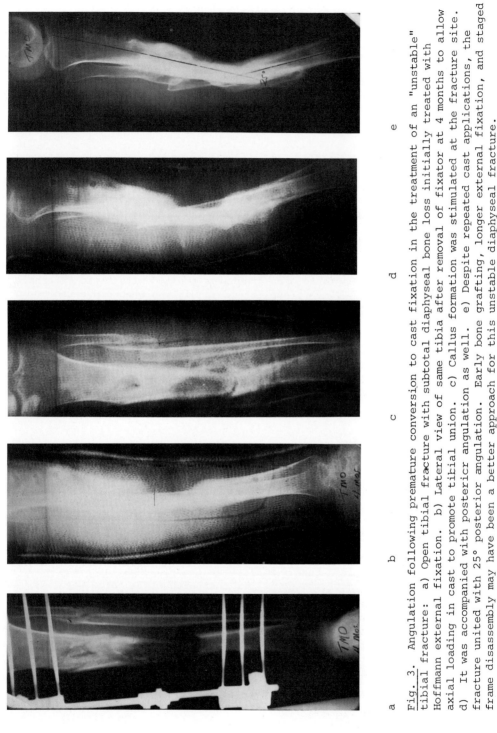

a   b   c   d   e

Fig. 3. Angulation following premature conversion to cast fixation in the treatment of an "unstable" tibial fracture: a) Open tibial fracture with subtotal diaphyseal bone loss initially treated with Hoffmann external fixation. b) Lateral view of same tibia after removal of fixator at 4 months to allow axial loading in cast to promote tibial union. c) Callus formation was stimulated at the fracture site. d) It was accompanied with postericr angulation as well. e) Despite repeated cast applications, the fracture united with 25° posterior angulation. Early bone grafting, longer external fixation, and staged frame disassembly may have been a better approach for this unstable diaphyseal fracture.

pin clamp produce excessive focal pressure at the pin bone interface and may be more subject to loosening. Furthermore, if insufficient numbers of pins are used relative to the size of the bone involved and to the anticipated activity level of the patient, each pin will be subjected to excessive forces. Excessive pressure at the bone-pin interface from any of these causes may result in local resorption of bone. Loosening will follow. If the loose pin is not promptly removed, pin tract infection is the expected sequaela.

Thermal necrosis

When drilling external fixation pins through cortical bone, the surgeon often encounters significant resistance. If excessive turning speed or pressure is required to penetrate the cortex, heat builds up and causes necrosis of the bone adjacent to the pins. The necrotic bone will either be sequestered or resorbed by the surrounding living tissue. In either case, loosening and, in time, infection generally follow. To minimize the risk of thermal necrosis during pin placement, we suggest predrilling pins when significant resistance to penetration is encountered. Use of a 3.2 mm drill bit before pin placement removes cortical material that would otherwise serve to increase friction between the cutting edge of the fixation pin and bone, thus producing heat.

Skin pressure

Another cause of pin tract infection is pressure necrosis of skin left "tented" by the fixation pins. Accordingly, any skin which does not move freely around the exiting pin following final fracture reduction should be released with a scapel. Continuous pressure by the pin against tented skin will produce focal ischemia, subsequent necrosis, and provide a medium for microbial growth.

Motion at the pin-skin interface

If skin is allowed to slide back and forth along the external fixation pin, a seal fails to develop and microbes easily invade the pin tract. Probably, for this reason, we find a higher incidence of pin tract infections where pins traverse fleshy tissue, as in the thigh, or where there is more skin motion over the bone, as in the humerus. On the contrary, pin tract drainage from pins properly positioned in the foot is uncommon. To some extent, motion at the pin-skin interface can be lessened by keeping sterile gauze wrapped between the pin clamp and skin to fix the position of the skin relative to the exiting pin (Fig. 4).

In reviewing the above list of factors predisposing to pin loosening and infection, we see that most are determined at the time of pin placement. Some of these factors, such as suboptimal pin placement or excessive motion, may not result in loosening and infection until patient activity levels increase weeks or months after injury. Loosening or infection from thermal necrosis, however, stretched skin, major focal overload at the pin-bone interface, or contamination are usually manifest within a few weeks after pin placement. Therefore, most pins that are destined to cause problems develop loosening or infection within the first two months. In a study of fractured tibias with associated tissue loss, which we carried out in 1979,

38

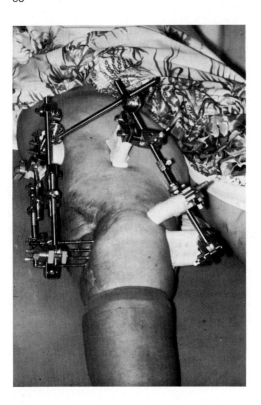

Fig. 4. Pin tract treatment
Sterile gauze is wrapped between the
pin clamps and skin to minimize motion at the pin-skin interface. This
is helpful when pins must traverse
fleshy tissues in the thigh.

we found the same percentage of draining pins in cases where the frame was
removed before 60 days as in cases where the frame was left in place for
more than 60 days (Edwards and Jaworski, 1979).

The majority of pin tract problems are probably due to factors determined
at the time of insertion. A certain incidence of pin-bone interface failure
with pin tract problems, however, will continue throughout the course of
treatment. This probably represents a small proportion of the pin tract
problems we see. Hence, although a factor, late pin tract problems should
probably not be one of the most important factors in deciding when to remove the fixator. One exception might be in the case of the femur where
greater loads and soft tissue girth are acting against the pin-tissue
interface.

Skin breakdown

The fourth major factor to consider in the duration of external fixation for
fractures of borderline stability is skin breakdown. The improved loading
and slight diminution of pin tract problems associated with early frame re-

moval must be balanced against the risks of angulation and skin breakdown following early conversion to cast fixation. Following major injury to soft tissues, extensive scarring within the tissues is usually observed. This may leave the overlying skin with less resilient subcutaneous fat and muscle. Consequently, the skin may be less able to withstand external pressure and shear stresses. All these factors are greatly aggravated when coverage has been achieved with split thickness skin grafting. In such cases, there is no subcutaneous fat padding, and there is reduced blood supply from subdermal scarring of the original granulation tissue. Accordingly, when areas of split thickness skin are placed under a weight-bearing cast, we frequently find skin breakdown even several weeks following graft maturation.

Other Approaches to The Management of Fractures of Borderline Stability

When treating an unstable open fracture, our goal is to achieve gradual physiologic loading without angulation or skin breakdown while minimizing pin-bone interface failure. Whereas rigid external fixation appears to be the optimum treatment immediately following major open injury, simply leaving the original frame in place without further intervention usually does not accomplish these goals. Replacing the frame with a cast or orthosis early in the course of healing also has major disadvantages for some injuries. The optimum management plan might represent a middle road between these two extremes. Such a course of action might include carefully selecting the frame configuration to be used, gradual disassembly of the frame as fracture healing proceeds, early grafting procedures, and possibly introducing sliding frame components.

Frame configuration

A frame configuration should be selected to achieve stable fixation of the injured soft tissues and bone without making the frame more rigid than necessary. For instance, the rigid Vidal quadrilateral frame may be optimum for severe trauma to the tibia with bone loss or comminution. A unilateral double frame using half pins, however, may provide optimum fixation for lesser tibial fractures requiring fasciotomy or for injuries to the humerus. For most foot injuries in which the Achilles tendon and plantar fascia remain intact, adequate fixation can be obtained from the simple tibio-metatarsal frame (Edwards, 1979; 1980) rather than the far more rigid bilateral triangular frame. Bicortical half pins can avoid some of the fleshy tissues traversed by transfixion pins. More flexible frames also permit greater physiologic loading during the latter stages of fracture healing.

Gradual frame disassembly

As discussed earlier, maximum stability is desirable initially. As soft tissues heal and early callus forms, however, bone formation is encouraged by physiologic loading (Wolf et al, 1981). As fracture healing progresses, connecting rods between the pin group proximal and distal to the fracture segment can be removed to increase frame flexibility. For example, the quadrilateral Vidal tibial frame can be converted to a unilateral double

frame by simply removing the lateral adjustable rods and cutting the transfixion pins off below the skin surface.

Early bone grafting

We find that over one-third of open tibias require bone grafting to achieve
union within reasonable time. Many more cases would profit from early
grafting to speed recovery. When there is any significant loss of bony substance or severe soft tissue injury with a delayed healing response, the
surgeon should consider early posterolateral cancellous grafting. Open
cancellous grafting (Papinou) is helpful for metaphyseal defects, but usually does not suffice for extensive diaphyseal bone loss. Where bone loss
is accompanied by soft tissue loss as well, myocutaneous flap coverage will
restore a more normal environment for healing bone. One edge of the myocutaneous flap can be raised to allow closed cancellous grafting for diaphyseal defects shortly after flap maturation. Early grafting accomplishes our
fixation goals in two ways: it speeds bone healing and, therefore, reduces
time in the fixator; and it stimulates the formation of peripheral callus.
As described earlier, this peripheral callus resists subsequent angulation
in a cast far better than the more central callus characteristic of fractures treated only with a rigid fixator.

Sliding frame components

Another approach to maximize physiologic loading later in the course of fracture healing, while preventing angulation, might be the introduction of sliding components between the pin groups on either side of a fracture. Further
fixator evolution and clinical experience will be necessary before we can
evaluate the degree to which this approach might address our treatment goals.

Epilogue

At present, we do not have the necessary data to provide a simple recipe or
formula for uniform success in the treatment of open tibial fractures. The
suggestions and methods outlined in this paper are based on laboratory data
and observations from our clinical experience treating open fractures with
external fixation. To make more specific recommendations and to further refine our management of patients treated with external fixation, we must learn
the answers to the following questions:

1) What is the optimum degree of rigidity for

    a) the initial healing of traumatized soft tissues,
    b) early callus formation, and
    c) callus consolidation?

2) What degree of callus rigidity and/or strength will resist angulation in
    a weight-bearing cast and how can this level of rigidity be most easily
    determined?

3) What is the relationship between frame design or rigidity and pin loosening? Would a frame that cushions impact or allows transmission of physiologic loads to the healing bone also reduce the incidence of pin loosening?

4) To what degree would electrical stimulation duplicate the effect of physiologic loading without introducing new problems? For instance, could a fracture be kept in a rigid frame while using electric fields to stimulate maximum healing rate?

To answer these questions and refine the general guidelines discussed in this paper, we must return to the laboratory and continue our clinical studies.

References

1. Adrey, J.: Le fixateur externe d'Hoffmann couplé en cadre. Étude biomechanique dans les fractures de jambe. Thesis, Montpellier. GEAD, Paris, 1970.

2. Bassett, C.A.L.: Current concepts of bone formation. J. Bone Jt. Surg. 44A, 1217, 1962.

3. Bradley, G.W., McKenna, G.B., Dunn, H.K., Daniels, A.V. and Statton, W.D.: The effects of mechanical environment on fracture healing. Trans. 23rd Orthopaedic Res. Soc. Mtg, 1977.

4. Clancy, G., and Hansen, S.: Open fracture of the tibia. J. Bone Jt. Surg. 60A, 118, 1978.

5. Crelin, E., and Southwick, W.: Mitosis of chondrycytes induced in the knee joint articular cartilage of rabbits. Yale J.Biol. Med. 33, 243, 1960.

6. Edwards, C.C.: New directions in Hoffmann external fixation. In, Vidal, J. (ed.), Proc. 7th Internat. Conf. Hoffmann External Fixation. Diffinco SA, Geneva, 1979.

7. Edwards, C.C.: Management of multi-segment injuries in the polytrauma patients. In, Johnston, R. (ed.), Advances in External Fixation. Yearbook Med. Publ., Miami, 1980.

8. Edwards, C., and Chrisman, D.: Articular cartilage. In, The Scientific Basis of Orthopaedics. Appleton-Century-Crofts, New York, 1979.

9. Edwards, C.C. and Jaworski, M.F.: Hoffmann external fixation in open tibial fractures with tissue loss. J. Bone Jt. Surg. Orthop. Trans. 3, 261, 1979.

10. Edwards, C.C., Jaworski, M.F., Solana, J., and Aronson, B.S.: Management of compound tibial fractures using external fixation. Amer. Surg. 45, 190, 1979.

11. Karlstrom, G. and Olerud, S.: Percutaneous pin fixation of open tibial fractures. J. Bone Jt. Surg. 57A, 915, 1975.

12. Latta, L.L., Sarmiento, A.A., and Tarr, R.R.: The rationale of functional bracing of fractures. Clin. Ortho., 146, 28, 1980.

13. Meyer, S., Weiland, A., and Willenegger, H.: The treatment of infected nonunion of fractures of long bones. J. Bone Jt. Surg. 57A, 837, 1975.

14. Nicoll, E.A.: Fractures of the tibial shaft, a survey of 705 cases. J. Bone Jt. Surg. 46B, 373, 1964.

15. Reudi, T., Moshfegh, A., Pfeiffer, K.M., and Allgower, M.: Fresh fractures of the shaft of the humerus - Conservative or operative treatment? Reconstruc. Surg. Traumatol. 14, 65, 1974.

16. Sarmiento, A.: Functional bracing of tibial and femoral shaft fractures. Clin. Orthop. 105, 202, 1972.

17. Sarmiento, A., Latta, L., Zilioli, A., and Sinclair, W.: The role of soft tissues in fracture stability. Clin. Orthop. 105, 106, 1975.

18. Sarmiento, A., Schaeffer, J., Beckerman, L., Latta, L., and Enis, J.: Fracture healing in rat femora. J. Bone Jt. Surg. 59A, 369, 1977.

19. Uhthoff, H.K. and Dubuc, F.L.: Bone structure changes in the dog under rigid internal fixation. Clin. Orthop. 81, 165, 1971.

20. Wolf, J.W., White, A.A., Panjabi, M.M., and Southwick, W.O.: Comparison of cyclic loading versus constant compression in the treatment of long bone fractures in rabbits. J. Bone Jt. Surg. 63A, 805, 1981.

21. Wolff, J.: Das Gasetz der Transformation der Knochen. August Hirschwald (Publ.), Berlin, 1892.

22. Woo, S.L., Akeson, W.H., Schmidt, D.F., Gonsalves, M., Coutts, R.D. and Amiel, D.: The effects of fixation plate stiffness on fracture healing. Trans. Soc. Biomaterials, 2, 58, 1978.

Complications of External Fixation

S. A. Green

In 1950, the American orthopedic community was surveyed to determine the
rightful place of external skeletal fixation in the armamentarium of
fracture management (Johnson and Stovall, 1950). The majority of surgeons
queried had tried and discarded external skeletal fixation because of
concern for the complications associated with external fixators. Nevertheless, there is currently a surge of interest among orthopedists for
external skeletal fixation. One reason for this is the increase of open
fractures caused by high-speed motor vehicle collisions, especially
among motorcyclists. Modern external fixators, while more rigid and
more versatile than their predecessors, have not eliminated the problems
associated with their use. On the contrary, the complications associated
with transcutaneous-transosseous pins are ever present and are common to
all fixators, past, present, or future.

Pin Tract Infections

It is difficult to determine from a review of the literature the exact
incidence of pin tract sepsis. The reported incidence ranges from
2 to 50%. In fact, even within the same institution it is difficult
(from a chart review) to determine which cases of pin sepsis were associated with clear drainage and which with frank purulence. For this reason,
the concept of major and minor pin sepsis has been introduced. A major
pin tract infection requires admission to the hospital, removal of the
involved pin, or removal of the entire fixator. A minor pin tract infection is any other type of pin reaction. This distinction was created to
simplify chart review: a treatment to deal with major pin sepsis will be
noted in a patient's record. Using these criteria, we have determined
at Rancho Los Amigos Hospital that 35% of the patients experience major
pin tract sepsis at some time during their fixator period. Almost 100%
of the patients show signs of minor pin tract problems at one or more
pin sites. Our observations correspond to those of Edwards (1979) in
Baltimore who notes that 11% of all pinbone interfaces demonstrate sepsis.

Certain factors are considered likely to contribute to pin tract infection.
These factors include: necrosis of tissue around the pin; excessive pressure at the pinbone interface; thermal damage to bone during pin insertion;
pin loosening or soft tissue motion around the pin (Fig. 1).

To reduce the likelihood of thermal damage to either bone or soft tissue, a
hand drill should always be used when inserting transcutaneous pins. Another way to avoid thermal damage is to predrill the bone hole with a
slightly smaller drill bit before pin insertion. Matthews and Hirsch (1972)
have demonstrated that predrilling a hole with a drill bit 1 mm smaller than

44

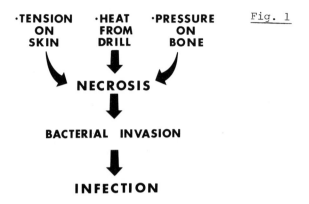

Fig. 1

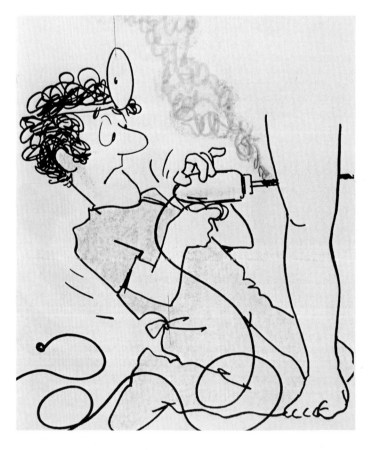

Fig. 2. A power drill may produce thermal necrosis.

the final bone hole size will reduce maximum temperature of drilling by approximately 50°C. This is especially important when drilling dense cortical bone in healthy young patients. (Fig. 2)

Necrosis of soft tissue around the pin can be reduced by releasing all tension with a scalpel blade. Undue pressure at the pinbone interface can be minimized by avoiding excessive compression with the fixator frame (Fig. 3).

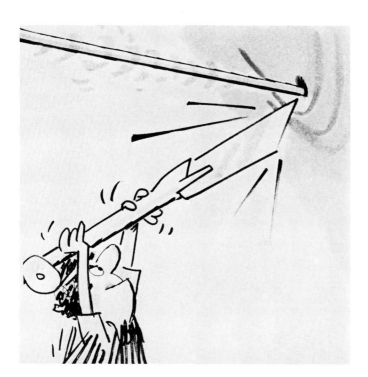

Fig. 3. Release all
tension after pin
insertion.

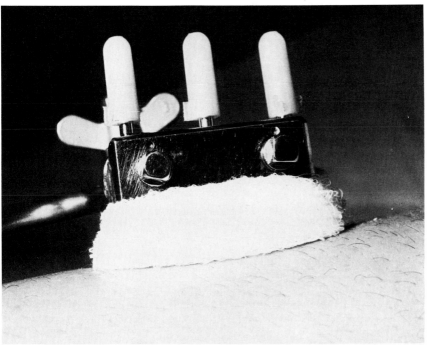

Fig. 4. Bulky wad around pins to stop skin irritation
(from Green, S.A., Complications of External Skeletal
Fixation; courtesy of Charles C. Thomas, publishers)

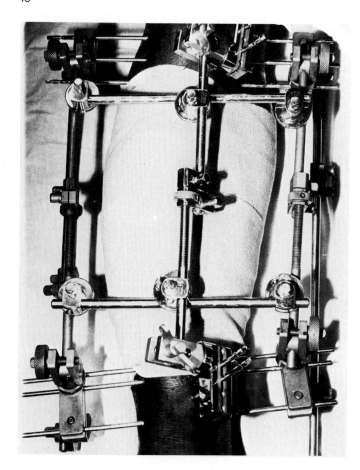

Fig. 5. A fifth (anterior) bar increases the rigidity of the frame configuration.

Motion of the pins within the bone can be diminished by employing only threaded pins. Excessive soft tissue motion around the pin can be reduced (but not eliminated) by wrapping the pin group with a bulky soft wad, filling the space between the pin-gripping clamp and the skin (Fig. 4).

Daily pin care routine should be directed at carefully cleansing the pin-skin interface at least once daily. My routine is to use hydrogen peroxide or soap and water around the pins to clean away the crust that accumulates.

Two most important measures to reduce pin loosening are: 1) biplanar fixation; and 2) elimination of weight-bearing stresses. Our most successful long-term (more than six months) applications have been in patients with biplanar frame configurations who have used crutches throughout the course of fixator application (Fig. 5).

Chronic Pinhole Osteomyelitis

A small but significant proportion of patients will demonstrate persistent drainage after removal of an infected pin. This distressing complication

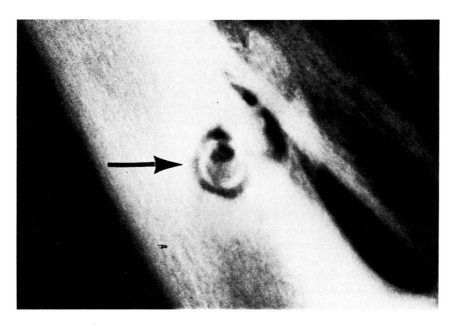

Fig. 6. The classic ring sequestrum.

usually requires a surgical procedure (debridement). The incidence of chronic pinhole osteomyelitis ranges between 1-4%.

Measures which appear to reduce this risk are: early removal of septic pins and avoidance of dense cortical bony ridges such as the anterior tibia.

The characteristic radiographic appearance of a chronic pinhole osteo-myelitis is the ring sequestrum (Fig. 6). This structure consists of a ring of dead bone floating in a radiolucent zone of soft granulation tissue which, in turn, is surrounded by viable cortex. In general, the dead bone must be curetted from the pinhole if persistent drainage is a problem after pin removal. On the other hand, a ring sequestrum-like structure, in the absence of sepsis, will probably resorb with the passage of time. Nevertheless, it is wise to follow such a lesion radiographic-ally even if no drainage is present. I am aware of two cases where a slow but indolent infection continued to erode the surrounding bone until a pathologic fracture occurred; yet, there was no evidence of external drainage.

Chronic drainage from a pinhole can occur in the absence of a ring seques-trum. In this situation, the walls of the pinhole represent a sequestrum which is in continuity with the shaft of the bone at the time of debride-ment. The walls should be curetted to bleeding bone.

Failure to Obtain Union

Failure to obtain union is a common problem with external skeletal fixation. The fixator, by retarding physiologic fracture motion, decreases the form-

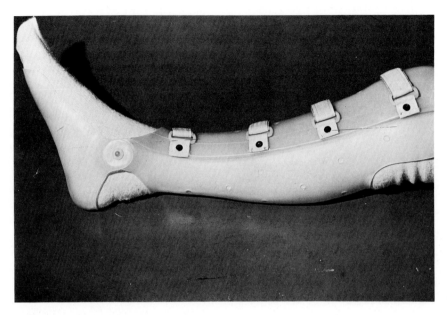

Fig. 7. Early fixation removal can be followed with a molded orthotic support. (from Green, S.A., Complications of External Skeletal Fixation; courtesy of Charles C. Thomas, publishers)

ation of fracture callus. Primary bone union is also delayed because an external skeletal fixation system is unlikely to prevent micromotion at the fracture site. Rigid internal fixation, on the other hand, permits interfragmentary compression to lock pieces together so that primary bone union can proceed across the fracture site (Perren, 1979). For these reasons, it is not surprising that delayed bone union is a problem with external skeletal fixation.

Many workers in the field of external fixation have developed strategies to deal with this problem. The most important of these is early bone grafting. Fresh autogenous cancellous bone graft can substitute for the inhibited fracture callus, thereby promoting bone union. Bone grafting should be accomplished early during the fixator application. If necessary, the cancellous bone graft can be repeated at four- to six-week intervals until union takes place. In the case of absolute bone loss, or bone resection secondary to a septic process, the bone graft should be applied as soon as the surrounding soft tissues are healthy enough to support the transplant.

It is unwise to insert a bone graft into dysvascular scar tissue, because a significant portion of the graft may not survive.

Another important strategy to prevent the problem of delayed bone healing is to remove the fixator early. Six to eight weeks after injury, an envelope of tissue will surround the fracture, stabilizing it enough to permit the fixator to be removed and the fracture to be managed with a molded orthotic device (Fig. 7). (When managing segmental bone loss, a solid mature bone graft will be necessary before the fixator can be removed.)

A gradual unloading of the frame is a concept that has evolved within the past few years. In this manner, an increasing proportion of the weight-bearing load is transferred to the healing fracture while elements of the fixator maintain alignment. When a quadrilateral frame configuration is used, upright bars are gradually removed at weekly intervals until all bars have been removed.

Elastic external fixation, promoted by Franz Burny (1979) of Belgium, is, in a sense, a continuation of Raoul Hoffman's original concept of fracture management. The fixator frame, consisting of a unilateral bar, is sufficiently flexible to permit the development of a moderate size fracture callus. Anatomic reduction is important in this concept. Interfragmentary compression of oblique fractures with a single lag screw applied across the fracture site is usually necessary.

Biocompression is a concept recently introduced by Zbikowski (1979), a Spanish orthopedic surgeon. He uses components of the Hoffman external skeletal fixation system but substitutes a telescoping bar for the compression bars. The telescoping frame permits up and down motion at the fracture site while maintaining overall alignment. Zbikowski's preliminary results are quite encouraging.

Electrical stimulation is another modality that has been used in conjunction with external skeletal fixation. Jorgensen (1972) has been applying electrical current to the pins of Hoffman's fixation system which, fortunately, are electrically insulated from the frame. His results indicate more rapid union when electrical stimulation is applied across the fracture site. Results using the external fixation with electromagnetically-induced current or percutaneous electrode systems have not yet been published. Such studies are currently in progress at various centers around the world.

Neurovascular Injury

Nerve and vessel injuries are, fortunately, quite rare after external skeletal fixation. Nevertheless, they do occur. Certain areas are especially dangerous. Loss of limb has been reported following pin insertion (Green, 1981).

In the lower leg, the region consisting of the lower portion of the third quarter and the upper portion of the fourth quarter is a danger area for transfixion of pin insertion; the anterior tibial artery and deep branch of the peroneal nerve cross the lateral surface to the tibia from the interosseous membrane to the front of the ankle joint. Another danger area is in the second quarter of the thigh where the deep femoral artery passes medial to (and then posterior to) the shaft of the femur. Likewise, at the junction of the second and third quarters of the femur, the superficial femoral artery passes the coronal plane of the bone to become posteriorly situated. In this region, it can easily be transfixed by pins.

In the upper limb, the radial nerve from the shoulder to the wrist poses a peril to orthopedic surgeons. It must be recalled that the radial nerve is

in intimate contact with the shaft of the humerus through the second and
third quarters of the upper arm and it winds around the radial neck in the
proximal forearm. In the distal forearm, the superficial branch of the
radial nerve can be likewise transfixed with a pin.

A zone system for pin placement has been developed for use by the surgeon.
The limb segments are divided into quarters by folding a surgical towel.
Orientation to easily palpable landmarks makes the system easy to use.
Details of the system can be obtained from the textbook, Complications of
External Skeletal Fixation (Green, 1981).

It is recommended that the surgeon use image intensification fluoroscopy
during pin insertion.

Persistent Wound Infection

The most common cause of persistent wound sepsis after application of an
external skeletal fixator is the presence of necrotic tissue in the wound.
Such necrotic tissue can be either soft tissue, which was not debrided
from the wound at the time of initial (or subsequent) debridement, or dead
bone.

To prevent wound sepsis, repeated wound debridement may be necessary. It
is difficult at the time of initial wound inspection to determine the margin of tissue viability. A reasonable approach is to remove all obviously
necrotic tissue at the time of initial wound debridement, followed by re-
evaluation of the wound 48-72 hours later. (The wound must be left open in
this situation.) If additional necrotic tissue is present, it should be
debrided. If the wound is completely clean, a delayed primary closure can
be carried out. If there is any question of viability, the wound can be
reassessed 48-72 hours later. This wound management technique greatly
reduces the likelihood of persistent wound sepsis.

Fixator Related Problems

The fixator frame itself may sometimes produce problems for the patient.
The most common fixator complication is pressure necrosis. This occurs
when one of the components of the fixator frame makes continuous contact
with the patient's skin, commonly in the proximal thigh (Fig. 8). The
surgeon should make sure to allow at least three fingerbreadths in this
region.

Component breakage has been reported, although rarely. Pin breakage is
unlikely to occur if the pins are used only once. The components of modern
external fixation systems are extremely well made and can be expected to
last for many years.

It is obvious that external skeletal fixation is associated with significant problems. Many can be prevented with proper care, but some seem to
strike capriciously. For this reason, external skeletal fixation should
be reserved for situations in which other techniques would not be satisfactory.

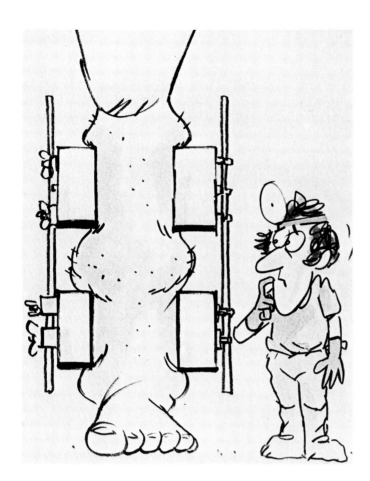

Fig. 8. Allow space
for swelling.

References

1. Burny, F.: Elastic external fixation of tibial fractures. Study of
   1421 cases. In, External Fixation, The Current State of the Art.
   Brooker, A.F., Jr. and Edwards, C.C. (eds.), Williams and Wilkins,
   1971.

2. Edwards, C.C., Jaworski, M., Solana, J., and Aronson, B.: Management
   of compound tibia fractures in the multiply injured patient using
   external fixation. Am.Surg. 45, 190, 1979.

3. Green, S.A., and Bergdorff, T.: External fixation in chronic bone and
   joint infections: The Rancho experience. Orthop. Trans. 4, 337, 1980.

4. Green, S.A.: Complications of External Skeletal Fixation. C.C. Thomas,
   Springfield, Illinois, 1981.

5. Johnson, H.F., Stovall, S.L.: External fixation of fractures. J.Bone
   Jt. Surg. 32A, 466, 1950.

6. Jorgensen, T.E.: The effect of electric current on the healing time of
   crural fractures. Acta Orthop. Scand. 43, 421, 1972.

7. Matthews, L. and Hirsch, C.: Temperatures measured in human cortical bone when drilling. J.Bone Jt.Surg. 54A, 297, 1972.

8. Perren, S.M.: Physical and biological aspects of fracture healing with special reference to internal fixation. Clin. Orthop. 138, 1975, 1979.

9. Zbikowski, J.L.: Biocompression. In, Proceedings of the 7th International Conference on Hoffmann External Fixation: Vidal, J. (Ed.), Geneva, Diffinco, 1979.

The Double-Frame External Fixator

J. Vidal and J. Melka

The external fixator is particularly helpful in the stabilization of bones of the extremities, the shoulder girdle, and the pelvis. Its use is primarily indicated for patients with extensive skin or soft tissue loss associated with fractures. In other words, it should be used in cases of fractures with a risk of serious infection. Furthermore, the external fixator is the treatment of choice when an infection is already present as in infected pseudarthrosis.

The major advantage of the external fixator of Hoffmann is ease of handling. Its basic design permits its use in any part of the skeleton without need for supplementary fixation (Connes, 1975).

We will describe in this paper the principal techniques of applying the external fixator of Hoffmann, restricting ourselves to a brief outline of its characteristics, technique of mounting, and the main indications for this procedure.

The Components of the Hoffmann System

1. Basic Elements: (Fig. 1)

Threaded pins. These are placed on both sides of the fracture. Two kinds of threaded pins exist: the transfixing (full pins) and the nontransfixing (half pins). Their use depends on the mounting and the location.

Universal ball joints. These are mounted on the pins.

Articulating couplings. They permit an orientation in all three planes of the rods which unite the couplings. These connecting rods can be simple or adjustable, permitting distraction or compression at the fracture site.

2. Tools required for installing frame:

Drill brace - to introduce the pins

Pin guide - for proper spacing and parallel insertion of pins

T-wrench - to tighten couplings and ball joints.

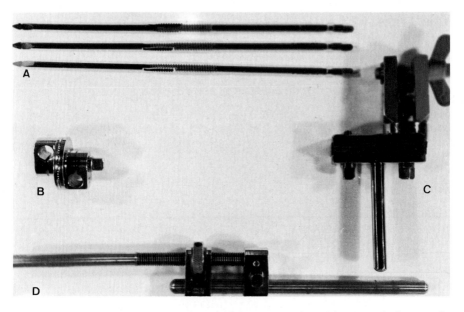

Fig. 1. The components of the Hoffmann system. A) threaded Bonnel pins; B) articulating couplings; C) universal ball joints; D) adjustable connecting rod.

Technique of Mounting Double Frame

We prefer the double frame (Fig. 2) for the leg. It constitutes the basic construction, and all other mountings can be modified depending on the anatomic site (Adrey, 1970; Connes, 1975). For this reason, we will describe the basic frame in greater detail.

The threaded transfixing pins are grouped at each side of the fracture. The spacing and parallelism of these pins, usually three, are regulated by the pin guide. Some points are of special importance. The pins should be inserted with a specially designed hand brace. The use of electrical or air-powered equipment is definitely not recommended since high speed rotation can cause burns, resulting later in osteolysis around the pins. We recommend that an incision, 1 cm long, be made before inserting the pins. This provides a certain mobility of the surrounding skin. The small incisions will remain open, preventing the development of hematoma which are not only painful but may cause infection. The pins should be inserted from the medial to the lateral aspects, thus assuring that the threaded parts do not cross the muscles of the anterolateral compartment. Two groups of three pins each are inserted at each side of the fracture.

Four universal ball joints are then placed on the pins, bringing them as close as possible to the axis of the diaphysis. Sufficient space, however, should be left in case edema develops and to permit observation of and skin care around the pins. A distance of 2 cm from the skin seems ideal.

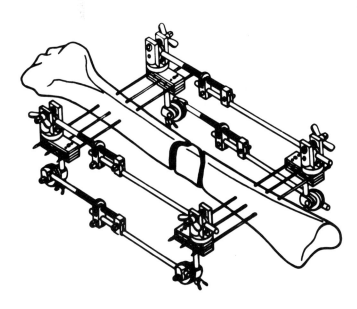

Fig. 2. The basic double frame. The four rods
permit a later correction in the sagittal and
frontal plane.

Once the fracture has been reduced, the threaded pins must be inserted perpendicularly to the diaphyseal axis. The reduction is carried out under
direct vision through the wound which can be opened more widely if required.
The universal ball joints, medially as well as laterally, are then connected
with two adjustable connecting rods, one anterior and one posterior. The
double frame is now complete (Fig. 2).

The four adjustable rods permit neutralization of forces at the fracture
site in cases of unstable fractures, compression in cases of stable fractures, or distraction for maintenance of length in cases of loss of bone
substance.

The adjustable rods even permit that certain corrections of the reduction
can be made later on in the frontal and saggital planes. Rotational deformities, which are more difficult to correct through simple adjustments of the
rods, should be corrected under general anesthesia. All eight couplings are
loosened and retightened after correction.

The mounting described above is the basic procedure. Additional anchorages
will increase the stability of external fixation. Additional parallel
anchorage with full pins and anchorage with oblique half pins is usually
used at the metaphyseal level if the fragment is too short to insert three

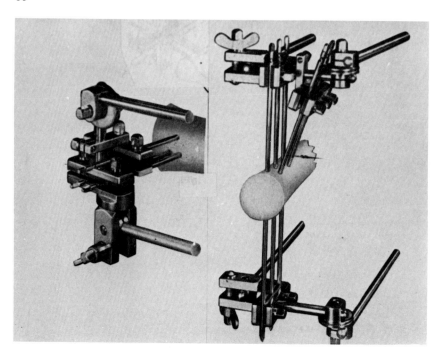

Fig. 3. Additional parallel anchorage with transfixing pins and additional anchorage with half pins
used to stabilize a small metaphyseal fragment.

parallel pins (Fig. 3). The stabilization of an intermediary fragment can
be achieved with a group of intermediary pins, full or half pins, depending
on the size of the fragment. These pins will be attached to the frame
either by a simple coupling, in cases of one pin, or by creating a two-
level double frame. Finally, in cases when the fracture is distracted we
have found insufficient stability with the double frame, especially when
exposed to bending forces. We were able to remedy this shortcoming, however, by adding a fifth anterior rod. A vertical anchorage is achieved
through pins as close as possible to the fracture site, attached to the
anterior rod. The half pins are therefore as far as possible from the full
pins (Fig. 4). This vertical mounting compensates totally the weakness
caused by a bending of the full pins.

Monitoring of the Hoffmann External Fixator

The leg with the external fixator is suspended on a support to prevent any
compression of the posterior compartment caused by the fixator's weight
(Fig. 5).

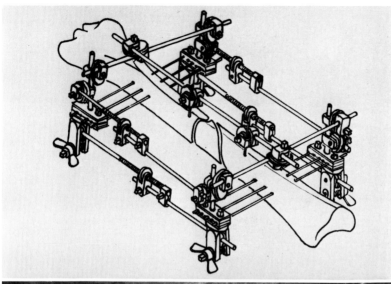

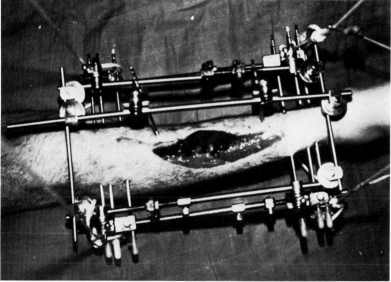

Fig. 4. Increase in rigidity of the double frame through addition of a fifth rod placed anteriorly and additional vertical anchorage.

Local skin care around the pins is of utmost importance. It is a simple but essential operation. The entry points of the pins must be cleaned daily with an antiseptic solution. No dressing is needed. Scabs should be removed to prevent accumulation of pus.

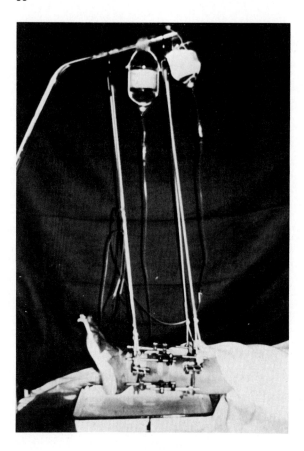

Fig. 5. Continuous open irrigation and suspension of the lower extremity through the external fixator.

An external fixator should not cause pain. If the patient complains of pain, either spontaneous or induced by skin pressure around the pins, subcutaneous pus should be suspected. The incision around the pins must be immediately enlarged to prevent osteitis developing around the pins.

The symptoms of osteitis are persistent drainage despite good skin care, confirmed by radiographs showing resorption around the pins. The affected pin should be removed immediately to prevent spread of osteitis and a possible pathologic fracture. If necessary, all pins of that group must be exchanged.

Osteitis is treated by local curettage. A mini-Papineau procedure is rarely indicated (Roy Camille, 1976).

Indications for a Double Frame

Generally, the ideal indication for an external fixator is a combination of severe bone trauma with extensive skin or soft tissue lacerations. Thus, all compound fractures, grade II and III according to the classification of

Cauchoix and Duparc, and infected pseudarthroses are treated by us with the double frame. Although mounting of the frame does not solve all the problems, it provides prime and steadfast support during the entire treatment period, thus permitting simultaneous handling of three problems: infection, skin lesions, and the fracture. The frame should not be used as a temporary means of fixation.

Treatment is divided into two stages whether for an open fracture or an infected pseudarthrosis. The initial stage must combine meticulous care of the fracture or pseudarthrosis with proper mounting of the frame, as described above. Continuous irrigation should be instituted and the wound kept open if closure cannot be achieved without tension.

During the second stage, additional treatment is instituted to obtain skin healing and fracture consolidation (ie, skin graft, bone graft). All types of bone grafts can be used with external fixation, particularly bone grafts not covered by soft tissues (Papineau, 1973); tibiofibular grafts; and free transfers with microvascular anastomosis (Melka, 1979).

Complications of External Fixation

1. Faulty mounting

Faulty mounting of the external fixator with half pins or full pins can injure delicate soft tissue, vessels, nerves, and tendons. Danger points exist at different levels. Here, it is advisable to insert the pins under direct vision, thus avoiding injury to nerves and vessels. Raimbeau et al (1979) drew attention to the risk of a compartment syndrome secondary to the insertion of pins. This complication may also be caused by the original trauma. We believe that it is due to the initial injury and the subsequent development of a hematoma.

Treatment consists of a large fasciotomy to decrease the pressure. The pins must be inserted from the medial to the lateral aspect to prevent any muscle or tendon damage by the threaded part.

2. Reactions

Immobilization causes thrombosis and sympathetic dystrophy. It is therefore important to mobilize the externally-fixed extremity and to move the adjacent joints (in cases of leg fractures: knee, ankle and toes). Weight bearing should be started as early as possible, to be increased gradually depending on the status of the bones. We recommend exercises twice daily in the form of compression through pressure (12.5 kg, 100 times, morning and evening, the amount of pressure to be increased slowly).

Osteolysis around the pins is caused by unstable mounting of the external fixator. Regular tightening of the screws of the external fixator is mandatory.

Osteitis around the pins can be prevented as already outlined above.

We have observed one postoperative aneurism of the humeral artery where the pin had pierced it. This complication was responsible for the healing of a pseudarthrosis which had been resistant to various kinds of treatment.

Fractures at pin site occur sometimes after removal of pins due to a weakening of bone secondary to an inadequately treated osteitis.

Internal fixation after external fixation represents a serious danger. We have insisted, repeatedly, that the use of an external fixator will lead to healing of all lesions which justified its use in the first place. Wrong indications and insufficient treatment must be avoided.

Conclusions

We believe that the complications of external fixation are due to faulty techniques or to wrong indications. If the external fixator is correctly mounted and strictly monitored with special care around the pins, and if stability is maintained, the external fixator should be well tolerated for periods of several months without adverse effects.

References

1. Adrey, J.: Le fixateur externe d'Hoffmann couplé en cadre. Etude bio-mécanique dans les fractures de jambe. Thése de Doctorat en Médecine. Université de Montpellier, 1970.

2. Cauchoix, J., Duparc, J., and Boulez, P.: Traitement des fractures ouvertes de jambe. Mem. Acad. Chir. 83, 891, 1957.

3. Connes, H.: Le fixateur externe d'Hoffmann. Techniques, indications et résultats. Edition Gead, Paris, 1975.

4. Melka, J.: Les pertes de substance osseuse des membres. Les transferts libres en micro-chirurgie face aux méthodes conventionnelles. Thése de Doctorat en Médecine. Université de Montpellier, 1979.

5. Papineau, L.J.: L'excision greffe avec fermeture retardée délibérée dans l'ostéomyélite chronique. Nouv. Pres. Med, 41, 2753, 1973.

6. Raimbeau, G., Chevalier, J.M., and Raguin, J.: Les risques vasculaires du fixateur en cadre à la jambe. Suppl. II. Rev. Chir. Orthop. 65, 77, 82, 1979.

7. Roy Camille, R., Reignier, B., Saillant, and Berteaux, D.: Résultats de l'intervention de Papineau (à propos de 46 cas). Rev. Chir. Orthop. 62, 347, 1976.

8. Vidal, J., Buscayret, Ch., Connes, H., Paran, M., and Allieu, Y.: Traitement des fractures ouvertes de jambe par le fixateur externe en double cadre. Rev. Chir. Orthop. 62, (433, 448), 1976

Hoffmann External Half Frame Fixation

F. Burny

The healing process of a fracture depends both on biologic and mechanical factors. It is now well proven that the amount of periosteal callus is closely related to the elasticity of the fixation. Callus formation also depends on an adequate capillary network of blood vessels. The possible influences of the type of fixation are presented in Table I.

It has become increasingly apparent that rigid internal fixation is responsible for disturbances of bone healing due to

- alterations of blood supply (large exposure of the fragments)
- overprotection of the underlying bone.

Elastic external fixation is an alternative to internal rigid fixation if we consider the duration of the primary healing process and the inherent complications of that technique (Burny et al, 1980).

Table I. Influence of treatment technique on healing

Treatment	Biologic Advantage	Mechanical Advantage	Total
Conventional open reduction	− −	+ ?	+ − ? −
Open reduction + associated internal fixation	− ?	+ +	+ ? + −
A *minima* opening	+ −	+ +	+ + + −
Closed reduction	+ +	? −	+ ? + −

Advantages of Hoffmann External Fixation (HEF)

From a review of the literature (Burny et al, 1965) and our own experience, we find many advantages in the use of the HEF.

One of its major advantages is the versatility of the material, providing adequate mounting for each fracture. The surgeon can select

- the type of pins (diameter, length, transfixation or not),
- the number and the location of the pins in each fragment and in each clamp,
- the number of fixation rods (half frame, triangular fixation, simple or double frame ...).

Any mounting can be built from the elastic half frame to the most rigid reinforced double frame.

Although the universally recognized indication for external fixation is the open fracture, we have extended this technique to simple fractures as well.

The treatment of simple fractures using HEF requires an absolutely accurate technique and rigorous postoperative care.

For tibial fractures, elastic external fixation (Fig. 1) is obtained when

- three pins are inserted in each fragment
- the clamps are tightened close to the bone
- the connecting rod is short (Burny et al, 1965, 1972, 1979).

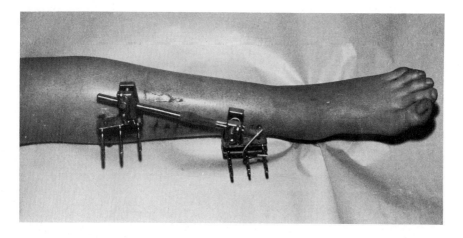

Fig. 1. Half frame external fixation following the mechanical principles.

Operative Technique

The advantages of the elastic external fixation are

-   the protection of the biologic and mechanical environment of the bone,
-   the mechanical stimulation at the fracture site leading to fast periosteal callus formation
-   the possibility of recording the mechanical characteristics of the callus, *in vivo* (Burny 1968, 1976, 1979).

Other advantages of the HEF are presented in Table II.

Table II. Advantages of the Hoffmann External Fixation frame

---

1. Easy treatment of associated soft tissue injuries
2. Reduction possible after pin insertion
3. No material at the fracture site
4. Early motion of the joints
5. Easy correction of possible secondary angulation
6. Good acceptance by the patient
7. Easy removal after healing

The HEF system is widely known. The required instrumentation for the half frame is restricted as presented in Table III.

Table III. Specific instrumentation

---

1   sharp, pointed scalpel
1   drill brace, with a 4 mm chuck
6   interrupted threaded pins, 12 cm Ø 4 mm
1   guide
2   clamps
1   T-wrench
1   set of connecting rods

The steps in the technique are presented in Tables IV, V, and VI.

Table IV. General Management

Anesthesia:	General
Patient Position:	Supine Leg in upper position
Special Equipment:	Image intensifier Radiolucent operating table
Draping:	No jersey

	Medium:	1 underneath the leg
	Split:	1 on the leg
	Large:	on the patient

Table V. Surgical Technique: A. Closed reduction

Patient supine
No tourniquet
Cleaning and draping of the leg
Longitudinal skin incision (1 cm)
    Pin drill in the proximal (5, 1, 3) and distal
    pins (1, 5, 3)
Fixation of the 2 clamps
Reduction controlled by image intensifier
Locking of the clamps on the connecting rod

Table VI. Surgical Technique: B. A *minima* opening

Insertion of threaded pins
Medial incision of the fracture site, 3 to 5 cm long
Exposure of the fracture
Visual reduction (without forceps)
Locking of the elements
Skin closure

Pin insertion

If possible, external fixation of the fractures should be carried out as
an emergency procedure. In the case of a closed fracture, the first pin
is inserted 3-5 cm of the fracture line at right angle to the medial
cortex in the proximal and distal fragments. Threaded pins spaced 12 cm
apart are usually used for tibial cortical bone; continuously threaded
pins can be used for epiphyseal or metaphyseal fixation.

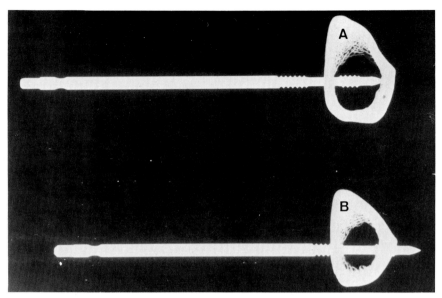

Fig. 2. a) Protection of the first cortical tape during pin insertion. b) Ideal position of the threads after insertion.

The advantage of pins with spaced threads is to protect the tapping of the first cortex when the pin reaches the second cortex (Fig. 2a). After insertion, both threaded parts must be in cortical bone (Fig. 2b).

Before placing each pin, a longitudinal skin incision, 1 cm long, on the medial aspect of the leg will prevent skin tension, secondary skin necrosis, and pin tract infection. The most proximal and distal pins of each set must be inserted first. Any other way of inserting pins may hinder the insertion of the peripherally located pins (Fig. 3).

Three pins are usually used in each fragment, equidistant to each other, except in patients with osteoporotic bone. Pin positioning can be checked by roentgenogram or image intensifier.

Reduction of the fracture

When possible, closed reduction of the fracture is obtained by means of an image intensifier. A possible closed reduction, if required after insertion of pins, is one of the advantages of the HEF. If a closed reduction cannot be easily obtained, surgery should be considered.

a) A minima opening. In case of tibial fractures, the superficial situation of the bone permits easy surgical procedure without devascularization of the fragments. The visual control of the reduction is possible, without

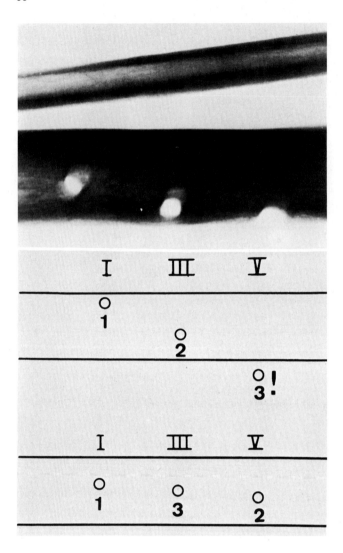

Fig. 3. Impossibility of proper insertion of peripheral pins because of misplaced intermediate pins.
I, III, V: position of the pins in the clamp.
1, 2, 3: succession of pin insertion.

bone clamps, using an *a minima* approach of the fracture site (4-5 cm long), exposing the fragments to be reduced.

b) *Associated internal fixation*. In long oblique or spiroid fractures, associated *a minima* internal fixation by screw is useful. The mechanical stability is then considered of primary importance.

Early postoperative care

Sterile dressing is applied around the pins until drying of the skin incisions (± 1 week); disinfection with alcohol is performed 2-3 times daily.

Suspension of the leg is recommended to prevent venous stasis. Early
physiotherapy of knee and ankle is started the day after the operation.
A drop foot splint is used for most of the patients' weight bearing.

The aim of the elastic external fixation is to provide some degree of
interfragmentary mobility to improve periosteal callus formation. One
must, however, take into account the general principles of internal fixation to avoid failure of implants or pseudarthrosis. Weight bearing
will then depend on the configuration of the fracture and on an eventual
associated fixation. Early weight bearing is possible in cases of stable
fracture or after associated *a minima* fixation.

For other types of fractures, we recommend delayed weight bearing based
on roentgenographic examination of healing, and on evaluation of the
rigidity of the callus by means of strain gauges.

Late postoperative care

After a hospitalization of one or two weeks, the patients are examined
every two weeks for pin tract reactions and measurement of the callus
rigidity as already mentioned.

In case of pin tract reactions, disinfection with alcohol usually controls
the situation without antibiotic treatment. Removal of the pins because
of infection is rarely required.

Every month, the amount of callus and the quality of the reduction are
observed by roentgenograms. In case of secondary angulation, correction
can be made by temporary disconnection of the fixation rod.

Removal of the external fixation

The treatment of external fixation is considered a definitive procedure,
and we do not use any auxiliary means of fixation (ie, plaster cast) after
removal of the material. The removal of the fixation apparatus is performed on an outpatient basis without anesthesia.

Complications

We will only consider the complications related to external fixation based
on a review of the literature (Burny et al, 1965) and our own experience.

Reactions around the pins

The causes of pin tract reactions are usually due to

- poor nursing care of the pin tracts
- weight bearing-induced friction between pins and soft tissues.
- eczematous conditions following improper dressing.

We did a prospective study of reactions related to the pins from 1975 to

68

Table VII. Pin tract reactions. Total number of
observations - Prospective study 1975-1980

Location of Pins	No. of Reports
Humerus	1,413
Radius	704
Cubitus	376
Metacarpal bone	335
Femur	312
Tibia	7,466
Calcaneus	211
Total	10,817

1980 (Burny et al, 1981). Four types of variables were considered: no
reaction; redness; infection; osteolysis.

The number of reports is presented in Table VII. Table VIII presents the
rate and type of reactions versus time for tibial fractures only (Fig. 4).

HEF of Tibia - Reactions around pins
(proximal + distal pins)

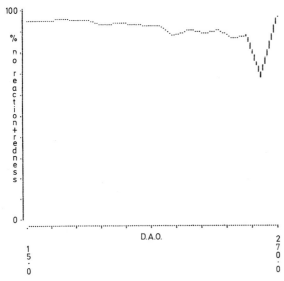

Fig. 4. Rate of pin tract reactions versus
time (tibial pins only) (D.A.O. - day after
operation)

Table VIII.　External Fixation - Reactions around pins

Tibia:Proximal Pins

| | | Reactions (%) | | |
D.A.O.*	Redness	Drain	Lysis	Observations
15	96.7	3.3	0.0	92
30	97.7	2.0	0.3	344
45	98.1	1.9	0.0	365
60	95.8	2.3	1.8	383
75	95.2	3.3	1.5	396
90	94.2	1.2	4.6	415
105	94.3	3.1	2.6	385
120	95.1	2.3	2.6	306
135	93.4	3.5	3.1	287
150	92.9	4.0	3.2	253
165	86.1	4.8	9.1	208
180	89.9	3.8	6.3	158
195	96.4	0.0	3.6	83
210	89.7	1.7	8.6	58
225	86.2	1.7	12.1	58
240	100.0	0.0	0.0	31

Tibia: Distal Pins

| | | Reactions (%) | | |
D.A.O.*	Redness	Drain	Lysis	Observations
15	94.8	2.1	3.1	97
30	93.8	5.4	0.8	355
45	94.9	5.1	0.0	355
60	95.1	4.6	0.3	391
75	95.3	4.7	0.0	406
90	92.2	5.4	2.4	410
105	92.8	5.5	1.8	400
120	90.8	6.3	3.0	303
135	91.1	6.4	2.5	281
150	92.0	5.4	2.7	261
165	87.8	9.2	3.1	196
180	91.5	5.9	2.6	153
195	80.7	13.3	6.0	83
210	90.3	3.2	6.5	62
225	87.0	4.3	8.7	46
240	76.5	2.9	20.6	34

(continued next page)

Table VIII. (continued)

Tibia: Total Pins

D.A.O.*	Redness	Reactions (%) Drain	Lysis	Observations
15	95.8	2.6	1.6	189
30	95.7	3.7	0.6	699
45	96.5	3.5	0.0	720
60	95.5	3.5	1.0	774
75	95.3	4.0	0.7	802
90	93.2	3.3	3.5	825
105	93.5	4.3	2.2	785
120	92.9	4.3	2.8	609
135	92.3	4.9	2.8	568
150	92.4	4.7	2.9	514
165	86.9	6.9	6.2	404
180	90.7	4.8	4.5	311
195	88.6	6.6	4.8	166
210	90.0	2.5	7.5	120
225	86.5	2.9	10.6	104
240	87.7	1.5	10.8	65

(* day after operation)

The reactions are treated by

- relative rest of the limb to avoid friction between pins and soft tissues,
- clearing and disinfection of the pins,
- general antibiotic treatment (seldom necessary).

Persisting drainage, after removal of the pins, was observed in 0.4% of cases. Simple curretage of the pin tract was successful in all cases associated with general antibiotic therapy.

Latent infection must, however, be taken into account if secondary internal fixation is planned.

Lack of rigidity

Elastic fixation means some degree of interfragmentary motion at the fracture site. Too much motion can lead to hypertrophic pseudarthrosis or to secondary displacements and malunion.

From a general statistical review of 1421 cases (Burny et al, 1979), we selected 450 cases of simple fractures (Burny et al, 1979). The rate of malunion (angular deviation of 10° or more) was 3.3%.

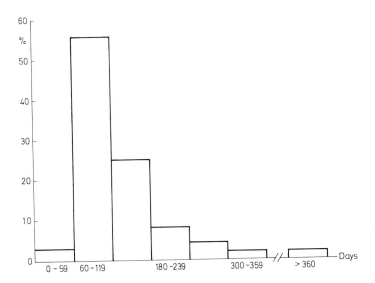

Fig. 5.Length of healing of 418 documented tibial
fractures.

Pseudarthrosis and delayed healing

External fixation was reported to be responsible for a high rate of pseudarthroses or delayed unions. In a review of 450 simple fractures, the rate
of pseudarthroses was 6.7%, occurring mostly in open grade I fractures
(11.5%) but less in closed, simple fractures (5.0%). A statistical analysis of the incidence of pseudarthrosis was conducted in 1979 (Burny et al,
1979). Based on a comparison with other means of fixation (Burny, 1972),
external fixation did not appear to be responsible for delayed union.

Fig. 5 is a graphic presentation of the healing time of 418 documented
simple tibial fractures (Burny et al, 1979).

Conclusion

Elastic external fixation of fractures appears to be more adapted to bone
physiology than rigid internal fixation.

The major advantages of Hoffmann External Fixation are the versatility of
the material providing adequate mounting for each fracture. The elastic
external fixation was therefore used for simple fractures as well.

The treatment of simple fractures by HEF requires a highly accurate technique:

-   accurate pin selection,
-   accurate pin insertion,

- adaptation of the method of fixation to the characteristics of the
  fracture
- *a minima* opening for anatomic reduction or *a minima* synthesis for unstable
  simple fractures,

and rigorous postoperative care.

The weight bearing will depend on the characteristics of the fractures and
the mounting. Pin tract reactions are not a contraindication for external
fixation.

This technique is a single, definitive procedure without requiring any
auxiliary instruments or materials.

References

1. Burny, F. and Deblois, G.: La fixation externe des fractures. Revue
    de la littérature. In, La fixation externe en Chirurgie, pp 31-56.
    Imp. Médicale et Scientifique, Bruxelles, 1965.

2. Burny, F., and Bourgois, R.: Etude théorique de l'ostéotaxis. In,
    La fixation externe en Chirurgie, pp. 109-119. Imp. Médicale et
    Scientifique, Bruxelles, 1965.

3. Burny, F.: Etude par jauges de déformation de la consolidation des
    fractures en clinique. Acta Orthop. Belg. 34, 917-927, 1968.

4. Burny, F., and Bourgois, R.: Etude biomécanique du fixateur externe
    de Hoffmann. Acta Orthop. Belg., 38, 265-279, 1972

5. Burny, F.: Traitement par ostéotaxis des fractures diaphysaires du
    tibia. Etude de 115 cas. Acta Orthop. Belg. 38, 280-300, 1972.

6. Burny, F.: Biomécanique de la consolidation des fractures. Mesure de
    la rigidité du cal in vivo. Etude théorique, expérimentale et clinique.
    Application à la théorie de l'ostéosynthèse. Thèse d'agrégation, U.L.B.
    1976.

7. Burny, F., El Banna, S., Evrard, H., Vander Chinst, M., Degeeter, L.,
    Peeters, M., Verdonk, R., Desmet, Ch., Fernandez-Fairen, M., Moeira, D.,
    le Rebeller, M., Martini, M.: Elastic external fixation of tibial frac-
    tures. Study of 1421 cases. In, External Fixation, The Current State of
    the Art, Chapt. 5, pp. 55-73. Williams and Wilkins Co., Baltimore, 1979.

8. Burny, F.: Strain gauges measurements of fracture healing. A study of
    350 cases. In, External Fixation, the Current State of the Art. Chapt.
    24, pp. 371-382. Williams and Wilkins Co., Baltimore, 1979.

9.   Burny, F., El Banna, S., Evrard, H., Vander Ghinst, M., de Geeter, L.,
     Peeters, F., Verdonk, R., Desmet, Ch.: Les fractures simples du tibia.
     Traitement par fixation externe élastique. 7èmes journées inter-
     nationales: la fixation externe d'Hoffmann. pp 60-77, Montpellier
     1980; Diffinco SA Ed, Genève.

10. Burny, F., Bourgois, R., Donkerwolcke, M.: Elastic fixation of frac-
     tures. In, Current Concepts of Internal Fixation of Fractures. Ed.:
     H.K. Uhthoff, Springer Verlag, pp 430-442, 1980.

11. Burny, F., Donkerwolcke, M., Saric, O., Coussaert, E.: External fixa-
     tion of fractures. The problem of the percutaneous implant. To be
     published, 1981.

External Fixation, Tubular ASIF Set

G. Hierholzer and A. Chernowitz

Introduction

External fixation is a method for clinically problematic cases; it is not
a standard method of fracture treatment (Codivilla, 1904; Hierholzer, 1978;
Hoffmann, 1942; Lambotte, 1908; Wagner, 1972). In pursuit of the best
program for injuries with severe bone and soft tissue damage, immobilization with a plaster cast is out of the question, and plating or nailing
entails a high risk of infection. Thus, external fixation does not compete with the standard method of internal fixation but is an alternative
which we need for certain special problems. It is of paramount importance
to find the correct indication for each patient.

Dealing with such problematic cases as

- open fracture III°
- open fracture II° admitted late
- fracture with polytrauma
- infected fracture and infected nonunion
- fracture or malunion associated with soft tissue damage
- arthrosis and arthritis

we have to consider the most important pathophysiologic factors: devitalization of tissue and instability of the injured area. In treating such a
severely injured limb, we need a technique which is able to bridge the
endangered area and to stabilize without disturbing the remaining vascularity of the bone.

Up to a few years ago, the stability of external fixation could not compete
with that of standard methods of internal fixation. Particular difficulties
were found in situations of severe damage without sufficient bone support.
Frequently, small metaphyseal fragments could not be stabilized adequately.
It seemed, therefore, necessary to improve both the operative technique and
the mechanical properties of the external fixator.

Clinical Consequence of Experimental Investigations and Classification of the Assemblies

In 1974 (Hierholzer, 1975; Kleining, 1975; 1976) we tested different assemblies based on the tubular system of ASIF (Association for the Study of
Internal Fixation). The tubular set, introduced by Robert Mathys, has a

bending stiffness of 2.5 to 3 times that of the threaded rod formerly used. This property permits us to bridge far greater distances. In engineering it is well known that a three-dimensional system provides higher stability than a two-dimensional one. For this reason, we constructed also a three-dimensional device using the tubular set.

The clinical relevance of previous experiments from our center (Hierholzer, 1975; Kleining, 1975; 1976) is as follows: In the diaphysis it is possible to achieve high stability with the two-dimensional device (the commonly known frame), even in cases of bone defect, by the application of at least two or three pins in each of the major fragments. In small metaphyseal fragments, on the other hand, where it is not possible to insert two or three parallel pins in one plane, we can achieve corresponding stability by using only one Steinmann pin and one Schanz screw with a three-dimensional device. This assembly consists of a frontal plane frame and anterior clasp which have to be connected by oblique pins. The simplicity of its application is also a matter for consideration.

It is important that for assembly of the different devices we need only a few components:

- tubes
- Steinmann pins
- Schanz screws
- one-adjustable clamps.

While the assemblies are still incomplete, the adjustable clamps permit correction of malalignment in the frontal or sagittal planes as well as malrotation (Fig. 1).

From our theoretical investigations and clinical experience we propose a classification of the application of the ASIF fixator into Types I, II and III (Fig. 2).

Clinical Versatility of the Assemblies of the Tubular ASIF Set

Type I (Fig. 3) is a clasp. We propose this type for the thigh because of anatomical topography and functional considerations. A typical indication is an open fracture of the femur in an adolescent with a near whole limb skin degloving. The clasp has to stabilize the fracture by bridging the endangered area without disturbing the epiphyseal plate. A second clasp can be used to temporarily immobilize the knee joint until split skin grafts have healed and mobilization is possible. The clasp is also suitable for a closed comminuted fracture in a patient with polytrauma; the external fixator preserves alignment and length of the bone without adding a large surgical insult to the existing trauma. Another indication is that of a severely infected femoral fracture, which also has to be stabilized by bridging the endangered area. Two lateral tubes are needed to build a stable assembly in the absence of continuous bony support.

77

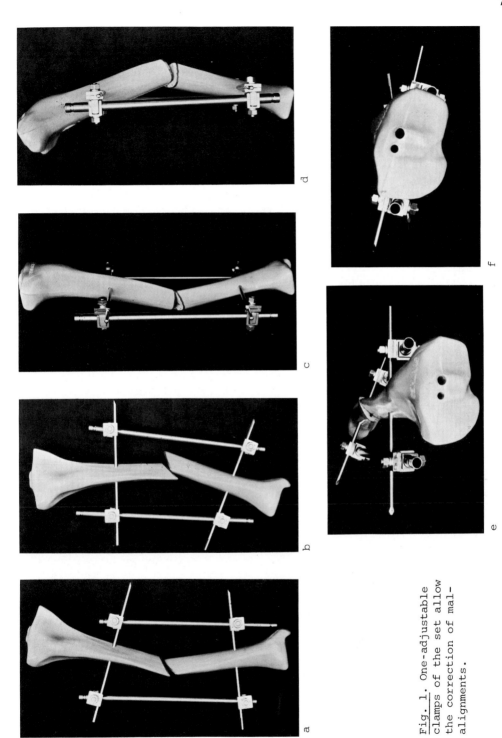

Fig. 1. One-adjustable clamps of the set allow the correction of malalignments.

TYPES OF CONSTRUCTION ASSEMBLY OF ASIF DEVICE

TYPE   I   CLASP

TYPE II   FRAME

TYPE III   THREE DIMENSIONAL DEVICE

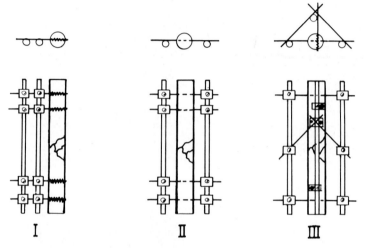

Fig. 2.   Assemblies Types I, II and III.

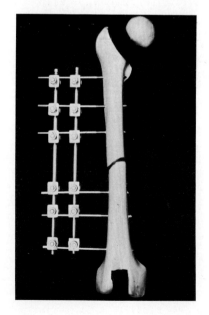

Fig. 3.   Bone model of assembly Type I.

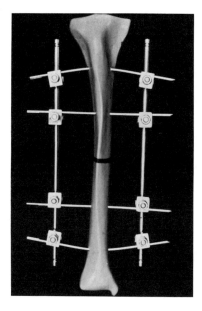 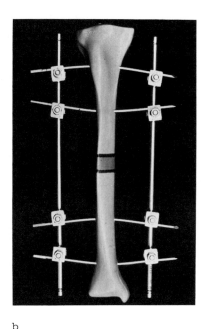

a   b

Fig. 4. Bone models of assembly Type II, a) with and b) without bone support.

Type II is the frame (Fig. 4). From our point of view, it is mainly indicated in the situation of broad bone contact. Under these circumstances we can take advantage of axial compression as in transverse fractures, in osteotomies (for example of the tibial head) or in arthrodeses of the ankle joint. In a short oblique open fracture, we may achieve the advantage of interfragmental compression with one or two lag screws without disturbing significantly the remaining vascularity. A single frame may then be sufficient and act as a neutralization apparatus. Some surgeons use the frame technique with several parallel pins even in patients with a bone defect; but here it is necessary to increase the stability of the assembly by compressing two pins, one to another, in each of the major fragments (Fig. 4b).

Type III is the three-dimensional assembly (Fig. 5). It can bridge great distances and can also fix a small metaphyseal fragment. In both situations, we need only one Steinmann pin and one Schanz screw in each of the major fragments plus a connection of the frontal frame to the anterior clasp by oblique pins (Fig. 5a, b). In each fragment the Schanz screw must be placed at a distance from the Steinmann pin to exert its stabilizing effect. When bridging external fixation is needed in the leg, we recommend Type III for stabilization. We would like to emphasize that of the three types, only Type III can bring stability to a short metaphyseal fragment. Another consideration is that Type III helps us to reduce

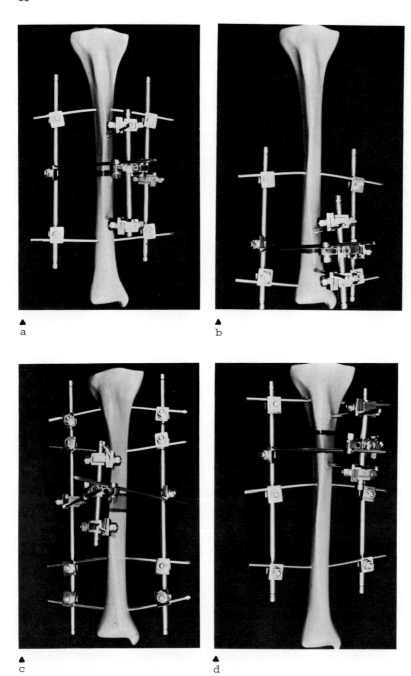

a

b

c

d

Fig. 5. Bone models of assembly Type III. Stabilization of a diaphyseal and metaphyseal fracture with (a and b) and without (c and d) bone support.

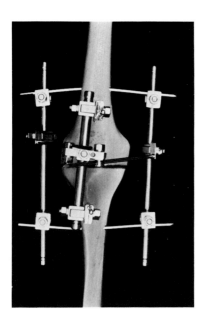

Fig. 6. Bone model of assembly Type III in arthrodesis of the knee joint.

the number of pins in the frontal plane which penetrate the muscles. An additional indication for the three-dimensional device is in arthrodesis of the knee joint (Fig. 6). The technique proposed by Müller (1955) with two frontal frames presents the difficulty of achieving sufficient distance between the assemblies, this distance being necessary to avoid bending instability. The single three-dimensional device neutralizes better the bending moment about the original axis of knee flexion and is certainly easier to apply.

Summary

Our experimental and clinical experience provides us with the opportunity to offer a classification of external fixator assemblies based on the ASIF set. Type I is recommended for the thigh; Type II for the leg under a condition of bony support; Type III to bridge great distances, to fix small metaphyseal fragments and for arthrodesis of the knee joint.

References

1. Codivilla, A.: On the means of lengthening in the lower limbs, the muscles and tissues which are shortened through deformity. Amer. J. Ortho. Surg. 2, 353, 1904.

2. Hierholzer, G.: Stabilisierung des Knochenbruchs beim Weichteilschaden mit Fixateurs externes. Langenbecks Arch. klin. Chir. 39, 505, 1975.

3. Hierholzer, G., Kleining, R., Hörster, G., and Zemenides, P.: External fixation. Arch. Orthop. Traumat. Surg. 92, 175, 1978.

4. Hoffmann, R.: Percutane Frakturbehandlung. Chirurg. 14, 101, 1942.

5. Kleining, R., Hierholzer, G., and Hörster, G.: Biomechanische Untersuchung zur Osteosynthese mit dem Fixateur externe. Vortrag: Dtsch. Sektion der Internat. Arbeitsgemeinschaft f. Osteosynthesefragen, 12, 4, 1975. Duisburg

6. Kleining, R., and Hierholzer, G.: Biomechanische Untersuchung zur Osteosynthese mit dem Fixateur externe. Act. Traumat. 6, 71, 1976.

7. Lambotte, A.: Sur l'osteosynthèse. Belg. Med. 231, 1908.

8. Muller, M.E.: Die Kompressionsosteosynthese unter besonderer Berücksichtigung der Kniearthrodese. Helv. Chir. Acta 6, 474, 1955.

9. Stader, O.: Treating fractures of long bones with the reduction splint. N.Amer. Vet. 20, 55, 1939.

10. Wagner, H.: Technik und Indikation der operativen Verkürzung und Verlängerung von Ober- und Unterschenkel. Orthopädie 1, 59, 1972.

External Fixation: The Dresden System

J. Hellinger

The Dresden system is not based on a particular form of a device, but comprises the systematic application of different devices for special indications. The basic classification into wire-fixed, pin-fixed and screw-fixed systems is essential for the future development of external fixation. Moreover, assessment of the value of these fixation sets is essential for their further improvement and more favorable results. We have therefore analyzed

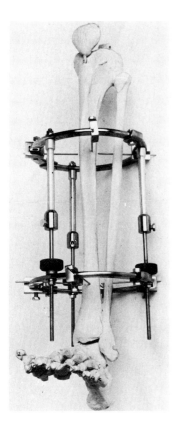

Fig. 1. Original Ilisarov device. Lower leg mounting demonstration on the model.

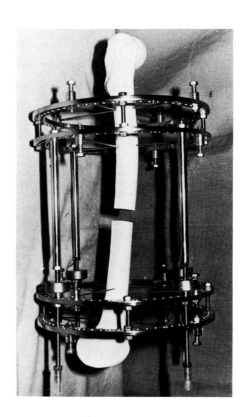

Fig. 2. Our own modified double-ring device with spatial fixation. The example shows the possibilities for distraction osteotomy on the femur.

our own technique for stability, infection rate, handling, mounting methods and comfort for the patient. Cost was also taken into consideration.

Since pin-fixed and screw-fixed models have been presented by other authors, I confine myself to the wire-fixed models. Generally, an Ilisarov device (Fig. 1, 2) with a crossed Kirschner wire fixation in the bone consists of a ring system connected by rods with threaded spindles. Our modification of this model consists of the basic double ring device and perforated rings allowing more versatile mounting possibilities. Half-ring mountings can be applied in the area of the pelvis and the shoulder as well as on the proximal femur.

From 1971 to 1979, we have treated 193 patients - 99 women and 94 men - with this external fixation method. Eighteen patients are still under treatment. The age distribution (Table I) is relatively even, including all age groups from infants to geriatric patients.

When distributing the material according to different diagnoses (Table II) we observe a high incidence of post-traumatic conditions. Acute traumata play a lesser role due to the current structure of our clinic.

Table I. Age distribution

Age	No. of patients
1- 6	6
7-14	23
15-20	23
21-30	33
31-40	15
41-50	21
51-60	34
61-70	32
71-80	6

Table II. Conditions necessitating external fixation

Diagnoses	No. of patients
Congenital malformations	35
Inflammatory changes	33
Degenerative diseases	54
Tumors and their sequelae	1
Post-traumatic conditions	70

A breakdown of diagnostic groups is shown in Tables III, IV, V and VI.

Table III. Congenital malformations

Diagnoses	No. of patients
CDH	10
Dysmelia	17
Ollier's disease (dyschondroplasia)	2
Recklinghausen's disease	2
Osteogenesis imperfecta	1
Meleorheostosis	1
Hemophilic arthropathy	1
Scoliosis	1

Table IV. Inflammatory changes

Diagnoses	No. of patients
Progressive-chronic polyarthritis	14
Poliomyelitis	12
Coxitis	2
Primary osteomyelitis	2
Gonitis	2
Scars after abdominal surgery	1

Table V. Degenerative diseases

Diagnoses	No. of patients
Varus gonarthritis	32
Valgus gonarthritis	13
Gonarthritis without deviation	7
Paresis after disc herniation	1
Paresis secondary to muscle dystrophy	1

Table VI. Post-traumatic conditions

Diagnoses	No. of patients
Pseudarthrosis	35
Deformities	23
Epiphyseal lesions	4
Delayed union	3
Osteomyelitis	3
Dislocations	2

We used 110 wire-fixed models, 109 pin- and screw-fixed models, and five combinations of pin- and screw-fixed fixators. Among the wire-fixed apparatuses, the Ilisarov ring model, especially our own version with double-ring mounting, was most frequently applied. Among the pin- and screw-fixed models the well-known AO-frame fixator was mostly employed (Table VII).

A knowledge of the different forms of application, depending on the indication, was also essential for the assessment. The application in correction and distraction osteotomies (Fig. 3, 4), arthrodeses, pseudarthrosis compressions and pseudarthrosis distractions prevailed in our series (Table VIII).

Table VII. Different devices used in the Orthopedic Clinic, Medical Academy Carl Gustav Carus

Device	Number
Wire-fixed models	110
modified ring system	77
Ilisarov system	29
joint-apparatus Wolkow-Oganesjan	2
Kalnber's device	1
Greifensteiner device	1
Pin- and screw-fixed models	109
AO-frame fixator	78
Polid/CSSR	9
Hoffmann-Vidal fixator	8
Wagner fixator	6
AO-tubular system	5
Miehle/GDR system	1
Halo-pelvic traction	2

Table VIII. Type of surgery with external fixation

Procedure	No. of changes
Corrective osteotomies	59
Distraction osteotomies	50
Arthrodeses	41
Pseudarthrosis compressions	21
Pseudarthrosis distractions	19
Iliofemoral distractions	8
Combined pseudarthrosis compression and distraction osteotomies	3
Fracture distractions	2
Fragmental alignments	2
Columnotomie	2
Fracture neutralization	1

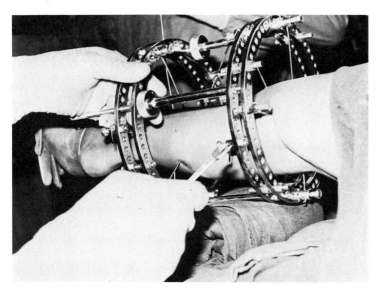

Fig. 3. Double-ring model during surgery on the lower leg.

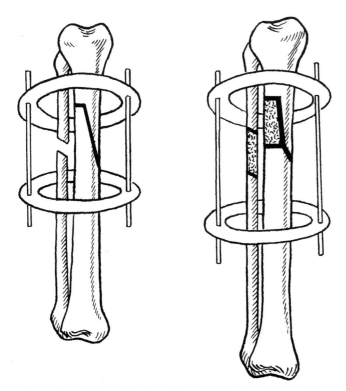

Fig. 4. Schematic drawing of distraction osteotomy with the Ilisarov device.

Table IX. No. of device changes

From double-ring device to	
Hoffmann-Vidal	3
AO-tubular system	2
Wagner	2
From AO frame fixator to	
Hellinger-Hoffmann	2
Hoffmann-Vidal	1
Ilisarov	1

The stability of the system is an important criterion of the assessment. Whereas on the one hand the stability is dependent on the construction of the device, it depends on the other hand essentially on the mode of anchorage in the bone. The quality of the bone, the gap that must be bridged, as well as the local and general mobility, must also be taken into consideration. Instability made changes mandatory in 11 of our 191 patients (5.7%). Table IX analyzes the modifications of the systems.

Perforation of the skin by pins, screws or wires contributes to infection. In evaluating 219 device mountings, we encountered 99 pin- or wire-site infections (45%). Out of 110 wire-fixed mountings, 66 infections occurred (60%). In the pin- and screw-fixed model series, 34 infections out of 109 mountings occurred (31%). We differentiate mild infections, requiring local treatment only, from severe infections, necessitating removal of wires or pins. The total number of infections consisted of 32% mild and 13% severe cases. The severest complication of pin-site infection was drill hole osteomyelitis, which occurred four times in our series. Sequestrectomy was immediately successful in three patients. One patient with intermittent drainage has not yet decided to undergo surgery.

Discussion

In the present development stage of perfecting the external fixation systems, we have made an evaluation of different models offered by many manufacturers. The stability of reduction is the major objective for the healing of bone whether fixed externally or internally. The kind of fracture healing depends on the degree of stability. The pin- and screw-fixed devices have the advantage of greater stability compared with the other devices. Also, in our series, more changes in the device had to be carried out, necessitated by instability, when wire-fixed devices had been used. The use of wire-fixed devices combined with the double ring system equipped with crossed Kirschner wires is definitely superior to the simple device.

With respect to stability, the wire-fixed model has the advantage that it can be used in small fragments near the joint or in epiphyseal positions for epiphyseal distraction. Instability-induced loss of tension can be easily corrected by simply exchanging the wires.

The stability of the system must be maintained during temporary removal of the connecting rods to perform additional surgery. Multilevel fixations with triangular mountings seem to be very useful in such cases. The problem of infection at the sites of skin perforation must not be underestimated. It occurs despite careful attention to essential details at the time of placing the device, including special care of the system.

We were able to control all infections and there was no permanent damage to the patients. We should like to point out, however, some of the disadvantages to the patients, such as prolonged hospitalization with the concomitant increase in cost. Since stability and infection of the pin- and wire-sites are very closely related, a comparison of both groups of our patient series reveals clear advantages of the pin- and screw-fixed models over the wire-fixed types.

The possibilities and limitations of mounting are also determined by the construction and the mode of fixation in the bone. In these cases the pin- and screw-fixed models have the definite advantage over other models since the application of universal clamp-fixator or the combination of clamp- and frame-fixator is only possible with screws fixed in the corticalis.

Triangular constructions, best performed with the AO-tubular system, offer optimal fixation of segmental fractures. Although we have performed iliofemoral distractions by means of wire-fixed mountings of our modified Ilisarov device, we are now using the pin- and screw-fixed models because of better mounting possibilities.

The construction advantages of the devices are essentially conditioned by the quantity of the articulated connections between the single bridging rods. The ball joint of the Hoffmann external fixator has proved to be extraordinarily useful in the types of devices used by us. The external fixator of the AO tubular system has nearly unlimited mounting possibilities with its pivoting jaws and hinges at highest stability. Threaded spindles or threaded rods are necessary for a universal application to allow initial or postoperative corrections.

External compression-distraction devices can also be classified according to their ease of handling. Their placement can be performed in a premounted or nonpremounted state. When using pin- and screw-fixed models, we prefer drilling templates to assure the exact position. The placement of the wire-fixed models is essentially more time-consuming since the guidance of the wires is more difficult when the device is mounted.

The insolation of transfixing pins or wires for electrical stimulation depends on the construction. Electrical stimulation can also be applied in the Hoffmann device.

The combination of external and internal osteosynthesis can also be considered. Frame mountings even with triangular construction offer better access and permit dorsal placement of the plate on the upper thigh and lower leg, on the condition that they are neither close to bone infections nor to contaminated sites around wires and pins.

External fixation requires greater cooperation from the patient. Since there are long periods of outpatient treatment, special attention has to be paid to the care of the wire and pin sites. The postoperative location of the patient and modes of available transportation later must be considered. The care of the system at risk of contamination by secretions is facilitated when uncomplicated systems are applied.

Having assessed the results in our patient groups with wire-fixed models, we now prefer the pin- and screw-fixed devices. In the light of these facts we should like to point out the advantages of the pin- and screw-fixed devices against the wire-fixed devices - stability, lower risk of infection, greater mounting versatility, and more comfort to the patient. These devices also have a wider application for a larger selection of indications.

Judet External Fixator

R. Judet, Th. Judet, M. Bisserié, N. Siguier, and B. Brumpt

As far back as 1932, Dr. Henri Judet and his sons, Jean and Robert, recommended the use of external fixators to maintain certain fractures and described a device which has existed in its present form since 1940. This device has been adapted to simple fixing of bone fragments, to compression of fractures and pseudarthrosis, and to gradual lengthening of bones.

Different constructions of this fixator have one factor in common: the material with which they are made is a U-shaped bar of stainless steel. The two sides of this bar are pierced with regularly-spaced holes, corresponding in pairs from one wing to the other. Bars with holes for 3, 4 and 5 mm diameter pins exist. The 5 mm bar is most in use, and the lengths vary between 16 to 60 cm. The pins pass through the holes of the bar and are screwed to the bone.

The fixator is designed to immobilize fractures already aligned and reduced; once the first pin is inserted, the straight longitudinal bar serves as a guide through which the other pins are placed.

Surgical Technique

The surgical technique is simple, but must follow certain principles:

- The operation is performed on a fracture table; the fracture is reduced and, if necessary, contained by bone clamps.

- All the pins are placed through the holes of the bar which is held parallel to the bone by the assistant.

- These pins must be placed either directly in the visible part of the bone in the wound, or at a distance through the soft tissues via a hole made by a scalpel.

- A motor-powered drill, guided by the holes of the bar-sides, prepares the holes in the bone. The drill bit has two calibers: the distal one, 3.5 mm diameter, penetrates the two cortices; the proximal, 5 mm diameter one, goes only through the first bone cortex.

- The pins, therefore, penetrate the first cortex with hard friction, but are screwed only into the second one where their correct position is felt by an increase of resistance to the screw insertion.

- Next, the bar is definitively fixed to the pins. It is important to place it as close as possible to the bone; that is to say, leaving a space between skin and bar just large enough for subsequent drainage.

- The fixation of the bar to the pins is obtained by metal-blocking plates which are placed between the corner iron and the rods, thereby insuring full rigidity of the junction bar/pin.

Stability and Solidity of Fixation

Maximum stability is an important factor in obtaining fracture union, particularly in cases of unstable fractures or bone defects. Laboratory studies performed by one of us have proved the superiority of rigid bars and 5 mm diameter pins. These studies have also brought certain precisions to the use of the device.

Length of the pins

As already mentioned, the distance between the bone and the bar must be as short as possible. This allows the use of small pins and, therefore, increases the comfort to the patient.

Position and number of pins

Best stability is obtained by spacing the pins to obtain the optimum leverage against the flexion forces: that is to say, by placing one or two pins

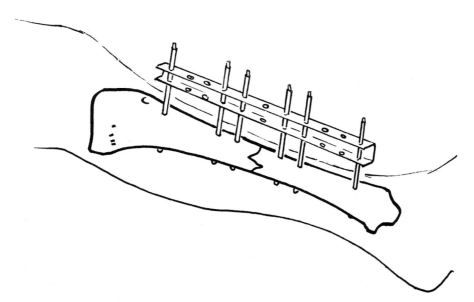

Fig. 1. Standard Judet fixator.

close to the fracture; one additional pin must be placed at a distance and acts as a pilot pin (Fig. 1). This procedure, with one single bar and three pins per fragment, is sufficient for stable fractures and all upper extremity fractures.

Maximum stability obtained by two bars -
Fixation in two different planes

Increased rigidity (necessary in cases of general fractures or tibial comminuted fractures) can be obtained by the use of a second bar with the pins so placed as to form an angle between 60° and 120° with the pins of the first bar (Fig. 2). Through each bar, two pins per fragment are placed: one close to the fracture, the other at a distance. No more than four holes are drilled in each fragment. Undesirable movements are thus strictly controlled both in the frontal and sagittal plane. Finally, the complete abolition of rotational movements is obtained by a coupling in a transverse fashion between a pin of each bar on both sides of the fracture.

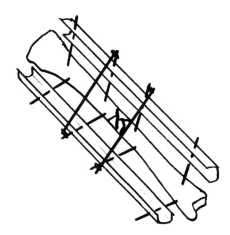

Fig. 2. Two-bar synthesis with transversal coupling.

Laboratory tests and our clinical experience have shown that this technique is, so far, the most solid that can be achieved by external fixation.

Adaptation of the Fixators for Fractures

The fixator is used in all patients with open or infected fractures.

The tibia

In the case of diaphyseal fractures, whether one or two bars are used, one rule must be strictly observed: one must not use a transfixing pin through the anterolateral compartment.

94

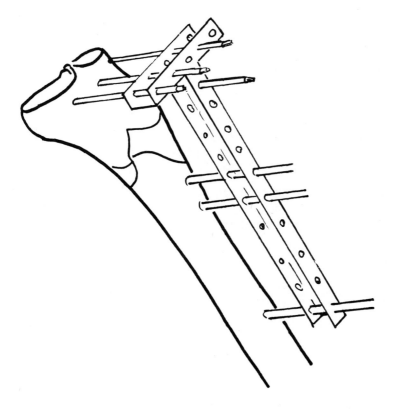

<u>Fig. 3</u>. T-shaped fixator inserted on an upper tibial extremity.

- A single bar should be placed right in the middle of the anteromedial side.
- When two bars are used, the sagittal pins should penetrate the shaft through the tibial crest, the frontal ones through the posteromedial edge of the bone.

In cases of high or low fractures, a T-shaped bar can be used (Fig. 3). In cases of intra-articular fractures of the ankle, this bar can bridge the joint and fix the foot to the leg at a right angle.

The femur

In femoral fractures, two bars are frequently used because of greater stresses at this level. The pins of the first bar are placed in the posterolateral plane of the lateral intermuscular fascia, the pins of the second bar reaching the bone in the anterolateral plane. This positioning permits early physiotherapy and preserves knee mobility.

For the proximal and distal metaphyseal regions, the T-shaped bar can be used. In cases of major lesions of the distal femur and/or the proximal tibia, the knee can be bridged by a long femorotibial bar.

Other Uses of the External Fixator

Compression fixator

In this device, the holes of half of one of the wings of the bar are oval shaped, whereas the holes of the other wing are circular. Possible oscil-

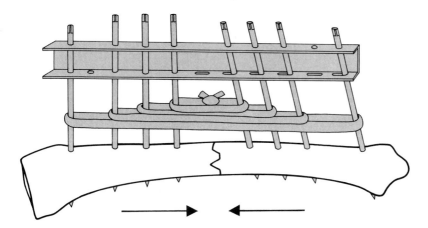

Fig. 4. Judet compression fixator

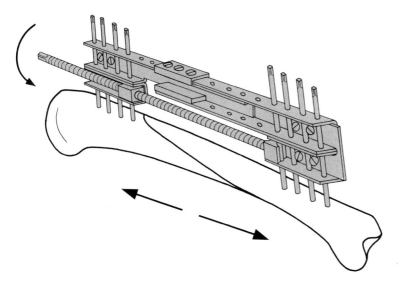

Fig. 5. Lengthening fixator inserted on a tibia.

lation of the rod permits applying elastic traction to compress a fracture
or pseudarthrosis (Fig. 4). This compression can be applied initially to
the treatment of pseudarthrosis or, eventually, in the process of healing
of a fresh fracture, simplifying the changing of the bar and applying
elastic traction. This compression is permanent even in cases of bone
resorption of the extremities.

Lengthening fixator

The lengthening fixator is composed of two elements of an ordinary fixator.
One, the male element, slides into the female element (Fig. 5). Four pins
are placed in each fragment of the bone to be lengthened. These pins go
through the sliding bar and two second short bars, set on each fragment, to
apply the progressive distraction by means of a long screw. Once the desired
amount of lengthening is obtained, a locking screw assures maintenance of
this position.

Geometrically variable fixator

This fixator is composed of two ordinary bars joined by a T-shaped element
with three vertical axes. With the geometrically variable fixator one can
align nonaligned bone fragments. It is particularly useful for the temporary
mounting of an iliotrochanteric coaptation. The two bars are fixed to the
iliac wing and to the femur (Fig. 6).

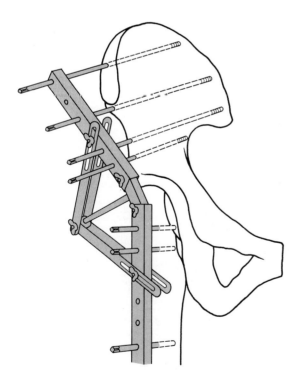

Fig. 6. Geometrically variable
fixator

The mobility given by the T-shaped device allows perfect positioning of the femur by permitting an angular mobility in the frontal plane and a medial transfer enabling the trochanter to be pushed as far as possible under the acetabular roof. The position thus obtained can be maintained by blocking the sliding grooves.

Conclusions

This set of fixators is made of very simple material widely used in various conditions. The rigidity of synthesis thus obtained has been tested by laboratory experiments. Furthermore, this device has the advantage of being neither heavy nor cumbersome, an important point when one remembers how long it takes for the bone lesions to consolidate.

Experiences with the Stuhler-Heise Fixator System

Th. Stuhler

The use of the external fixator is the accepted method today for serious injuries to soft tissues, infected fractures, pseudarthroses, tibial valgus or varus osteotomies, and arthrodeses.

On the basis of these surgical indications, the general requirements for the construction of an external fixator are the following:

1) use of simple, precisely designed elements;

2) limitation of the specific elements to a minimum of functional and easily obtainable parts;

3) standardized application for every surgical situation;

4) easy accessibility for primary or secondary correction;

5) mechanical durability;

6) a balanced ratio of weight to stability.

The fixator we are describing here consists of a three-dimensional construction, bringing the spheres into contact with rods, Steinmann pins or Schanz screws. Here, an increasing number of elements likewise reduces the degree of freedom in the x-y-z axes.

A solution was found in the form of hemispherical compression elements. To save space and material, they were changed into disc-like compression elements. For most applications, a so-called compression block consists of a compression element with an 8 mm boring and a central thread boring, an intermediate disc, 0.5 mm, and a compression element with 5 mm borings and a central boring without a thread (Fig. 1). All parts can be fixed in every desired position with a hexagonal screw. In the 5 mm and 8 mm borings, Steinmann pins, Schanz screws or rods project a few tenths of a mm. Under increasing compression loading, all parts are clamped. If a hexagonal screw is slightly loosened, Steinmann pins or rods are adjustable without disengaging them.

The 0.5 mm intermediate disc not only increases stability but also provides protection for the surfaces of the compression elements. Adjustments in the direction of the third dimensional axis are made possible by the use of intermediate discs of differing thickness.

If compression blocks have been forgotten or if additional reinforcements are warranted, 8 mm compression elements with a groove and a thread - marked "oben" (upper) - can be fitted into any other mounting.

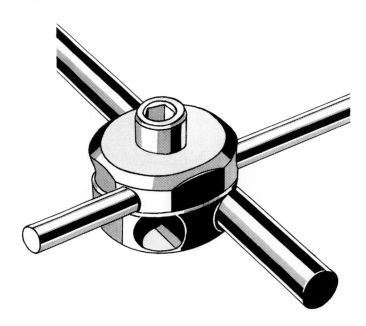

Fig. 1. Generally, the fixing blocks are assembled from the following parts: Fixing element with two 8 mm holes and central tapped hole; spacer disc 0.5 mm; fixing element with two holes 5 mm each and central untapped hole; bolt with hexagonal recess.

In numerous situations, preconstructed compression elements can be fitted on. It is sometimes more practical to clamp the single parts one after the other, for example:

- sliding of compression elements onto the rods and Steinmann pins;

- insertion of an intermediate disc or other essential compression elements, or 0.5 mm intermediate discs, as the case may be;

- final tying up of ends with the hexagonal screwdriver.

For separate indications requiring joints, extensions or triangular struts, the compression elements are laid out the other way around, ie, 5 mm compression elements with a central threaded opening and 8 mm compression elements without a thread. Thus, for example, two 8 mm compression elements can be combined to make a joint or an extension. In the same way, several 5 mm compression elements can be added for a tent strut.

The combination of two or three 5 mm compression elements with an 8 mm compression element or with intermediate discs permits a staggered insertion of the Steinmann pins parallel to the joint axis; for example, at the head of the tibia in alignment, fractures, or near an epiphysis.

Two different compression clamps are at our disposal for compression and distraction. The so-called "Bow" apparatus can be applied in every position and fixed to the rod by means of a clamp. In this way, compression elements which closely follow one another can be moved without difficulty. The small compression apparatus can be slipped on or put on.

We will demonstrate the application of this external fixator by the following examples:

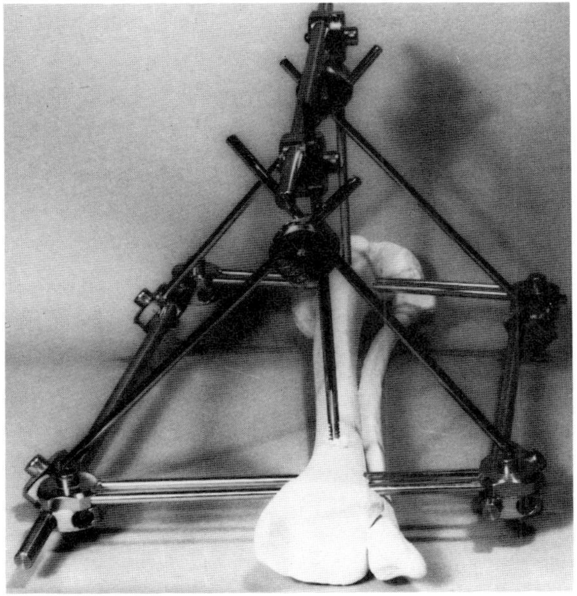

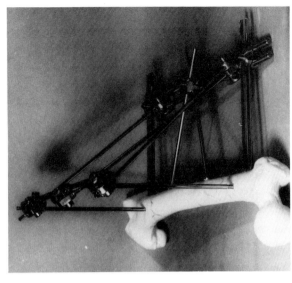

Fig. 2

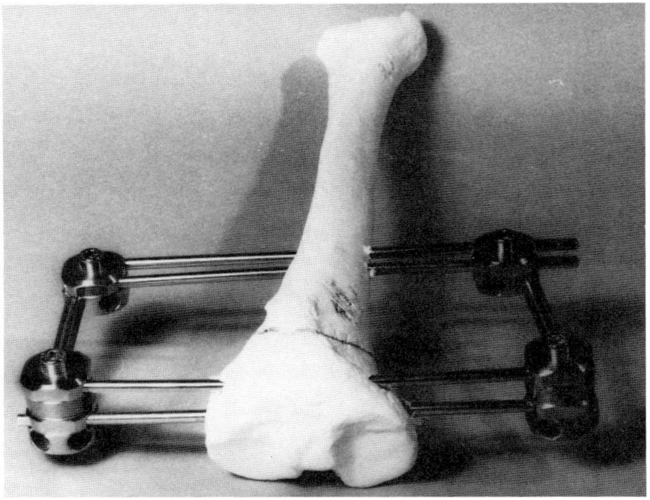

Fig. 3

Fig. 4

Fig. 5

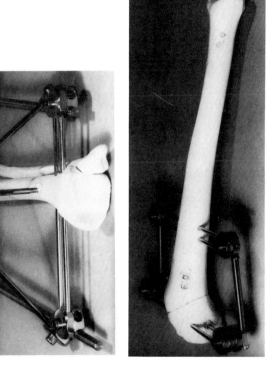

Fig. 2-5. Examples: thigh, realignment of the tibia joint; lower leg.

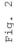

- Steinmann pins which, after insertion, do not lie parallel and in addition rise or decline in the z-plane do not need to be reinserted. The differences are compensated by the capacity to revolve or by the interposition of intermediate discs.

- Steinmann pins which spatially deviate provide an increased stability.

- By positioning the compression blocks above or below the rods, Steinmann pins can be purposely staggered (eg, arthrodesis of the knee).

If positional corrections in the frontal or sagittal plane seem necessary, especially where rotation is concerned, the loosened compression elements can be readjusted. Where greater distances are involved other intermediate discs can be inserted.

For many types of fixing, eg, complicated fractures of the lower leg, the following procedure is recommended: if a frame structure has been set up, by means of which a provisional correction can be made, the final stabilization is made easier. The screws are loosened for necessary positioning or rotational correction. All parts can be moved in relation to each other. If larger adjustments are necessary, further intermediate discs can be added to the compression elements for compensation. The insertion of further Steinmann pins is not required in the new position.

In extreme situations, where a repeated axial or rotational correction becomes necessary, compression blocks can be used as a joint or double joint. Here, we must at first set the proximal and distal fragments and reposition the whole. Afterwards, we can add a joint or a rod medially and laterally with a double joint.

The illustrated models show examples which assure a swift stabilizing of fractures in emergency cases. If secondary corrections are necessary, the Steinmann pins can also be left in. Through further insertion of Steinmann pins or Schanz screws in the x-y-plane, and corresponding screws in the z-axis, completing the three-dimensional mounting, additional reinforcement can be obtained. The required compression elements should be put onto the rods at the beginning. If some elements have been forgotten, it is still possible to add a supplementary strut by the use of so-called "open"-elements.

No problems concerning stability have so far resulted in practice. Measurements currently being carried out on distance-osteosyntheses made by Bloemer and Ungethüm (1981) have shown that the stability of the described model can be classified as being between the Hoffmann and the AO systems.

We can furthermore demonstrate different applications in models:

- stabilization of the upper or lower arm;

- stabilization in the pelvis;

- fractures of the thigh and lower leg;

- readjustment at the level of the thigh or below the knee;

- arthrodeses of the knee, ankle or subtalar-talonavicular-calcaneocuboid joint. (Fig. 2, 3, 4, 5)

We have applied this system in 103 patients without encountering any problems. Furthermore, the surgical team at the University Clinic at Göttingen, West Germany, has applied this fixator system in 20 patients with open fractures of the lower leg with good results.

In our clinic, the system has been used in 23 arthrodeses of the knee, five supracondylar realignments, 41 high tibial realignments, eight pseudarthroses of the lower leg, as well as for six ankle and triple arthrodeses.

References

1. Bloemer, W. and Ungethüm, M.: Measurements on distance-osteosyntheses. (in preparation) 1981.

2. Stankovic, P.: Personal communication, University Clinic, Göttingen

3. Stuhler, Th.: Fixateur externe Stuhler-Heise. Aesculap Information, 1981, Publ: Aesculap Werke AG, 7200 Tuttlingen.

A Review of the Day Frame as External Fixation for Trauma

J. King and B. Day

Introduction

Lambotte (1907) was the first surgeon to lend his name to a form of external fixation. In 1938, Hoffmann described the external fixation device
which bears his name and which was later popularized by the work of Connes
and Vidal (1975).

In the last six or seven years, many alternative methods of stabilizing
bones by the so-called method of external fixation have been reported,
varying from the demanding fixator of Müller (1976) to the simplistic technique described by Denham (1978).

The ideal frame should be cheap and simple to sterilize and apply. It
should stabilize the fracture to the extent that no other method of fixation (internal or external) is required, while allowing free uninterrupted
access to the wound. Moreover, it should be possible to apply it before
reduction of the fracture.

This report describes a four-year experience in one centre with the Day
external fixator. This frame was designed initially to facilitate the
problem of arthrodesis of the knee and ankle following failed surface
replacement. Its usefulness in fracture work was immediately apparent and
it has been used mainly in this context.

Description

Any pin over 3.5 mm diameter can be used for this frame, but we usually use
Steinmann pins of 4.5 mm diameter or Denham pins of a similar size, of which
two are placed above and two below the fracture. The clamp is designed to
accommodate a significant degree of unparallelism of these pins and can
accommodate a spread of 9 cm.

The importance of the nonparallelism of the pins is twofold:

1) The frame is frequently used on severe, comminuted fractures, during
   evenings or nights, by relatively junior staff who may experience
   difficulties in setting the pins parallel, or indeed where local anatomy
   may make it unfeasible.

2) In fact, lack of parallelism is an advantage in that once the pins are
    firmly clamped at each end they cannot shuttle to and fro through the
    bone, thus preventing pin movement and associated infection.

The clamps are secured by means of recessed, hexagonal nuts, and are connected above and below the fracture by external bars of 10 mm diameter,
again fixed by recessed hexagonal nuts. The clamp bars interlink in a
sphere-type held between two plane surfaces, each with a hole, so that up
to the moment of tightening this particular joint the operator has complete
flexibility in terms of angulation, rotation and translation. At that point,
four nuts only have to be tightened to achieve complete stability. These
clamps begin plastic deformation at loads around 1000 kg in an anteroposterior direction. The average failure load of a drilled tibia is 990 kg.

A portable device is applied to the bar and clamp which allows compression
or distraction to be applied as appropriate. One set, right and left, can
be carried and used on any number of frames in the hospital. The overall
weight of the frame is 1.4 kg.

For more complex indications, such as in the pelvis, bar benders and prebent
bars are available with an attachment that can be fixed to the bars for
middle fragment fixation in segmental fractures.

Insertion Technique

For the management of fractures, pins are placed above and below the fracture
site. They may be in any plane, ie, sagittal or coronal, and do not have to
be absolutely parallel. They are inserted through stab skin incisions into
the bone with a hand drill, since power tools produce considerable overheat-
ing and bone necrosis. In young, very hard bone, it is possible to predrill
with a twist drill and then use the tissue protector as a guide to relocate
the hole. Because it is not necessary initially to reduce the fracture,
skin ridging is frequently found against one side of the pin once the limb
has been normally aligned. It is necessary then to incise this ridge to
prevent high pressure contact between the skin and the pin; otherwise, pressure necrosis of the skin may occur. These pins may be transfixing, as is
usual in the tibia, or single pins simply entering the bone as in pelvic
fractures and certain femoral shaft fractures.

Once the pins are in situ, the clamps are applied to the pins and then interconnected by the bars which are firmly clamped on to the bar holders. At
this stage there is complete freedom to reduce the fracture in all three
planes of angulation, rotation, and translation, and once that is achieved
the four locking nuts are tightened.   This can be done under the image intensifier, or by eye and checked by radiograph. Fine adjustment of angulation or distraction/compression can be done with the appropriate use of the
distractor/compressor applied, either symmetrically or to one side alone, on
the ward without discomfort to the patient.

Clinical Applications

The most common application is in tibial fractures with associated soft tissue damage necessitating stabilization of the bone for the protection of the overlying soft tissues. The usual arrangement is two pins above and below the fracture site at a distance from the damaged soft parts.

The greater the spread of the pins, the nearer to the fracture they can safely be inserted. Furthermore, the better the quality of the reduction the more the rigidity of the system is improved, as with any type of fixator.

It is possible to use the same frame on a segmental fracture using a middle fragment set with Schanz screws into the middle fragment. For comminuted fractures of the distal tibia with skin loss, it is sometimes necessary to insert a pin, or pins, through the talus if it is impossible to put two pins in the same horizontal plane in the distal tibial fragment. It is important to get the talus rather than the calcaneum, in that the immobilization is then restricted to the ankle rather than including the subtalar joint.

The frame has been used in the femur where, for example, an injury necessitated plating of a closed fracture of the tibia, repair of a compound patella fracture, and a penetrating wound of the femoral fracture. In these cases, transfixing pins are inserted across the distal femur and Schanz screws are inserted from the lateral and the anterior aspects of the proximal femur. Bars join the medial distal pins to the anterior screws, and the lateral distal to the lateral screws, the two bars being interconnected for rigidity.

The frame has been used in pelvic fractures for two basic indications:

1) for the control of pain in elderly or obese patients who would otherwise be expected to get basal pneumonia and painful coughing due to immobility. This has allowed them to get out of bed early and to cough without pain. The system involves inserting Schanz type pins into the wings of the iliac crest. We recommend carrying out this procedure under direct vision. The bars are then connected with appropriate bending across the front of the abdomen.

2) for the restoration of alignment. Theoretically, this may diminish blood loss but it certainly reduces the risk of extensive urethral stricture (Glass et al, 1978). The patient's comfort is at the same time improved.

The frame has also been used in a simple form to close the duckbill fractures of the calcaneum under compression with good results. It has been used in fractures of the upper limb, particularly the humerus, but this indication is rare. The use at this level is exclusively with nontransfixing Shanz screws. With modifications it has been used for the cervical spine.

Complications

We have encountered remarkably few complications since we began using this frame four years ago.

In the beginning, we encountered some skin necrosis around the pins; but once the technique of incising the skin was perfected to prevent pressure on the skin edges, this problem has been overcome. In more than four years, with 24 frames in use averaging four pins per tibia, two recorded cases of pin infection have occurred necessitating late surgical drainage. Loosening of the pins in the bone has not been a significant problem.

The main problem noted in the treatment of the tibial shaft fractures has been delayed healing, presumably caused by the rigidity of the frame. McKibbin (1978) has described the various forms of bone union and rein-forced the concept that certain types of healing are dependent upon some motion and others are intolerant to it. When one compares similar tibial shaft fractures treated by a Day frame or by *os calcis* traction, it is quite striking that in patients treated with the rigid frame no primary bridging callus response is seen. It seems on the basis of observation of these fractures that to obtain healing involving external bridging callus it is necessary to remove the frame before six weeks. If this is not done, healing apparently takes place mainly by medullary callus. While the lack of primary callus response may suggest that the rigidity is capable of leading to primary bone union, we have not yet felt it justifiable to leave on a frame for the length of time necessary to confirm this type of healing.

This rigidity, of course, has not presented a problem in arthrodesis where two large, well vascularized surfaces of cancellous bone are in intimate contact. It is possible to diminish this problem either by the use of an isolated bar or by using a less rigid material for the linkages.

Discussion

The Day frame is very versatile, permitting easy application under difficult circumstances, and is not technically demanding. Up to the moment of secur-ing the last four nuts, there is freedom of movement in the three modes of rotation, angulation, and translation.

In practice, the weight of the frame has not been a problem in fracture work (although it is too heavy for an elbow arthrodesis in rheumatoid arthritis, for example). We have not had one clamp failure in four years nor evidence of wear, and hence no loss of rigidity, as has been observed with certain other types of designs.

The major problem we have encountered is delayed fracture healing. We accept that the majority of the fractures treated are the severe type, perhaps seg-mental fractures and extensive skin loss; but it has been possible to match these fractures with similar ones treated with less rigid fixation, and there certainly appears to be a difference in the healing characteristics. This observation accords well with the theories of bone healing as expressed by McKibbin (1978), in that it is the change seen with immobilization. We now accept that if the frame has to be used for more than six weeks, healing will be slowed, but there has not been a recorded case of nonunion in all the tibial fractures treated in the frame.

Summary

This report records four years' use of an external frame (the Day frame), which has proved versatile in its application to bone injury, technically undemanding for its insertion, and capable of application to the pelvis, the femur, the tibia and the calcaneum. The complications are described, mainly relating to delayed healing, possibly due to the rigidity of the fixation.

References

1. Lambotte, A.: L'intervention opératoire dans les fractures. Ed. Lambertin, Bruxelles, 1907.

2. Connes, H.: Le fixateur externe d'Hoffmann. Edition Gead, Paris, 1975.

3. Bulletin, A.O.: The External Fixation Device, November 1976.

4. Edge, A.J. and Denham, R.A.: External fixation of complicated tibial fractures. Proc. First Sympsoium on Fracture Fixation, Biological Engineering Soc., June 1978.

5. Hoffmann, R.: Rotules à os pour la réduction dirigée, non sanglante des fractures (osteotaxis). Cong. Swiss Chir., 1938. Helv. Med. Acta 1938, pp 844-850.

6. Glass, R.E., Flynn, J.T., King, J.B., and Blandy, J.P.: Brit.J.Urol. 50, 578, 1978.

7. McKibbin, B.: Biology of fracture healing in long bones. J. Bone Jt. Surg. 60B, 150, 1978.

Kronner System

R. L. Buechel

Introduction

The Kronner apparatus is a method of external fixation using pericutaneous
transfixion pins attached to a frame. The frames are lightweight, carbon-
reinforced nylon material. The frames offer considerable variability with
either circular frames, 4-bar compression frames, or a combination. The
unique advantage of this system, compared with others, is that it offers
either rigid or flexible fixation. The difference between rigid and flexible fixation is in the use of either a circular 5-bar frame with transfixion pins or a 3- or 4-bar system with half pins. In the treatment of
well vascularized bone, a flexible frame may offer advantages for stimulation of periosteal new bone formation (Burny, 1978). With severely comminuted fractures or infected fractures, rigid fixation may be required to
permit primary endosteal fracture healing (Fig. 1). Once stable, rigidly
aligned fractures may be converted to a more flexible fixation (Fig. 2).

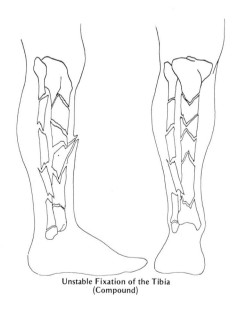

Unstable Fixation of the Tibia
(Compound)

Fig. 1.

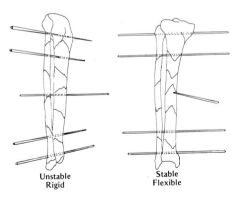

Unstable   Stable
Rigid   Flexible

Fig. 2.

Indications and Contraindications to External Fixation

Indications (Mueller et al, 1970)

1. Closed or comminuted fractures which are not applicable to standard forms of treatment, or fractures which have failed to heal with other forms of therapy due to infected nonunion, pseudarthrosis, or infection in presence of implants (Weber and Cech, 1976).

2. Compound fractures, especially Type III, involving the diaphyseal and metaphyseal area of the bone.

3. Fractures associated with severe soft tissue damage to the neurovascular structures, muscles, ligaments, periosteum and skin. Multiple procedures may be necessary such as grafts and neurovascular repair.

4. To facilitate arthrodesis either primarily or following removal of failed prosthesis where a large amount of bone defect is present.

Contraindications

Fractures that will heal with noninvasive conservative management or fractures which can be best treated with standard internal fixation devices.

Possible adverse effects

1. Loosening of pins or drainage from pin tracts, especially if non-threaded pins are used.

2. Bone sequestrum secondary to necrosis from rapid drilling of cortex.

3. Breakage of pins due to stress.

4. Entrapment of muscle, nerve, or penetration of large vessels by pins.

5. Failure to pin bone segments properly, thus leading to failure to manipulate the fracture into proper position.

6. Pressure on skin from component parts.

Proper use of the system should help to avoid the above adverse effects. Each complication should be recognized and corrected promptly. Appropriate treatment of the complications should lead to proper healing without the necessity of removing the entire external fixation device. An example is the removal of an infected or loose pin with reinsertion if necessary in an adjacent site. Dermatologic consultation for superficial pin tract infections is extremely valuable because of unusual bacterial contamination.

Material

The Kronner external fixation device is a method of stabilizing, either with rigid or flexible fixation, fractures in the mid to lower femur, about the knee, in the tibia, and about the ankle (Kronner, personal communication).

Multiple segments of bone may be treated by combining U rings with the circular system or the 4-bar system. Using the circular frame with a 5-bar system, rigid mobilization is obtainable. Using the full pins, the circular frame can be combined with the 4-bar type system. For treatment of well vascularized bone, a flexible frame may offer advantages for the stimulation of periosteal new bone formation (Burny, 1978).

With the severely comminuted fracture or infected fracture, rigid fixation may be required to allow for primary endosteal fracture healing (Burri, 1975; Rittmann and Perren, 1974). Additional advantages of this system are:
1) large areas of bone may be spanned in the femur or tibia; 2) the material is lightweight and autoclavable; 3) the frame is radiolucent; 4) the frame may be reused; 5) the frame is easy to construct and may be assembled before or during application; 6) the soft tissue is easily accessible, and vascular and nerve repair can be performed with the frame in place; 7) multiple adjustments are easily accomplished, such as distraction, compression, angulation, rotation, and correction of offset in any plane; 8) the rigid fixation permits partial or full weight bearing and adjacent joint motion.

Description of Frame

The frame is of lightweight carbon-reinforced material, either made as a circular frame or a 4-bar system (Fig. 3, 4)

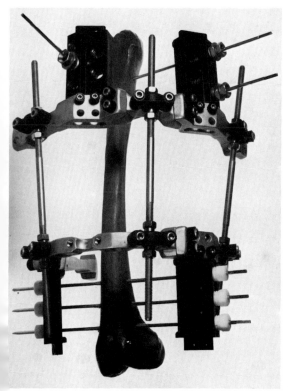

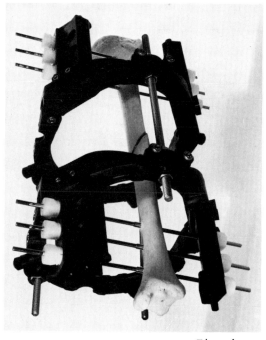

Fig. 4

Fig. 3

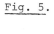

Fig. 5.

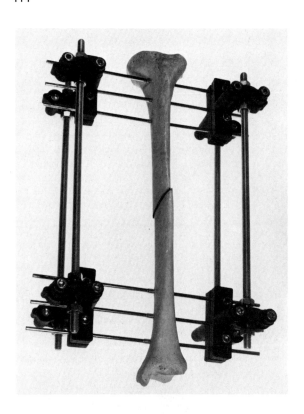

Two to six bars which consist of a 5/16" threaded rod with nylon balls and 1/2" hex nut are used to connect the circular or 4-bar system. This permits ease of manipulation with traction, distraction, or rotation by tightening or loosening of the component parts.

Nylon plates are attached to the circular frame for pin fixation. Four plates may be used with the circular frame if necessary, the pins locking into the plates with collets.

The pins are either full pins with a raised self-tapping thread or half pins, preferably 3/16" in size. A pin guide is used for ease and correction of placement. The only instruments necessary are a hand drill, pin guide set, T-handled Allen wrench, and 1/2" wrenches.

With the circular frame, the hinges should be placed on the same side so that the frame can be hinged open. The rear segment of the frame may be removed in bed or for additional surgical procedures. The frame may be modified to span short or long distances and to stabilize any area from the ankle to the midfemoral area. With this system, the surgeon can accomplish either temporary supportive care or immobilization for the entire period of fracture healing. Partial to full weight bearing may be allowed with this system without casting.

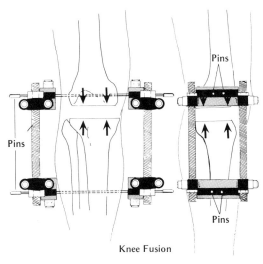

Fig. 6. Knee Fusion

The 4-bar frame may be used with either parallel or perpendicular pin placement (Fig.5).

Biomechanical Analyses

Biomechanical analysis was undertaken to ascertain the strength of various
types of external fixators (Briggs et al, 1979). A comparison was made of
the Hoffmann, Roger Anderson, Kronner, and Volkov-Oganesian fixators.

Five testing modes were established: compression, distraction, AP bending,
lateral bending, and torsion. On a tibial model, the results showed that
the Kronner 5-bar system showed the highest ratings in torsion and lateral
bending compared with all the other models tested. In compression and distraction, the Kronner 5-bar apparatus rated highly, second only to the
Hoffmann apparatus. All frames were weak in AP bending. The Kronner
apparatus was second compared with all the other tested frames.

Overall stiffness can be increased by increasing the number of pins, increasing the pin diameter, and by decreasing the side bar distance.

Management and Treatment

In the severely comminuted fractures, external fixation is the treatment of
choice. With large gaping wounds, extensive debridement, wound care, and
skin grafting can be performed while stability at the fracture site is still
maintained. Once primary or secondary wound healing has occurred and the
soft tissue edema subsided, the external frame may be removed and standard
weight bearing type casts applied. Crush injuries to the lower and upper
tibial area can also be treated with external fixation to reduce the fracture and maintain alignment. In vascular injuries, repair can be made with
the external fixation device in place.

External fixation is beneficial for mid and distal femoral fractures, proximal mid and distal tibial fractures. Gaping areas of bone loss may be
treated with bone grafting. Failed arthroplasties may be converted to
arthrodesis with the use of the external fixation device. (Fig.6)

In patients with severe polytrauma, external fixation is extremely beneficial, mobilizing various injured limbs while preserving position of the
fractures (Brooker and Edwards, 1979). In the treatment of osteomyelitis,
external fixation offers good stability with compression. Extensive debridement, skin grafting, bone grafting, and wound care can be carried out
until satisfactory healing at the fracture area occurs.

Summary

A description of the Kronner apparatus has been presented and its advantages
and disadvantages discussed. The most distinct advantage of this system is
that rigid immobilization over a large area of bone damage can be carried
out, thereby stabilizing more than one segment of bone simultaneously without an open, invasive surgical procedure. Both rigid and flexible fixation
are possible through this system by varying the transfixion pins and the
method by which they are fixed to the support structure.

Weight bearing can be allowed and adjacent joint function preserved while the
appropriate soft tissue procedures are being carried out. Compression, distraction, angulation and rotational changes can be easily accomplished with
adjustment of several bolts and hex nuts.

References

1. Briggs, B.T., Chao, E.Y., McCoy, M.T., et al: External fixators: Bio-
    mechanical and clinical analysis of the Hoffmann, Roger Anderson, Kronner,
    and Volkov-Oganesian fixators. Scientific Exhibit, American Academy of
    Orthopaedic Surgeons, San Franciso, CA, February 22-27, 1979.

2. Brooker, A.F., and Edwards, C.C.: External Fixation. The Current State of
    the Art. Williams & Wilkins, Baltimore, 1979.

3. Burny, F.: Strain gauge measurement of fracture healing; a study of 350
    cases. Sixth International Conference on Hoffmann External Fixation.
    Williams & Wilkins, Baltimore, 1978.

4. Burri, C.: Post-Traumatic Osteomyelitis. H.Huber, Bern, p. 181, 1975.

5. Kronner, R.: Personal communications.

6. Mueller, M.E., Allgoewer, M. and Willenegger, H.: Manual of External
    Fixation. Springer-Verlag, New York, p. 284, 1970.

7. Rittmann, W.W. and Perren, S.M.: Cortical Bone Healing After Internal
    Fixation and Infection. Springer-Verlag, Berlin, p. 58, 1974.

8. Weber, B.G. and Cech, O.: Pseudarthrosis. Grune & Stratton, New York,
    p. 67, 1976.

An External Fixation System Using Formable Plastic Rods

W. M. Murray

Introduction

An epoxy plastic rod replaces the customary set of mechanical linkages
in the external fixation system to be described. The rod is applied
in a flexible state to the fixator pins, and then becomes a rigid interconnecting element.

The system design philosophy was to provide a frame of extreme simplicity,
compactness, and security following application, while at the same time
allowing maximum freedom in orientation, spacing, and number of pins
incorporated into the fixator.

An adjustable temporary holding bridge facilitates optimization of fracture alignment before plastic rod application. Following rod hardening,
the frame is no longer freely adjustable and is thus tamper-proof. Compression or distraction, however, may be applied at any time.

As a course of fracture treatment proceeds, clinical union may be repeatedly assessed quantitatively by a technique involving the use of
rapid-disconnect pin clamps.

Stiffness of the plastic rods results in frame rigidity against transverse bending and torsion exceeding that of conventional fixators
(Lundeen et al, 1980). A bilateral frame, however, may be reversibly
destabilized to allow a limited arc of minimally restrained motion at
the fracture site.

Alternate Frame Configurations

Since the plastic element of a frame structure may be of virtually any
shape or length, the number of possible configurations is unlimited.
Some illustrative examples will be described below. Generally, it is
best to use the simplest and most compact frame which permits optimal
management of a particular case.

a   b

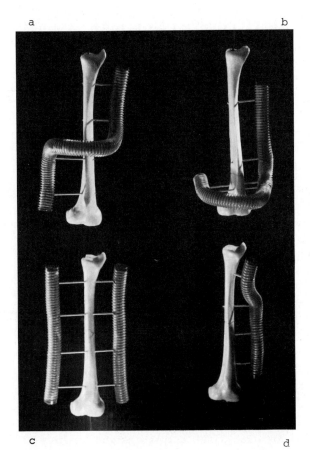

c   d

Fig. 1.   a) unilateral frame;
b) bilateral frame;   c) J-
frame;   d) crossover frame.

Unilateral frame (Fig. 1a).   The use of half-pins renders this frame much
less rigid than a bilateral frame of similar dimensions (Chao et al, 1979).
Rigidity can, however, be maximized by wide spacing of pins and placement
wherever minimal soft tissue thickness is overlying the bone.   Thus, it
can be suitable for treatment of tibial shaft fractures where pins can be
placed along the subcutaneous portion of the tibial crest.

Bilateral frame   (Fig. 1b).   This frame is capable of a high order of
rigidity.   In treating an extremity with extensive soft tissue damage, it
has the added advantage of facilitating suspension without using slings.

J-frame (Fig. 1c).   This design is useful in the treatment of fractures
near the end of a long bone.   Here, whole-pins in the shorter fragment may
be necessary because of the lesser rigidity associated with pins closely
spaced in softer metaphyseal bone.   Wide spacing of pins in the long
fragment makes moderate rigidity possible with half-pins.

Crossover frame (Fig. 1d).   This is one of many variants of the unilateral
frame which can be useful with particular patterns of soft tissue injury.

Frames can be shaped to give free access to selected areas, or to facilitate placement of pins away from areas of infection or questionable viability.

Materials Required for Fixator Construction (Fig. 2)

Epoxy plastic resin and hardener are supplied in a cartridge in which they are mixed at the time of use. Each cartridge provides 240 ml of plastic, sufficient for a rod up to 35 cm long. When mixed at 22°C, the plastic solidifies 15 minutes after the start of mixing.

Corrugated flexible polyethylene tubing, having an inside diameter of 2.5 cm, is used to contain the liquid plastic in the shape of a rod. Before use, it is cut to the required length.

Filling caps, made of vinyl, are snapped onto tubing ends before filling with liquid plastic. After rod hardening, they are discarded.

Steinmann pins, 4.8 mm by 30 cm, are threaded along their entire lengths. The thread design incorporates a flattened bottom which increases pin stiffness and resistance to breakage by cyclical stress.

The components described above are sized for treatment of lower extremity and pelvic fractures. A set of smaller components (3.2 mm pins, and 1.6 cm tubing) is in preparation.

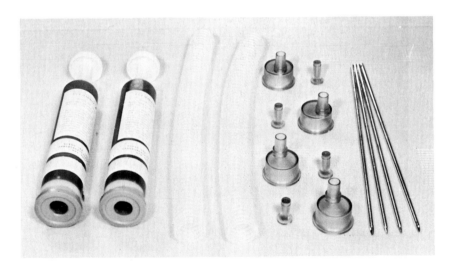

Fig. 2. Materials for constructing bilateral frame; left to right: epoxy cartridges, polyethylene tubing; filling caps, Steinmann pins.

Method of Use

The following discussion is directed at the treatment of tibial and
femoral fractures. The basic techniques, however, and the general
principles exemplified are applicable to treatment at other sites of
injury.

Open fracture debridement and exploration, and debridement of other
contiguous wounds, are best completed before proceeding with external
fixation. With a fresh wound, it may be desirable to maintain access
to the fracture site to facilitate reduction. On the other hand, it
may be advisable to carefully occlude an old infected wound.

The next step before fixation is to approximately reduce the fracture.
The use of a fracture table is recommended since it will help greatly
in holding the reduction. At this point, minor fracture angulation is
of no consequence. The length to be finally accepted should be obtained
with traction and any rotational displacement corrected. In most cases,
this will result in a nearly perfect reduction. Occasionally, a closed
fracture will be irreducible because of interposed soft tissue; if so,
it is mandatory that the operator recognize the condition at this point
so that the necessary open reduction be accomplished before proceeding
with external fixation.

After reduction appears satisfactory, spinal needles are placed at the
sites selected for Steinmann pin placement. Roentgenograms are then
obtained to assess both the reduction and the locations selected for
pins.

The Steinmann pins may be driven into place after adequate reduction
(except for minor angulation) and suitability of the selected pin sites
have been confirmed. It is recommended that pins be advanced through
very short incisions (barely large enough to admit each pin) rather than
the large relaxing incisions usually advocated. The resulting snug entry
sites will help to minimize oscillatory soft tissue motion with respect
to each pin shaft. Since fracture reduction has already been attained,
no tenting of soft tissue will occur as long as the operator keeps each
pin centered at its entry site while drilling into bone. Sterile dressings are now applied to each pin site.

A temporary holding bridge may now be used to interconnect the fixation
pins. Even where a bilateral frame is being constructed, a single bridge
on one side will usually suffice. The bridge should be secured closely
against the dressings, so that the plastic rod can be placed at the
recommended 2.5 cm distance from the skin (Fig. 3). With the bridge
tightened, roentgenograms are taken to check final fracture reduction
and pin placement (including pin depth, in the case of half-pins).

When fracture alignment and pin depth have been determined to be satisfactory, pins are trimmed so that a 5 cm length protrudes beyond the
skin. Any remaining open wounds should now be occlusively dressed.

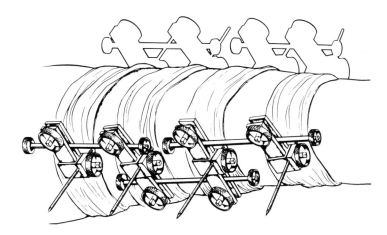

Fig. 3. Temporary holding bridge used to stabilize
fracture.

For each plastic rod to be made, a length of ribbed tubing is cut to
length and a filling cap applied at each end. A cartridge of plastic
is mixed and dispensed into the tubing. The filled tubing is mounted
on the pins by passing each pin end through a hole in the tubing wall
which has been made using an awl.

After plastic hardening is complete, temporary holding bridge hardware
may be removed and traction discontinued.

Fracture Remanipulation after Frame Hardening

Fracture malposition will seldom occur if the steps outline above are
followed in obtaining reduction before plastic rod application. Free
remanipulation, however, may be done if necessary. The plastic rods
are removed by cutting all pins, the stumps of which are relengthened
with the help of rapid-disconnect clamps. Following remanipulation,
new rods can be mounted.

Application of Compression or Distraction

At any time following plastic hardening, compression or distraction may
be applied, using compressor-distractors as illustrated in Fig. 4. The
devices act by flexing the Steinmann pins. The bone fragments may be
moved axially as much as about 6 mm to or from each other. With a bilateral frame, compression of more than 50 kg is possible.

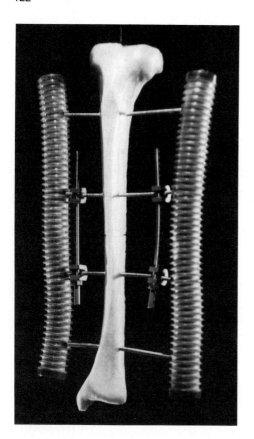

Fig. 4. Compressor-distractors
used to close 6 mm gap (note
bending of pins)

Evaluation of Fracture Consolidation

Roentgenographic evaluation of the union of fractures treated by external
fixation is frequently unreliable. A method is therefore described for
quantitatively testing fracture stiffness. The relationship of stiffness
to strength of union has been extensively studied (Jorgensen, 1972).

Using a pin cutter developed for this purpose, a 6 mm section of fixator
pin is removed between the rod and pin dressing. All pins on one side of
the fracture site are severed in this way; with bilateral frames, these
pins must be severed on both sides of the limb.

Since cutting the pins as described will disconnect the frame from the
major fragment attached to these pins, the frame no longer will immobilize
the fracture. Bending moments, or other selected stresses, may be applied
to the limb. Calibration of the applied force is generally unnecessary.
Angulation of the fracture, or other motion, will be apparent from dis-

placement of the pin segments attached to the frame, with respect to the segments attached to bone. For example, at a pin located 10 cm from the fracture site, motion of 1.6 mm (about 1/3 of the pin diameter) will correspond to 1° fracture angulation.

After testing of consolidation, pins may be rigidly rejoined with rapid-disconnect clamps. The clamps may be repeatedly removed and reapplied.

Frame Destabilization

It is recognized that a rigid external fixator can retard fracture healing through excessive immobilization and stress shielding (Mears, 1980). Using clamps which rejoin cut pins to allow a limited arc of motion between the severed ends, a bilateral frame may be modified to allow motion of low amplitude at the fracture site with little restraint. A section is removed from each side of the pins immediately proximal and distal to the fracture, and the pins are then rejoined using destabilizing clamps (Fig. 5). Clamp dimensioning permits fracture angulation of ±1° in the anteroposterior plane, and ±2° in the mediolateral plane. At the time of writing, early clinical experience with frame destabilization is sufficient to confirm its feasibility, but not to permit conclusions as to its effectiveness.

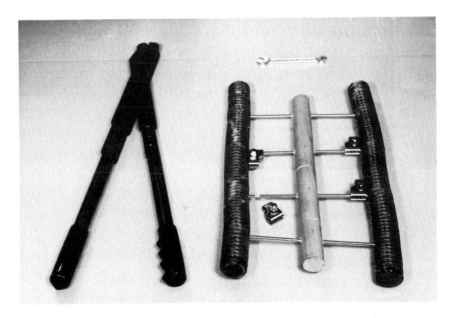

Fig. 5. Special pin-cutter; mock-up with destabilizing clamps (one removed to show gap in pin).

References

1. Chao, E.Y.S., Briggs, B.T., and McCoy, M.T.: Theoretical and experi-
    mental analyses of Hoffmann-Vidal external fixation system. In:
    External Fixation, The Current State of the Art, pp 345-370. Brooker
    and Edwards (eds.), Williams and Wilkins, 1979.

2. Jorgensen,T.E.: Measurements of stability and crural fractures treated
    with Hoffmann osteotaxis. Acta Orthop.Scand. 43, 188-218 and 264-291,
    1972.

3. Lundeen, M.A., Jones, R.E., Mooney, V., and Murray, W.M.: Complex open
    tibial fractures treated by external fixation. Presented at the Annual
    Meeting of the American Academy of Orthopaedic Surgeons, Atlanta, GA,
    1980.

4. Mears, D.C.: Editorial Review, Clinical results of the triangular
    external fixation device in serious lesions of the lower extremity.
    Orthop.Surv. 3, 354-355, 1980.

An External Fixation Device Made of Polymer Materials

R. Spier

The advantages of the treatment of fractures by external fixation are well known today. These advantages apply as well to an external fixator made of polymer materials. According to clinical experiences, the indications are the same as for any other known external anchorage. The external fixation device made of polymer materials has been used in numerous mounting assemblies for:

- open fractures

- infected pseudarthroses

- arthrodeses of large joints.

The external fixation device made of polymer materials consists of five carbon- or fiberglass-reinforced basic elements, the parts of the system being connected by socket pieces. Fig. 1 shows the plastic parts formed by injection die-casting: the screw-connection and the protective cap, which also serves as a brace for the bone screws. Also shown is the socket piece, the ball star, and a connecting rod of special roentgen-transparent

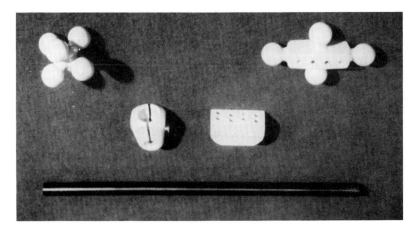

Fig. 1.

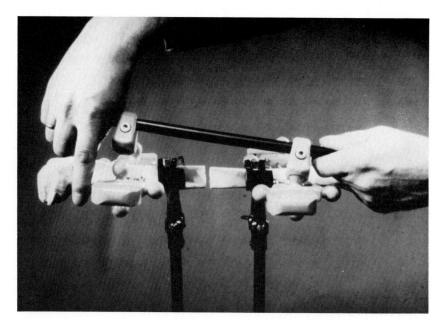

Fig. 2.

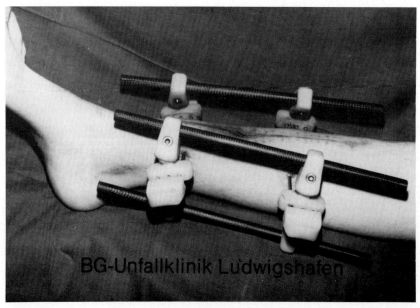

Fig. 3.

To build such a device, a connecting rod must be mounted on the socket piece and connected to the ball head of the screw-connecting part (Fig. 2). The ball joint allows the components to move in all directions. The rough surface of the plastic material prevents slipping. When the desired position is reached, it is fixed with only one socket head cap screw. The protective caps serve as a protection for both textiles and tissues, and firmly fix the screw-connecting parts on the bone screws.

The few examples below will describe some applications for this device. To begin with, Fig. 3 shows a double frame construction for an infected pseudarthrosis on the lower leg, which is the most common indication for this device. The system is fixed by means of only six screws. If necessary, compression and distraction forces are exerted by an attachable metal clamp, which can be removed once the desired position has been obtained. It also permits, subsequently, precise measurable corrections of the position.

One-bone stabilization in the case of an infected defect pseudarthrosis of the ulna is shown in Fig. 4. Flexion and extension of the elbow are possible.

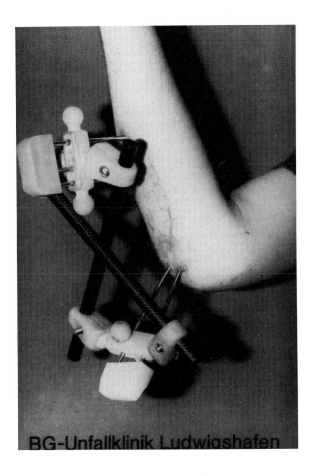

Fig. 4.

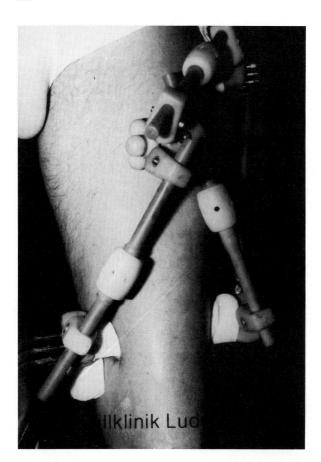

Fig. 5.

Fig. 5. demonstrates the external fixation device made of polymer materials positioned on the thigh. Because of the danger of damaging a blood vessel or a nerve, the proximal bone screws should not pass beyond the inner cortex of the bone. Consequently, in this case multipoint fixation is required. Across the front spherical heads, an additional rod may be added without adding bone screws.

The mounting for arthrodesis of the ankle joint is shown in Fig. 6. In this case, the planes of the sets of screws are almost vertical to one another. These sets can be connected to one another using the front spherical heads of the screw-connecting parts without any additional constructional pieces. Adequate compression can be achieved in the region of the arthrodesis. In roentgenographs the compressive force becomes evident by the considerable deformation of the bone screws.

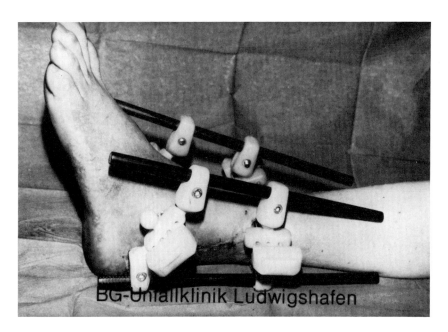

Fig. 6.

Before being used in a clinical setting, the stability of the whole system
and the strain on the individual parts were tested. In extensive studies
comparing its stability with that of clinically proven, conventional fixation systems, it was found that the stability of the external fixation
device made of polymer materials met all the necessary requirements. These
findings have been confirmed so far by our clinical experience.

It should be mentioned here that the compressive forces produce a visible
deformation of the carbon-reinforced connecting rods. This deformation is
due to the elasticity of the polymer materials. It does not cause loss of
stability and seems to guarantee a lasting compression.

The external fixation device made of polymer materials was used in 39 cases
during the past three years in our clinic: 5 times on the lower arm;
4 times on the upper leg; twice on the knee; 23 times on the lower leg;
and 5 times on the ankle. During this time the device met all the necessary
requirements. Its outstanding advantages are:

-   ease of handling combined with adequate stability comparable to other
    systems;

-   possibility of multiple, even three-dimensional mounting variations;

-   roentgen transparency;

- heat resistant and resistant to plastic deformation;

- a weight reduction up to 70% compared with other systems.

Patients previously treated by an external fixation system made of metal describe the feeling of the new polymer materials as exceptionally pleasant.

The Stability of Different Systems. A Comparative Study

R. Kleining and A. Chernowitz

Introduction

In the study of existing and potential new models for external fixation we must keep in mind what we expect from these devices - above all, ease of application and success in stabilization. We should also take into consideration the capability of the surgeon; that is to say, within what limits should we expect him to align the fragments before application of the fixator. The question is important since a fixator with a great capacity for late adjustment of fragment position is necessarily a complex device. We suggest that the surgeon should be able to control rotation within acceptable limits by clinical inspection and to bring frontal and sagittal plane alignment fairly close to the anatomic. That means that the fixator should allow for correction in the range between the accuracy of a reasonable clinical inspection and the exact measurement obtained by radiography.

Our mechanical analyses have shown that the main weakness of existing systems lies in the compliance of the pins and screws which are inserted into the bone. The reason is limitations of their size. The construction of a three-dimensional assembly has overcome much of this weakness but at the continuing expense of using pins that penetrate thick layers of soft tissue and, particularly in the leg, the anterior compartment muscles. The soft tissue is irritated by the pins, this irritation being greatest in the actively moving tissue of muscle. Infection follows pin tracts to the bone and leads to loosening. The care of pin seepage is an untidy and unpleasant chore for patient and staff.

We have been working on a design which we hope will overcome the problems created by transfixation and pin compliances. There is no reason for the portion of the pin which does not pass through bone to fall under the size limitation for bone defects. Also, if a clasp of sufficient rigidity can be constructed, fixation is possible without transfixation. Furthermore, a screw thread that is self-tapping and conical can be retightened in bone without setting it into a new hole (which means another operation).

As a binding clamp we are trying out a ball (with a slot to allow compression and grip on the screw) which will allow adjustment of position in the limited range discussed above.

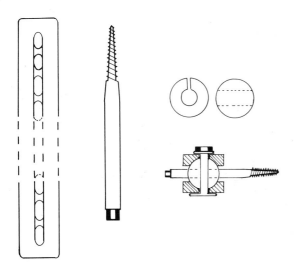

Fig. 1. Elements of the prototype; the right lower drawing is
an end-on schema of the fixator
bars holding the ball which, in
turn, holds the bone screw.

For the connecting rod, we have chosen carbon fiber-reinforced (and radiolucent) plastic so that the assembly will be lightweight and the metal will
not hide the bone during roentgenograph follow-up (Fig. 1).

Method

To compare assemblies we made bone models of wood and constructed the various fixators on the models, holding the distances from frame to model constant, insofar as possible, given the differences in design. The testing
was done under a condition of no bone support and all binding clamps were

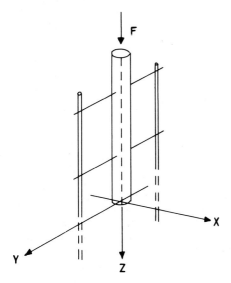

Fig. 2. Proximal fragment of model with
axes in which displacements were measured
after application of force F.

tightened to the same torque (8 Nm). Displacements were measured in a Schenck testing machine with controlled travel and measurement of applied load. The axial, frontal, and sagittal displacements of the proximal fragment were measured by induction gauges (Fig. 2) and all data assembled electronically while the distal fragment was held by a vise on the test stand.

Results

The load deformation curves of four common assemblies (AO, Stuhler, Hoffmann and Fischer) as well as that of our prototype showed almost no displacements in the plane perpendicular to the bending plane (Fig. 3) with one exception. The Fischer fixator had almost equal displacements in frontal and sagittal planes. This is caused by unequal diameters of the pin on the two sides of its threaded midportion.

The bending plane displacements varied among the different models but were smaller than the z-axis displacements. Z-axis displacement was always the largest observed (Fig. 4 and 5).

In the load range reported (0-500 N) for the bending plane, the most rigid system was our prototype and the least rigid the Fischer. For z-axis stability the same pattern was obtained.

The load deformation curve of the prototype shows a loss of rigidity above 400 N. This progressive weakening was the result of loss of rotational fixation of the balls and not the result of pin bending. We expect that the forthcoming model, which was not ready in time for the tests reported here, will show improved rigidity in the binding clamps. Assuming that the binding clamp's instability can be resolved through improved materials, we suggest that the dotted line extrapolated on the graph can be realized. We expect further that a carbon fiber-reinforced plastic connecting rod will increase the friction and give the desired result.

More important than the technical details of the prototype model, however, is the demonstration that a clasp assembly can give at least as much sta-bility as a frame which depends on transfixation. In addition to avoiding problems of transfixing pins, the prototype offers a substantial weight reduction and requires less screws to fix the assembly.

Summary

A comparison of four common types of external fixator with our prototype has shown that the prototype can stabilize fragments without bone support as well as the assemblies of the AO, Hoffmann and Stuhler. The Fischer ex-ternal fixator allows the greatest deformations in all axes under axial load. The prototype requires only bone screws and no transfixing pins at the tibia.

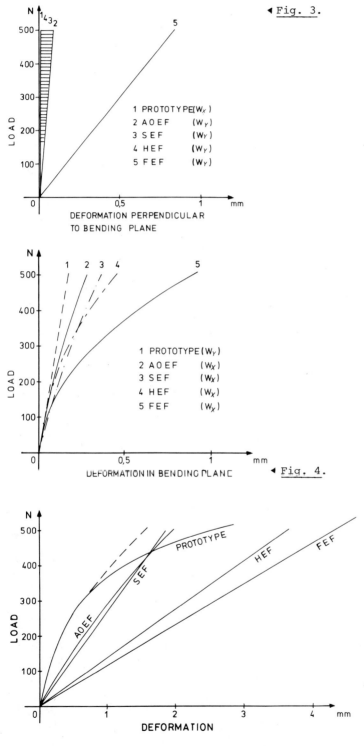

◄ Fig. 3.

1 PROTOTYPE (W_X)
2 AOEF (W_Y)
3 SEF (W_Y)
4 HEF (W_Y)
5 FEF (W_Y)

DEFORMATION PERPENDICULAR
TO BENDING PLANE

1 PROTOTYPE (W_Y)
2 AOEF (W_X)
3 SEF (W_X)
4 HEF (W_X)
5 FEF (W_X)

DEFORMATION IN BENDING PLANE ◄ Fig. 4.

◄ Fig. 5. Load deformation curves for the z-axis (axial displacement).

Table I.

EXTERNAL FIXATOR TYPE		WEIGHTS (g)	SCREWS (n)
HOFFMANN	(HEF)	2200	24
STUHLER	(SEF)	1410	14
AO	(AOEF)	1300	15
FISCHER	(FEF)	1220	40
PROTOTYPE STEEL		930	6
PROTOTYPE CFRP		580	6

In comparison with the other four assemblies (Table I) the prototype is lightweight, has less elements and screws, allows late adjustment of fragment position, and is simple to apply. We hope that our model under development will prove straightforward in application for the surgeon, and at the same time more tolerable and comfortable for the patient.

Stability in the Absence of Contact in the Lower Limbs

K. H. Müller

The external fixator is indicated for two biomechanically antithetic types
of osteosynthesis - on the one hand, compression osteosynthesis, and on the
other, gap osteosynthesis (Fig. 1)(Boltze et al, 1978; Hierholzer et al,
1978; Labitzke and Henze, 1978; Müller, 1981; Müller et al, 1979). In the
first case, interfragmental compression can be applied because the area of
bone contact permits axial loading. The compression stress, which is effective for longer periods according to the principle of a soft spring, guarantees increased interfragmental friction; it therefore also assures the
stability of the external system (Fig. 1b)(Müller et al, 1979). In the
second case, absence of contact between the bone fragments precludes compression (Fig. 1c, 2, 4, 5, 6). The stability achieved using an external
fixator (ie, the state of relative nonmovement of the individual fragments
with respect to each other) is therefore based solely on the outer stabilizing construction (Labitzke and Henze, 1978; Müller, 1981). In other
words, external gap osteosynthesis is a fixation using an external supporter
which absorbs externally applied forces. The stability of gap osteosynthesis
relies exclusively on the rigidity of the external support.

Individual external construction forms are required in each case because of
the many anatomic, structural, and pathogenic characteristics of the defect.
Nevertheless, certain basic principles generally hold for external gap
osteosynthesis (Fig. 1). The following remarks pertain to the tubular
system of the AO-Group:

- smallest possible support-width (support-width: distance between the
  tubular rod and the bone);

- maximum distance between the Steinmann pins in the same fragment;

- minimum distance between the two Steinmann pins located on either side
  of the defect;

- the Steinmann pins of a single fragment are stressed at the time of
  insertion.

One can refer to the distance between the two pins close to the defect as the
free bending stretch of the system (Fig. 1b). The free bending stretch is
the sum of the defined width of the defect and both distances existing between the defect and the pin close to it. The greater the free bending
stretch, the smaller the rigidity of the system (Burger et al, 1977; Hoffmann
et al, 1977; Kleining and Hierholzer, 1976; Labitzke and Henze, 1980). One
can thus say that a short osseous defect only leads to a more stable system

when the Steinmann pins closest to the defect are not too far apart. The following variant of gap osteosynthesis can occur: external fixation with fragment contact without interfragmentary compression (Fig. 1c). A fragment contact which will not tolerate compression, such as shattered areas or partial osseous defects with small areas of contact, causes frictional resistance. This rather small interfragmentary mechanical contact changes at least in theory the character of the external osteosynthesis. When fragments which are not brought under compression have contact with one another, the stability of this external osteosynthesis does not rest solely on the rigidity of the external supporter; the role played by the interfragmentary friction depends on its magnitude. Here, fragments are externally splinted in the sense of a neutralization. Nevertheless, even such a system behaves like a case of gap osteosynthesis. On the one hand, the mere friction caused by contact can be ignored when compared with other loads supported by this system; on the other hand, although the width of the gap is reduced to zero, a free bending stretch nevertheless exists because of the distance between the Steinmann pins and the contact area. This is a characteristic feature of gap osteosynthesis. In actual practice, we see this in the displacement of an oblique fracture to which compression pressure has been unsuccessfully applied. The prognosis for such contact situations is, however, generally more favorable because biologic stabilization by a bony union occurs more rapidly.

Given a certain defect width, the stability of osteosynthesis depends on the mechanical data of the individual construction elements, on the stability between the bone and the outer system, and on the rigidity of the entire construction. The individual elements are the bone, the Steinmann pins, including the Schanz screws, the tubular rods, and the clamps. The holding power of the pins depends on the morphologic condition of the bone at the anchoring site (eg, type of the injury causing the defect, osteoporosis, age) and its location. Thus, diaphyseal bone sections show greater strength than metaphyseal. The Steinmann pins are placed perpendicularly to the bone axis and connect the bone with the outer system. The Steinmann pins are the most essential and also mechanically the weakest element of external fixation (Fig. 3) (Labitzke and Henze, 1978; 1980; Müller, 1981; Müller et al, 1979). As cross pins, they are mainly loaded in bending (Fig. 1a, 2, 4, 7). Since the possibilities of improving pin strength by using improved materials have been largely exhausted, their section modulus could be improved by design changes (Müller et al, 1979).

Greater rigidity could be achieved by diagonal tubular rods with a larger outer diameter or with an altered profile. To date, profiles which are not round have caused surgical problems which have either not been solved or not yet tackled. Increasing the number of pins improved the purchase in bone and simultaneously the rigidity of the entire system. In principle, the number of pins which can be used for external fixation is limited by biologic requirement to use the smallest number of implants possible (Labitzke and Henze, 1978). In view of the above-mentioned general problem of achieving rigidity when gap osteosynthesis is carried out, the section modulus of the tubular rods and clamps is sufficient. When the purchase of the Steinmann pins in bone diminishes, mechanical instability of the external gap osteosynthesis accompanied by fragment movement will result (Fig. 3) (Müller, 1981).

Our own experimental investigations of external compression osteosynthesis
have shown that for these forms of osteosynthesis only biologic interdepen-
dencies can be seen as the cause of pin loosening, provided surgical and
mechanical errors during insertion of the pin were avoided (Müller et al,
1979). Even when bone necrosis due to heat and necrosis due to stress
peaks could be avoided, inflammation in the soft tissue and pin tract
leading to loosening in principle cannot be avoided (Fig. 3c). It has
already been said that Steinmann pins in a given fragment should be stressed
at the time of insertion. On the other hand, the danger of inflammation is
reduced because there is less relative motion around the pin (Fig. 2a, 3)
(Boltze et al, 1978). Finally, should an inflammation cause widening of
the pin tract, this can initially be compensated by prestressing the pins
without significant loss of stability. Partially-threaded pins also improve
the hold in the bone.

In addition to the basic rules discussed above, an optimal construction is
important for the stability of the external gap osteosynthesis (Fig. 4, 7, 9)
(Hierholzer et al, 1978; Hoffmann et al, 1977; Hoffmann et al, 1980; Kleining
and Hierholzer, 1976; Kraus et al, 1977; Martineck et al, 1980; Müller et al,
1981). The construction itself depends on the location and size of the defect and on the topographic limitations present in the individual limb segment (Fig. 1c, 8, 9). As outlined in the following remarks, it is necessary
to differentiate between gap osteosynthesis of the tibia and of the femur.

The anatomy of the lower leg permits the use of a frame fixator whose sym-
metric design is advantageous from a mechanical standpoint (Fig. 1, 2)
(Boltze et al,1978; Hierholzer et al, 1978; Labitzke and Henze, 1978). The
rigidity of the frame fixator is improved by a three-dimensional arrangement
(Fig. 4, 9a). Here Schanz screws are anchored in the anterior tibial surface perpendicularly to the frame, and braced against the frame (Fig. 4).
A large number of experimental investigations have tested and analyzed the
stability of various forms of application to the tibia (Boltz et al, 1978;
Burger et al, 1977; Hierholzer et al, 1978; Hoffmann et al, 1977; Hoffmann
et al, 1980; Kleining and Hierholzer, 1976; Kraus et al, 1977; Labitzke and
Henze, 1980; Martineck et al, 1980). For diaphyseal defects, a standard
application using four Steinmann pins and two to four Schanz screws has
proved a success (Fig. 1c, 4a, 5). Fixation of defects close to a joint
using a Steinmann pin and a Schanz screw, which should be placed close to
the defect, combined with three-dimensional bracing has proved to be sufficiently rigid for clinical purposes (Fig. 4b)(Kleining and Hierholzer,
1976).

Occasionally, the individual anchoring possibilities and topographic location
of a defect close to a joint do not allow a three-dimensional arrangement
using a frame (Steinmann pins) and its bracket fixator (Schanz screws) perpendicular to the frame. In such cases, the principle of the reinforcing
diagonal rod offers further three-dimensional construction possibilities for
improving the stability of a simple frame (Fig. 4d, 4e)(Müller, 1981). In a
fragment of the proximal tibial epiphysis, two Steinmann pins can be introduced, one behind the other, parallel to the axis of movement of the knee
joint (Fig. 4c). For large comminuted defects close to a joint, a fixation
which bridges the joint is necessary. Depending on whether an arthrodesis of
the afflicted joint or only a temporary fixation bridging the joint is planned,
different application methods are required.

The anatomy of the femur does not allow external fixation with a frame (Labitzke and Henze, 1978; Labitzke et al, 1980; Müller, 1981). The considerable static weight load of the body and dynamic forces acting on the femur limit, in an absolute and temporal sense, the stability of external fixation. Considering these biomechanical and anatomic requirements, internal plate osteosynthesis guarantees the relatively safest form of stabilization, even for extensive bone defects, as well as a good functional result (Fig. 6, Müller, 1981). Our own clinical and experimental investigations using static and dynamic stress have shown that internal fixation with a plate and neutralization with an additional external bracket fixator result in the greatest rigidity for defects of the femur (Fig. 6a, 6c) (Müller et al, 1981).

When biologic priorities permit only external fixation of the femur, mechanical and functional disadvantages of the external fixing system must be accepted (Fig. 7, 9b). Osteosynthesis of the infected femur with an external fixation device is always indicated when plate osteosynthesis is out of the question. Such a situation can exist when the plate is unreliably anchored, when severe infection is present, when endosteal (due to a medullary nail) and periosteal (due to a plate) disturbance of blood circulation exist, and when irreversible damage of the extensor muscles and of the knee joint has occurred (Fig. 8). In view of the relatively large support-width of the femur and the small number and small section modulus of the Schanz screws, a lateral bracket fixator can only inadequately neutralize axial loads, much less bending and torsional loads, in the absence of contact (Labitzke and Henze, 1980; Labitzke et al, 1980; Müller, 1981). For this reason, the lateral bracket fixation (Femur Fixator Type 1) is not suitable for defects of the femur (Fig. 7a). The three-dimensional extension of the bracket fixator using a diagonal tubular rod which does not touch the soft tissue on the extensor side (Femur Fixator Type 2) affords sufficient rigidity for total osseous defects when knee function is to be retained (Fig. 7b, 8). A three-dimensional system using a lateral bracket fixator and a bracket fixator through the extensors (Femur Fixator Type 3) is only indicated for femur defects in conjunction with advanced damage to the extensor muscles and to the knee joint (Fig. 7c, 9b).

We recommend extending this three-dimensional femur fixation by bridging the joint to the lower leg (Femur Fixator Type 4) for defects close to the knee complicated by infection, in the presence of irreversible damage to the knee, for other complex injuries, or for cases where the survival of the leg is threatened (Fig. 7d, 9b)(Müller, 1981). Other authors have reported improved rigidity of femur defects using the so-called drawbar fixator ("Zugstangen-fixateur"), a modified lateral bracket fixator (Labitzke et al, 1980).

In summary, stability tests permit the unequivocal conclusion that the rigidity of external gap osteosynthesis in its various construction forms does not provide sufficient stability of the defect area in the lower leg and much less stability at the level of the thigh. Especially at the femur, even small loads under conditions of nonweightbearing occurring during torsional motions and active movements of muscles and neighboring joints, can influence the entire system; for instance, displacements of up to a few millimeters in the area of the defect can be observed. Nevertheless, assuming correct utilization of techniques, the stability of gap osteosynthesis is adequate - as clinical experience has sufficiently demonstrated - provided further surgical measures including bone grafts are carried out to stimulate biologic processes resulting in increased stability (Fig. 1c, 5, 6, 8).

References

1. Boltze, W.H., Chiquet, C., and Niederer, P.G.: Der Fixateur externe (Rohrsystem) Stabilitätsprüfung. AO-Bulletin, Spring 1978.

2. Burger, H., Kraus, J., Hild, P., and Hoffmann, D.: Festigkeitsuntersuchungen am Fixateur externe unter Biegebeanspruchung bei Defekten am Bruchspalt. Unfallchir. 3, 221, 1977.

3. Hierholzer, G., Kleining, R., Hörster, G., and Zemenides, P.: External fixation. Arch. Orthop. Traumatol. Surg. 92, 175, 1978.

4. Hoffmann, D., Burger, H., Kraus, J., and Hild, P.: Festigkeitsuntersuchungen am Fixateur externe unter Biegebeanspruchung bei Defekten am Bruchspalt. Unfallchir. 3, 147, 1977.

5. Hoffmann, D., Hild, P., and Burger, H.: Untersuchungen zur Leistungsfähigkeit des Fixateur externe. Hefte Unfallheilk. 148, 521, 1980.

6. Kleining, R., and Hierholzer, G.: Biomechanische Untersuchungen zur Osteosynthese mit dem Fixateur externe. Akt. traumatol. 6, 71, 1976.

7. Kraus, J., Hild, P., Hoffmann, D., and Burger, H.: Festigkeitsuntersuchungen am Fixateur externe unter Biegebeanspruchung. Seitliche und exzentrische Belastung bei Defekten am Bruchspalt. Unfallchir. 3, 227, 1977.

8. Labitzke, R., and Henze, G.: Biomechanik des Fixateur externe. Unfallheilkunde 81, 546, 1978.

9. Labitzke, R., and Henze, G.: Klinisch experimentelle Untersuchungen zur Stabilität des Fixateur externe. Hefte Unfallheilk. 148, 519, 1980.

10. Labitzke, R., Henze, G., and Towfigh, H.: Stabilisierung ausgedehnter infizierter Femurschaftdefekte. Lecture Österreichische Gesellschaft für Unfallchirurgie, 16. Conference, Salzburg, October 1980 (in press).

11. Martineck, H., Egkher, E., and Wielke, B.: Experimentelle Grundlagen zur optimalen Montageform äußerer Spanner. Hefte. Unfallheilk. 148, 516, 1980.

12. Müller, K.H., Exogene Osteomyelitis von Becken und unteren Gliedmaßen. Springer, Berlin-Heidelberg-New York, 1981 (in press).

13. Müller, K.H., Bowe, K.H., and Witzel, U.P.: Experimentelle Untersuchungen & klinische Erfahrungen der Osteosynthese von Femurdefekten durch Platte und neutralisierenden Klammerfixateur. To be published in Arch. Orthop. Traumat. Surg. 1981

14. Müller, K.H., Stratmann, P., and Rehn, J.: Grundlagen zur kontinuierlichen Spannungsmessung am Frakturspalt nach Fixateur-externe-Osteosynthese. Unfallheilkunde 82, 183, 1979.

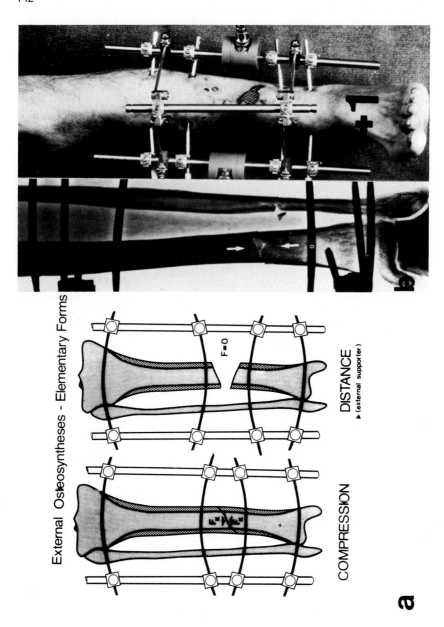

External Osteosyntheses - Elementary Forms

COMPRESSION

DISTANCE
▶ (external supporter)

F=0

a

Fig. 1. Comparison of external compression osteosynthesis and gap osteosynthesis.
a) Schematic representation of the mechanical differences. b) Clinical example of an external compression osteosynthesis for a compound tibia fracture; the interfragmental compression load is measured at the tubular system using strain gauges.

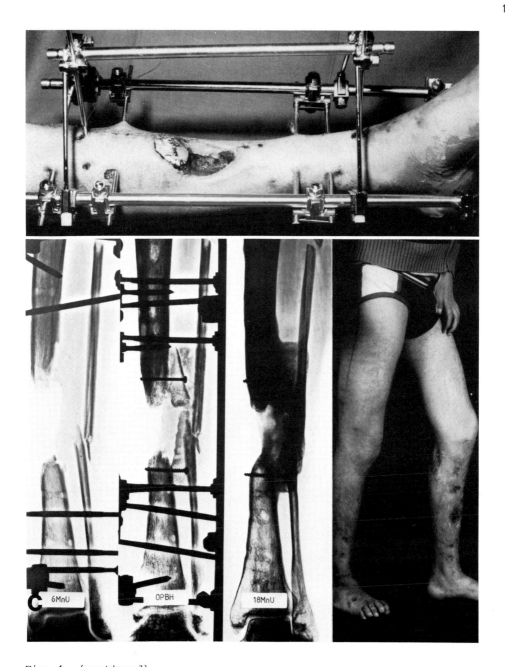

Fig. 1. (continued)
c) Clinical example of an external gap osteosynthesis for an 8 cm
long defect in the tibia; polytraumatized 26-year old motorcyclist;
osseous bridging by means of fibulotibial synostosis.

External Distance Osteosynthesis - application of a frame

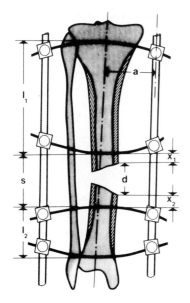

a ▸ support - width

d ▸ max. osseous defect stretch

s ▸ free bending stretch

l_1
l_2
{ distance between pins in the fragment

x_1
x_2
{ min. distance between defect and pin

a

External Distance Osteosynthesis - free bending stretch (s)
Rigidity: 1 » 2 , 1 ~ 3 , 3 » 2

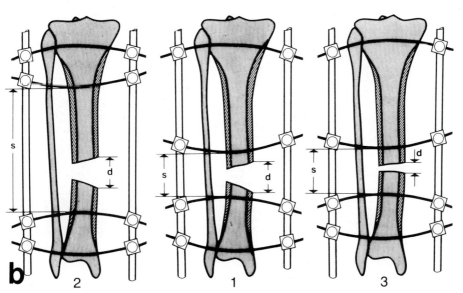

b 2 1 3

Fig. 2. Schematic representation of external frame osteosynthesis for tibial defects. a) Characteristic mechanical data. b) Rigidity of the frame system as a function of the position of the Steinman pins close to the defect and of the various defect lengths.

External Distance Osteosynthesis -

osseous contact not resistant to compression

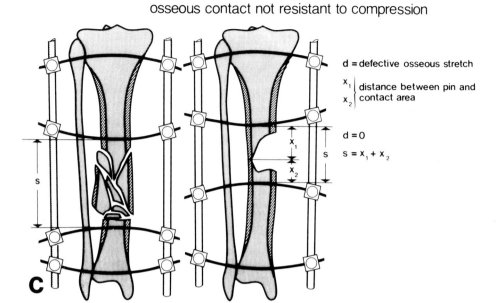

d = defective osseous stretch

$\left.\begin{array}{l} x_1 \\ x_2 \end{array}\right|$ distance between pin and contact area

d = 0

$s = x_1 + x_2$

Fig. 2. (continued)
c) External osteosynthesis when the fragmental contact is not pressure resistant. The free bending stretch without interfragmental compression makes this system behave mechanically like a case of gap osteosynthesis.

Fig. 3. (see next page): Loosening of the Steinmann pins. a) Schematic representation. Row 1: pins which were not prestressed already loosen when minor widening of the pin tract occurs (1b); Row 2: prestressed pins only loosen when advanced widening of the pin tract no longer guarantees three-point anchoring (2c); Row 3: partially threaded pins improve anchoring with respect to lateral shifting (compare the difference between 2b and 3b).
b) Prestressing of both Steinmann pins on one fragment side in relation to each other, using as an example an extensive tibial defect. c) Sequestrum in the presence of osteomyelitis at a Steinmann pin tract, in situ and as a specimen.

146

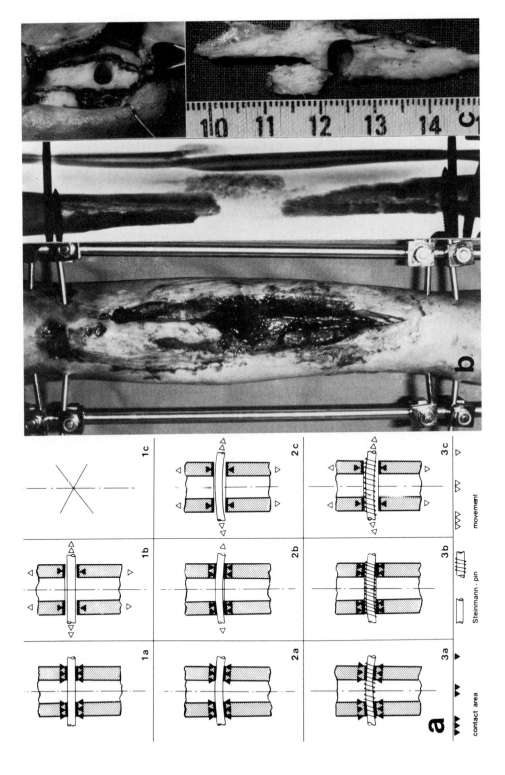

Fig. 3

External Distance Osteosynthesis Tibia

Shaft defect: spacial application distal defect (close to joint):
                                      spacial application

proximal defect (close to joint)
spacial application

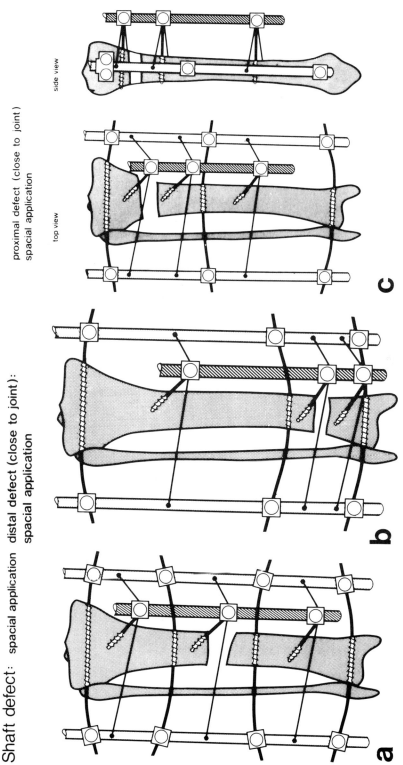

side view

top view

a

b

c

Fig. 4. Three-dimensional applications of external gap osteosyntheses in a tibia as a function of the location of the defect. a) Diaphyseal defect: three-dimensional application combining a frame system with 4 Steinmann pins and a bracket fixator with 3 Schanz screws. b) Defect close to the ankle joint: three-dimensional application using 1 Steinmann pin and 1 Schanz screw in the fragment close to the joint. c) Defect close to the knee joint: three-dimensional application with 2 Steinmann pins introduced into the fragment of the tibia head one after the other.

148

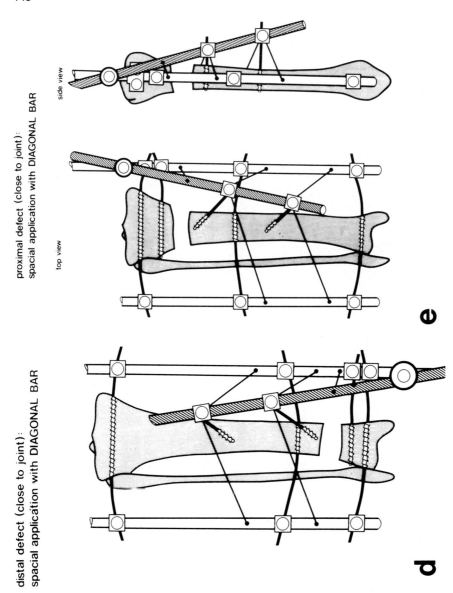

distal defect (close to joint):
spacial applicátion with DIAGONAL BAR

proximal defect (close to joint):
spacial application with DIAGONAL BAR

top view

side view

d

e

Fig. 4. (con=inued) d) and e). Three-dimensional applications for defects close to a joint using a supporting diagonal rod; these methods are used when unfavorable bone and soft tissue conditions prevent use of the standard applications.

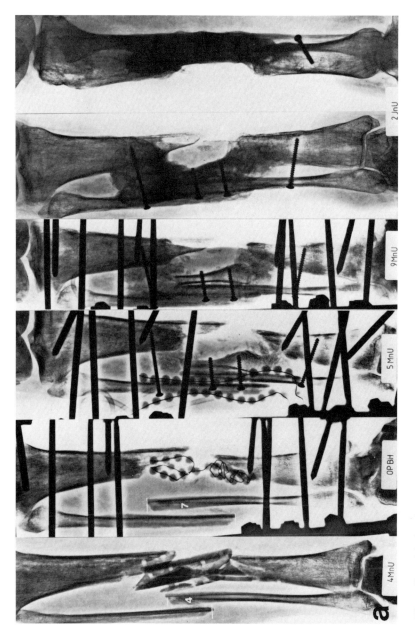

Fig. 5. Clinical example of an infected pseudarthrosis following plate osteosyntheses; the patient is a 53-year old woman. a) Roentgenograph series: sequestration of the middle tibia fragment and progressive reconstruction of the defect using fibulotibial synostosis; the leg is shortened.

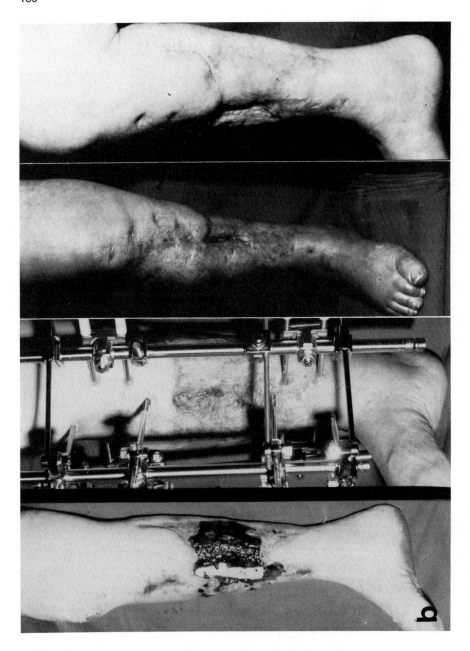

Fig. 5. (continued)
b) Clinical picture upon admission, following external stabilization and following perfect bone consolidation.

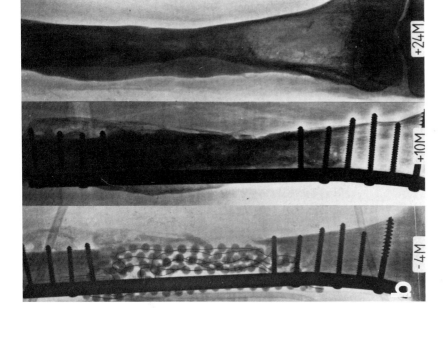

Internal Distance Osteosynthesis Femur

plate osteosynthesis
+
bracket fixateur
(for neutralization)

plate osteosynthesis

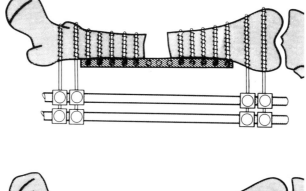

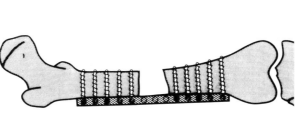

a

Fig. 6. Internal gap osteosynthesis of the femur. a) Schematic representation: adequately dimensioned plate osteosynthesis and increased rigidity using an additional external bracket fixator. b) Roentgeno-graph series: stabilization and bridging of a 12 cm long infected defect in the femur using plate osteosyn-thesis and autologous cancellous bone grafting.

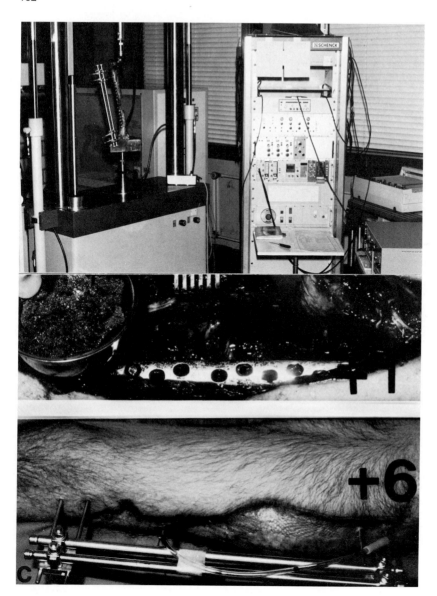

Fig. 6. (continued)
c) Experimental testing of the rigidity of internal gap osteosyntheses in the femur shaft for dynamic cyclical loading.

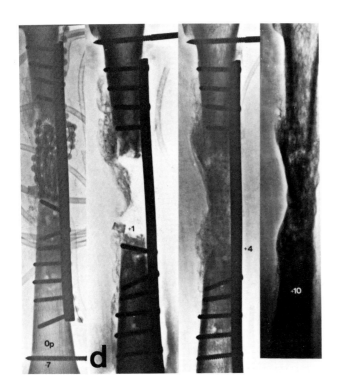

Fig. 6. (continued)
d) Clinical example on a roentgenograph series
of an infected pseudarthrosis in the femur;
stabilization using internal plate osteosynthesis, and neutralization of this system
using an external lateral bracket fixator.

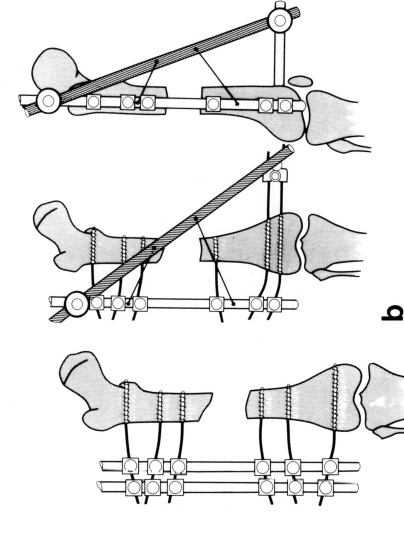

External Distance Osteosynthesis Femur

bracket fixateur (femur fixateur Type I)

Bracket fixateur and diagonal bar
(femur fixateur Type II)

top view

side view

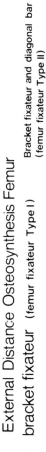

a

b

Fig. 7. Forms of external gap osteosyntheses in the femur (Type I-IV). a) Lateral
bracket fixator (Type I); insufficient stability when the defect is complete and without bone support. b) Three-dimensional external application using a diagonal rod
(Type II); improved rigidity without long-lasting disturbance of the extensors and

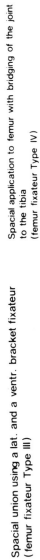

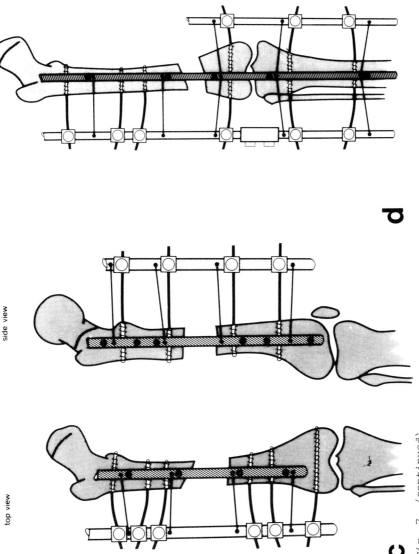

Spacial union using a lat. and a ventr. bracket fixateur
(femur fixateur Type III)

top view

side view

Spacial application to femur with bridging of the joint to the tibia
(femur fixateur Type IV)

c

d

Fig. 7. (continued)
c) Bracing with a lateral and an anterior bracket fixator (Type III); only indicated when the knee joint is already damaged, since the extensors are blocked. d) Three-dimensional external fixator which bridges the knee joint (Type IV); for use with femur defects close to a joint.

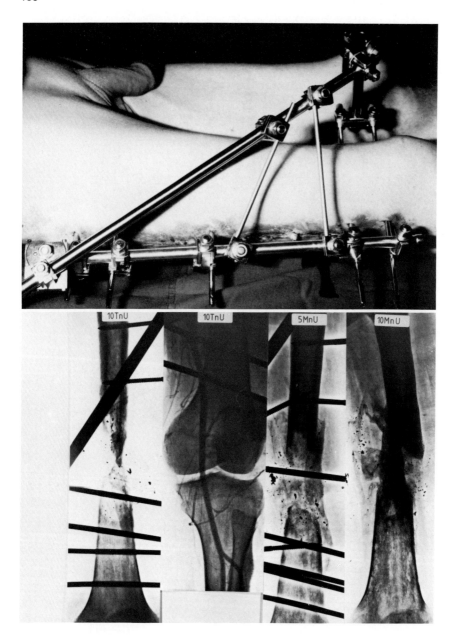

Fig. 8. Clinical example and roentgenograph series of a femur fracture caused by a gunshot, with an infected femur defect; stabilization using the femur fixator Type II.

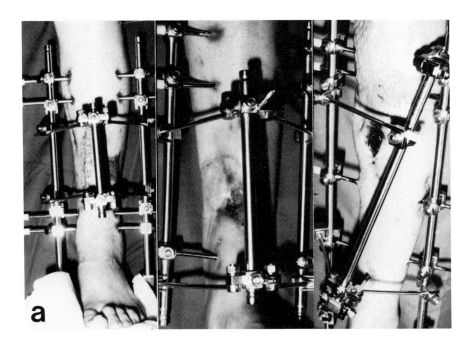

Fig. 9. Clinical examples of the forms of external gap osteosyntheses of the lower limbs. a) Three-dimensional application in
the shaft area of the tibia (standard application, cf Fig. 4a),
close to the ankle joint (cf Fig. 4b), and close to the knee joint
with a supporting diagonal rod (cf Fig. 4e).

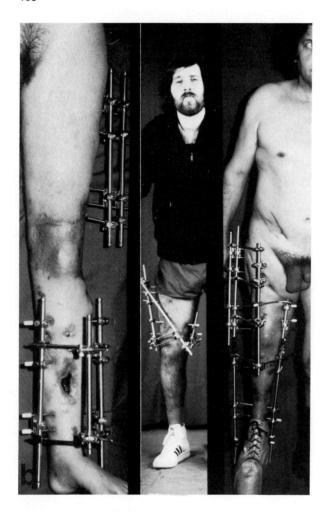

Fig. 9. (continued)
b) Applications in the femur, femur fixator
Type I (cf Fig. 7a), femur fixator Type II
(cf Fig. 7b), and femur fixator Type IV,
which bridges the joint; here indicated because loss of leg is threatened due to an
18 cm long infected bone defect and simultaneous infected tibial pseudarthrosis.

Elastic External Fixation of Tibial Fractures: Influence of Associated Internal Fixation

F. Burny, M. Donkerwolcke, and O. Saric

An osteosynthesis is a means of fixation of bone fragments with direct anchorage of the material to the bone. Due to muscular function and daily living activities, the osteosynthesis is subjected to mechanical forces.

If we consider the normal biologic environment, we may assume that fracture healing is dependent on mechanical conditions. Callus formation depends on mechanical conditions: under a given threshold of mechanical stimulation (interfragmentary motion) (Burny, 1979; Burny et al, 1980), primary bone healing occurs without periosteal callus formation (Nunamaker, et al, 1980;

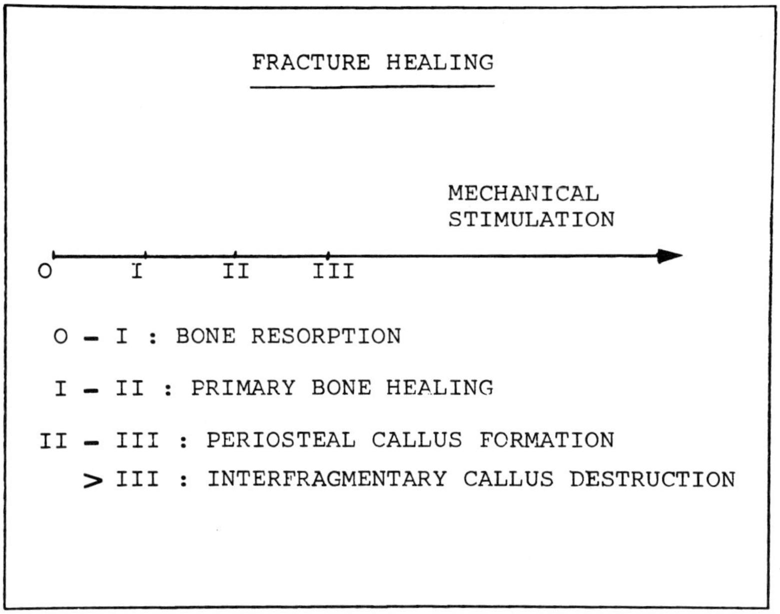

FRACTURE HEALING

MECHANICAL
STIMULATION

O   I   II   III

O - I   : BONE RESORPTION

I - II : PRIMARY BONE HEALING

II - III : PERIOSTEAL CALLUS FORMATION

   > III : INTERFRAGMENTARY CALLUS DESTRUCTION

Fig. 1. Steps in the mechanical stimulation of the bone or of the surrounding tissues. Steps I, II, III represent thresholds of mechanical stimulation; their exact position on the axis remains to be determined.

Perren et al, 1980). Conversely, excess mechanical stimulation leads to the destruction of interfragmentary blood vessels and to hypertropic pseudarthrosis (Fig. 1).

Materials and Methods

Our study was conducted on tibial fractures treated by elastic external fixation based on

- half frame configuration
- short fixation rod (10 cm)
- 3 pins distant to each other in each clamp
- clamps tightened at 1 cm from the skin.

In the case of a stable fracture, early weight bearing is recommended leading to early healing with periosteal callus (Fig. 2). For an unstable simple fracture, early function after treatment by elastic half frame fixation could be responsible for loss of alignment and pseudarthroses.

Our hypothesis, based on general statistics on tibial fractures (Burny et al, 1979; 1980) was that associated *a minima* osteosynthesis (screw, cerclage, etc) is useful for the stabilization of simple fractures.

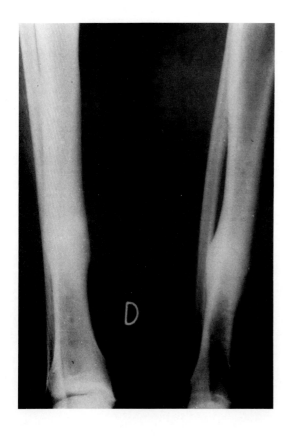

Fig. 2. Periosteal callus formation after elastic external fixation.

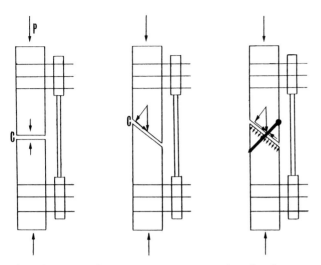

Fig. 3. Interfragmentary compression by lag screw, neutralizing shearing stress.

This technique

- avoids motion at the fracture by neutralization of shearing forces by compression (Fig. 3);

- avoids splitting of the fragments if damaged by the trauma (Fig. 4).

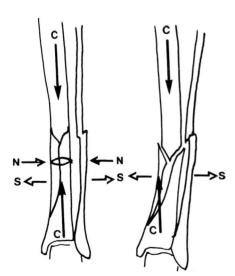

Fig. 4. Cerclage avoiding possible splitting of the fragments.

162

Table I. Combined external-internal fixation.
          Inclusion criteria

Tibial fractures –

   noninfected; closed; without skin contusion;
   oblique; spiral; butterfly.

Table II. Location of the fracture

	Combined Ext. and Int. Fix.		Ext.Fix. only	
Proximal shaft	4	7.5%	15	5.6%
Midshaft	27	50.9%	148	55.4%
Distal shaft	21	39.7%	85	31.8%
Distal metaphysis	1	1.9%	10	3.8%
Other	–	–	9	3.4%
TOTAL	53		267	

To satisfy the inclusion criteria of this retrospective study, presented in
Tables I and II, only patients with fractures usually considered to be unstable were admitted. Fifty-three fractures had been treated with combined
external and internal fixation, and 267 by external half frame fixation only.

As part of the study we did an evaluation of interfragmentary motion in some
patients of the two groups. We used fixation rods equipped with a strain
gauge. In all cases, the strain gauge was located in a sagittal plane on
the anterior aspect of the rod (Fig. 5). For a given load, the registered

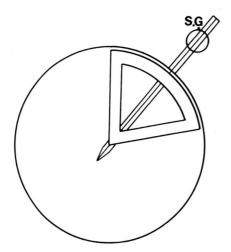

Fig. 5. Position of the strain gauge
(S.G.) in a sagittal plane.

deformation was related to the interfragmentary mobility. We then compared the deformations observed at 14 ± 3.4 days for the two groups of treatment.

Results

We selected 267 fractures treated by external fixation only and 53 fractures with combined external and internal fixation.

We compared the rate of skin complication (Table III) and of sepsis (Table IV), the anatomic results at the end of the treatment (Table V), the healing time (Tables VI, VII; Fig. 6), and the rate of pseudarthroses (Table VIII).

Table III. Skin complications

	Combined Ext. and Int. Fix.		Ext. Fix. Only	
No	46	86.8%	256	95.9%
Yes	2	3.8%	7	2.6%
Unknown	5	9.4%	4	1.5%
TOTAL	53		267	

Table IV. Sepsis

	Combined Ext. and Int. Fix.		Ext. Fix. Only	
No	46	86.8%	256	95.9%
Yes	4	7.5%	7	2.6%
Unknown	3	5.7%	4	1.5%
TOTAL	53		267	

Table V. Axes - final result

	Combined Ext. and Int. Fix.		Ext. Fix. Only	
Very good	51	96.2%	245	91.8%
Good	-	-	7	2.6%
Poor	-	-	2	0.7%
Unknown	2	3.8%	13	4.9%
TOTAL	53		267	

Table VI. Cumulated percentage of healing delay

%	Combined Ext. and Int. Fix.	Ext. Fix. Only
10	90 days	65 days
25	100	75
50	125	95
75	150	125
90	180	180
97.5	210	225

Table VII. Percentage of healing.

After (days)	Combined Ext. and Int. Fix.	Ext. Fix. Only
90	5.6%	31.9% $(p<1.10^{-7})$
120	36.1%	65.3% $(p<0.001)$
150	63.9%	79.0% $(p<0.08)$
180	86.1%	86.7% (NS)
210	94.5%	92.7% (NS)

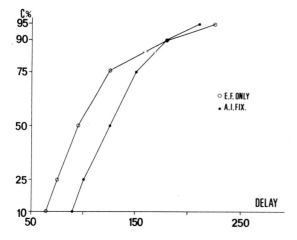

Fig. 6. Difference of healing between the two groups (cf Table VI). Ordinate: percentage of healed fracture. Abscissa: delay (days).

Table VIII. Pseudarthroses

	Combined Ext. and Int. Fix.		Ext. Fix. Only	
No	47	88.6%	215	80.5%
Yes	3	5.7%	12	4.5%
Unknown	3	5.7%	40	15.0%
TOTAL	53		267	

In this retrospective study, the time to partial and total weight bearing was not reliable and we had to disregard this variable.

The results of the extensometry with strain gauges are presented in Table IX. Considering the reading of the strain gauges as an indication of interfragmentary mobility, we observed that associated *a minima* internal fixation decreased the mobility by one-third.

Table IX. Deformation of the fixation rod at
           the first measurement

	Mean time of first measurement: 14 days	
	Combined Ext. and Int. Fix.	Ext. Fix. Only
Deformation	64.3 ± 36.1	212 ± 22.6
	Sign. +ı+	

Discussion

Used as the only means of osteosynthesis, screws, bolts, and cerclage are inadequate to insure the stability of a fracture. They must be considered as auxiliary treatment and be combined with other fixation procedures (plates, nails, etc.).

A *minima* internal fixation of simple unstable fractures (spiral, oblique, butterfly . . .) combined with half frame external fixation could represent the treatment of choice for such fractures because of

- minimal interference with the biologic processes of fracture healing,
- possibility of early joint motion,
- early weight bearing,
- anatomic axes' restoration.

Table X. Conclusions (on documented cases)

	Combined Ext. and Int. Fix.	Ext. Fix. Only	Sign.
Skin complications	4.2%	2.7%	++++
Sepsis	8.0%	2.7%	++++
Final axes	100.0%	96.0%	+++
Pseudarthroses	6.0%	5.3%	(-)

An analysis of the two series demonstrates some complications (Table X).
An increased rate of skin complications and sepsis is significantly related
to the associated internal fixation. These complications, however, will
not impair the final result (rate of pseudarthroses) and a better anatomic
result is obtained.

As demonstrated by the strain gauge study, combined internal and external
fixation provides higher rigidity and minimal callus formation (Fig. 7).

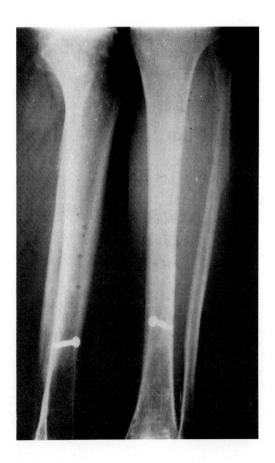

Fig. 7. Reduced periosteal
callus formation after more
rigid fixation.

The 3.5 time increase of stability (Table IX) does not cause pseudarthroses (Table X) and significantly increases the healing time during the first five months (Table VII).

Conclusion

A *minima* internal fixation combined with half frame elastic external fixation leads to better final anatomic results than external fixation alone in unstable, simple tibial fractures. The rate of septic complications, however, and skin infections increases.

Increasing stability by 3.5 times significantly decreases the healing time, thus demonstrating the superiority of elastic fixation of fractures.

References

1. Burny, F., El Banna, S., Evrard, H., Vander Ghinst, M., De Geeter, L., Peeters, M., Verdonk, R., Desmet, Ch., Fernandez-Fairen, M., Moreira, D., Le Rebeller, M., Martini, M.: Elastic external fixation of tibial fractures. Study of 1421 cases. In, External Fixation: The Current State of the Art. Williams and Wilkins Co., Baltimore, 1979.

2. Burny, F.: Mechanical problems of fracture treatment: Theoretical and clinical study. In, Bioengineering Seminar. Berkeley, 1979.

3. Burny, F., El Banna, S., Evrard, H., Vander Ghinst, M., De Geeter, L., Peeters, F., Verdonk, R., Desmet, Ch.: Les fractures simples du tibia. Traitement par fixation externe élastique. 7èmes journées internationales: la Fixation Externe d'Hoffmann, Montpellier 1980; Ed., S.A. Diffinco. Geneva, 1980.

4. Burny, F., Bourgois, R., Donkerwolcke, M.: Elastic fixation of fractures. In, Current Concepts of Internal Fixation of Fractures. Ed., H.K. Uhthoff. Springer-Verlag, Heidelberg, 1980

5. Nunamaker, D.M., Perren, S.: Pure titanium plates in sheep: The effect of rigidity and compression. In, Current Concepts of Internal Fixation of Fractures. Ed., H.K. Uhthoff. Springer-Verlag, Heidelberg, 1980.

6. Perren, S., Cordey, J.: The concept of interfragmentary strain. In, Current Concepts of Internal Fixation of Fractures. Ed., H.K. Uhthoff. Springer-Verlag, Heidelberg, 1980.

External Fixation in Lower Extremity Trauma: Cook County Experience

A. M. Pankovich

Introduction

At Cook County Hospital, before 1973, pins and plaster were the only components of external fixation for the treatment of certain acute tibial and
femoral fractures. Our first experience with a commercially available
device was with the original AO external fixator. It was used for an
infected nonunion following an open tibial fracture. Subsequently, it
became the external fixation device of choice for almost all open fractures in lower extremities. The reason for using the AO external fixator
was its low cost. In our institution, replacement of such devices is
difficult and their loss is not uncommon: when patients are transferred
out or go for follow-up elsewhere; when rods are abused and bent, removed
and lost; or when they have been discarded after being used three to four
times. Other devices are much more expensive. Over the years, external
fixation in lower extremities was used for a number of indications.

Open Tibial Fractures

Our rationale for using external fixation in open tibial fractures:

1. Open fractures are frequently the result of severe injury accompanied
by soft tissue damage, particularly 2nd and 3rd degree lesions (Gustilo
and Anderson, 1976). These wounds must be treated by thorough debridement
of all devitalized tissues which include bone, muscle, and skin. Closure
of such wounds is contraindicated in our view because it increases the
risk of infection. It is thus convenient to have easy access to these
extensive wounds by immobilizing the extremity with an external fixator.

2. Open fractures are frequently comminuted, generally unstable, and difficult to hold in good alignment in a plaster cast. An external fixator
usually takes care of this problem very effectively.

3. Moving the patient in and out of bed is greatly facilitated by immobilization of the limb with an external fixator when compared with cast immobilization. This is particularly true with the original AO external fixator which
is light and not too bulky, an important factor in polytraumatized patients.

4. Early motion of the knee and ankle is possible. This is another advantage, particularly important when an ipsilateral femoral fracture is present.

5. Early elevation of the limb, and early muscle contractions with an external fixator in place, probably increase venous drainage and consequently
diminish the incidence of venous thrombosis (Olerud, 1979).

6. Early bone grafting is possible with the device in place without disrupting the alignment of fracture fragments.

7. When a muscle pedicle graft is anticipated, unicortical placement of the pins and the rods can be planned.

8. Early weight bearing is allowed after the wounds are healed and swelling has subsided.

Technique

It is extremely important to understand that the Steinmann pins must be inserted in nearly perfect position since with the original AO device correction of malposition of fracture fragments is limited for varus-valgus deformities and impossible for rotational deformities. The fracture fragments must therefore be anatomically reduced which is often difficult when smaller or larger fragments are missing. Radiographic or fluoroscopic control should be liberally used to position the pins correctly.

Usually two or three of the largest threaded Steinmann pins are inserted above and below, and at some distance from the fracture site whenever possible. When the fracture is close to the tibial plafond, one pin is inserted in the distal tibial fragment and the second in the same line in the *os calcis* (Fig. 1a, b).

Postoperatively, the limb is either elevated on a pillow or suspended with strings tied to the fracture frame. Once the wounds are healed and swelling has subsided, the patient is allowed to walk progressing from partial to full weight bearing, whenever possible. Since the original AO external fixator is light, usually applied close to the skin, and is not bulky, ambulation and weight bearing are possible for most patients.

The external fixator is usually removed within three months after application and, whenever possible, replaced with a short leg walking cast. This is deemed necessary particularly in cortical diaphyseal fractures when little or no callus is observed on roentgenograms at eight to ten weeks. In the metaphyseal part of the tibia, the device is removed at about two months if the fracture line is visible to allow for impaction of the fragments and healing (Fig. 1c, d). If the fracture line is obliterated, the device is left in place for another month and removed. Further immobilization is then not needed.

Cancellous bone grafting is necessary in cases of bone loss. Although immediate bone grafting is desirable, it is often necessary to wait until the soft tissue healing is advanced enough. This stage is usually reached when healthy, easily bleeding granulation tissue covers the bone. Open or closed bone grafting is then done depending on the condition of the skin. Bone grafting should not be needlessly delayed hoping that it will not be necessary and that the fracture will heal by itself.

Complications in our series attributed to the external fixator included:
Pin tract drainage which was usually the result of skin tenting over the

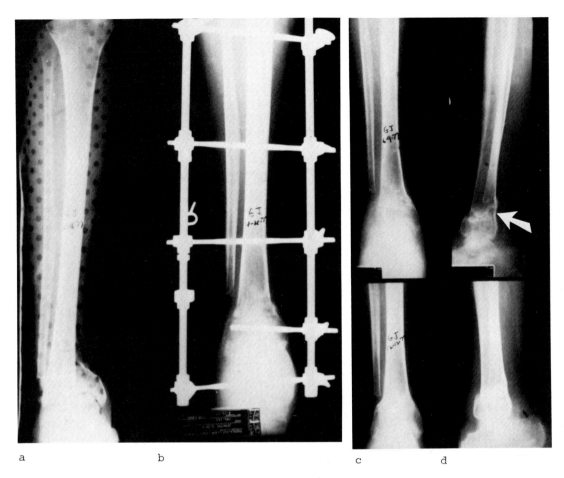

a   b   c   d

Fig. 1. An open fracture in the distal tibial metaphysis with the open wound over the distal fibula. a) Roentgenogram on admission: about $2\frac{1}{2}$ cm of the fibula was missing. b) Postoperative roentgenogram; there was space for only one Steinmann pin above the tibial plafond, and the second pin was inserted through the *os calcis*. c) The external fixator was removed after 2 months; note some resorption at the fracture site (arrow). d) Short leg cast was applied allowing for impaction of the fragments. The fracture was healed 6 weeks later.

pin and formation of a local abscess in some cases, yet usually subsiding after release of the tented skin.

Malrotation, as a result of improper technique, required reinsertion of pins. This complication could have been avoided by careful reduction of fragments before insertion of pins.

Nonunion developed in some cases in which the fixator was used for extended periods, although these were also type III open injuries with soft tissue damage and it is possible that nonunion would have developed even with other treatment modalities.

Obese Patients

A number of very obese patients with tibial fractures were managed with external fixation instead of a long leg cast which would be ineffective and difficult to apply. Similarly, we used external fixation in bilateral closed or open tibial fractures. The tendency was to keep external fixators on longer, at least until a short leg cast would be adequate. These fractures are now treated with Ender-type flexible intramedullary nails.

External fixation was also found useful in a very obese patient necessitating postoperative immobilization of a dislocated knee (Fig. 2). Again, the patient became mobile early while the external fixator effectively immobilized the repaired knee. For this purpose, we used unicortically-inserted pins which were removed at three months and no further immobilization was needed. Clinical result was excellent.

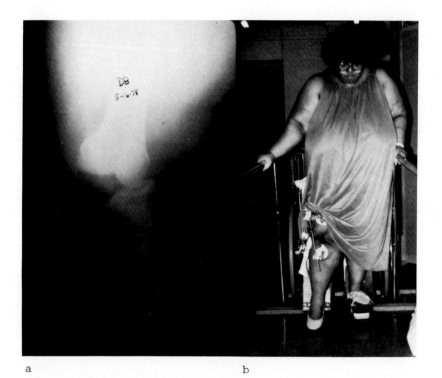

a   b

Fig. 2. A very obese young woman with a dislocation of the right knee. a) Roentgenogram on admission. b) One week after repair and application of Hoffmann apparatus the patient is walking in parallel bars.

Vascular Injuries

Vascular injuries are not uncommon in femoral fractures, particularly those produced by gunshot and shotgun injuries. These are frequently fractures of the femur in its distal third, the arterial injury involving the popliteal artery. The object of treatment is to facilitate repair and healing of the injured vessel. Although some authors recommend traction following surgical repair of the artery and vein (Connolly et al, 1971), it is more practical to stabilize the bone before undertaking repair of the vessels. An effective and quick stabilization procedure makes vascular repair easy (Lim et al, 1980).

The procedure is usually done as follows: The patient is placed on a fracture table and the femoral fracture is reduced under control of an image intensifier. An arteriogram is taken to determine the type and level of vascular injury and the possibility of multiple injuries. Preliminary leg fasciotomies are done whenever required. A large threaded Steinmann pin is inserted from the lateral aspect of the thigh and through both cortices,

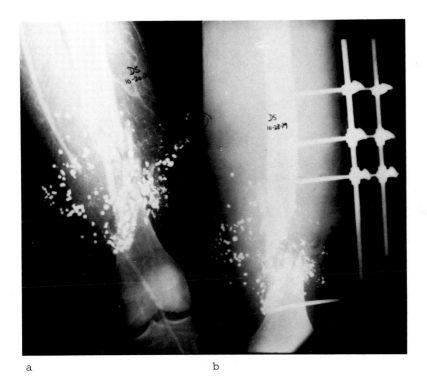

a   b

Fig. 3. Shotgun fracture of the distal femur. a) An angiogram shows interruption of flow of the superficial femoral artery. b) Roentgenogram after debridement and immobilization of the fracture with an AO external fixator. The most distal pin does not show on this film.

usually in the distal portion of the femur. Two AO external rods are positioned on this pin. All other pins are inserted through the rest of the clamps on the rods as guides (Fig. 3). Medial approach for repair of the injured vessels is then undertaken by the vascular team. Postoperatively, no special precautions are needed. Patients may walk in about two weeks. The external fixator is removed and replaced with a long leg cast in about two months. Although our experience has been primarily with the original AO external fixator, other types of external fixators could be used just as effectively in these situations.

Adjunctive Fixation in Ender Nailing

The AO external fixator has also been used as an adjunctive fixation system to Ender nailing of femoral shaft fractures with bicortical comminution (Pankovich, 1981). Usually, the fracture is reduced anatomically on a fracture table and fixed with two Ender nails. Then, a large threaded Steinmann pin is inserted from the lateral aspect above or below and at some distance from the fracture site. Using this pin as a guide, another four or five pins are inserted through appropriately positioned clamps as guides. Insertion of the Steinmann pins is difficult if the medullary canal is narrow.

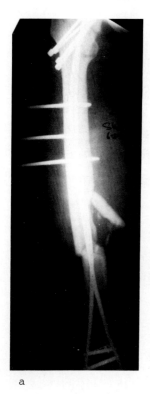
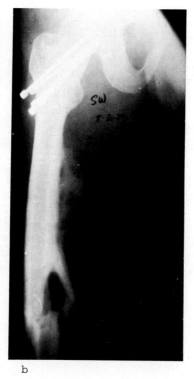

a   b

Fig. 4. The external fixator was used to prevent shortening after insertion of Ender nails in this triple fracture of the femur involving the neck, the midshaft, and the distal part. a) Post-operative roentgenogram. b) The appearance of the femur one year later.

The rationale for this procedure is to prevent shortening of the femur when bicortical comminution is present, since the fracture fragments tend to slide along the Ender nails, as in all other intramedualllary nails, until the main fragments reach each other, thus producing shortening commensurate to the length of the bicortical comminution. The AO external fixator serves the purpose effectively and is removed in about two months. By that time, sufficient healing takes place **without further shortening. (Fig.4)**

The main disadvantage of this system is fixation of the *vastus lateralis* by multiple Steinmann pins and consequent limitation of knee motion until the pins are removed. Permanent loss of knee motion can occur.

Osteomyelitis

Our experience has been particularly gratifying in acute post-traumatic osteo-myelitis (Burri, 1975) in which the periosteum had been supposedly retained. After diaphysectomy to remove all infected bone, the remaining periosteum contributed to restoration of continuity of the tibia (Pankovich et al, 1980).

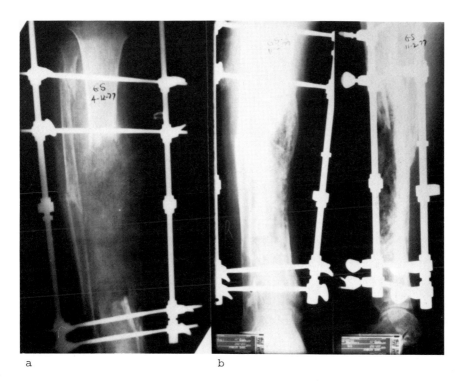

a   b

Fig. 5. The external fixator was used to immobilize the re-maining tibia. During debridement more than half of the in-fected tibial diaphysis was excised. a) Postoperative roent-genogram. b) Seven months after debridement, continuity of the tibia was restored.

One case is shown in Fig. 5. So far, 15 patients have been treated: tibia in 12 patients; femur in two patients; and both femur and tibia in one patient. In all patients, continuity of the bone was restored. Periodic drainage has recurred in four patients, requiring debridement in two.

In one patient with femoral osteomyelitis, a pseudoaneurysm of the deep femoral artery developed six months after application of the external fixator at the tip of a proximal Steinmann pin which was protruding from the medial cortex (Pankovich et al, 1981.)

In chronic osteomyelitis, with or without nonunion, more problems developed, particularly with respect to reconstitution of the resected portion.

References

1. Burri, Caius: Post-Traumatic Osteomyelitis. Hans Huber Publishers. Bern, 1975.

2. Connolly, J.F.; Whittaker, P.; and Williams, E.: Femoral and tibial fractures combined with injuries to the femoral or popliteal artery. A review of the literature and analysis of fourteen cases. J. Bone Jt. Surg. 53A, 55, 1971.

3. Gustilo, R.B., and Anderson, T.J.: Prevention of infection in the treatment of 1,025 open fractures of long bones. J. Bone Jt. Surg. 58A, 453, 1976.

4. Lim, Leonardo T.; Michuda, Maryanne S.; Flanigan, D. Preston; and Pankovich, Arsen: Popliteal artery trauma. Arch. Surg. 115, 1037, 1980.

5. Olerud, Sven: The management of open tibial fractures. A short review. In, External Fixation, The Current State of the Art, pp 51-53. Williams and Wilkins Co. 1979.

6. Pankovich, Arsen: Adjunctive fixation in flexible intramedullary nailing in femoral fractures. A study of twenty-six cases. Clin. Orthop. (in press).

7. Pankovich, Arsen; Perry, Clayton; and Miskew, Don: Open bone grafting in post-traumatic osteomyelitis. Proc. Inst. Med. Chgo. 33, 67, 1980.

8. Pankovich, Arsen; Shivaram, Mysore; and Lim, Leonardo: Infected late false aneurysm of the deep femoral artery. Clin. Orthop. 154, 208, 1981.

Unilateral External Fixation Experience with the ASIF "Tubular" Frame

F. Behrens and K. Searls

About 70% of all external fixators are currently used for the management of severe open or infected lower extremity lesions. Following the suggestions of Adrey (1970) and Vidal et al (1976), most are applied as bilateral frames (Fig. 1). This means that two or more parallel transfixion pins inserted into each major bone fragment are connected by parallel rods on each side of the leg.

Despite their present popularity, bilateral frames have serious mechanical and clinical shortcomings:

- They are weakest in the sagittal plane where most of the clinically relevant forces apply (gravity if the patient is supine; ground reaction forces when walking)(McCoy et al, 1980).

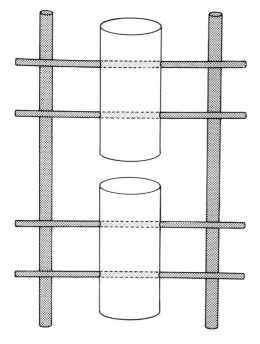

Fig. 1. Diagram of a bilateral frame.

- Transfixion pins can cause compartment syndromes (Raimbeau et al, 1979) and injuries to the anterior tibial artery (Burny, 1975; Raimbeau et al, 1979).

- The impalement of musculotendinous units in the distal part of the leg is inevitable, and frequently leads to fibrosis and a permanent decrease of ankle motion.

- Bilateral rods can interfere with wound access.

- Transfixion of soft tissues and a cumbersome frame rarely permit full weight bearing.

After careful consideration, we concluded that most of the shortcomings of bilateral frames can be alleviated with unilateral designs (Fig. 2). We felt that more rigid pins and rods would prevent some of the difficulties experienced with the original Hoffmann frame and, therefore, chose components of the ASIF "tubular" fixator.

To test these concepts, we applied unilateral frames to all severe knee and tibial lesions admitted to St. Paul-Ramsey Medical Center over a 17-month period. During this time, 32 unilateral fixators were applied. All lesions are now healed. The final analysis excludes one patient who was lost to follow-up before the final measurements were made. The remaining 31 patients form the basis of this report. Twenty of the fixators were applied to Type II (5) and Type III (15) open tibial fractures which were complicated by 38 associated injuries. The remaining 11 fixators were used for closed

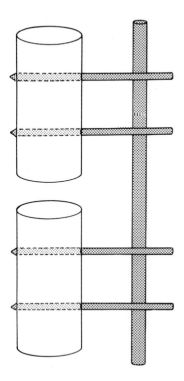

Fig. 2. Diagram of a unilateral frame.

fractures after other methods had failed (4), nonunions (4), knee fusions (2), and one ligamentous injury of the knee with soft tissue loss.

Results

Frame configurations and adjustments

The instrumentation was simple. For most frames, we limited ourselves to one longitudinal rod in an anterior or anteromedial position (Fig. 3). We managed comminuted, proximal metaphyseal fractures by inserting parallel half pins in the transverse plane from the medial or lateral side. Over two rods, these pins were then connected to two or more anterior or antero-medial half pins in the distal fragments (Fig. 4, 5, 6). Two bar half-frames were also preferred for lesions with segmental bone loss. We felt that the higher frame rigidity would reduce the incidence of pin loosening which can be a serious problem in patients who need external fixation for longer than six months.

Early in the study, the lack of universal joints occasionally prevented adequate reduction. The alignment of four of the 31 fractures was ini-tially unacceptable and had to be corrected by replacement of one or more pins. Experience and the use of an image intensifier have since largely solved this problem.

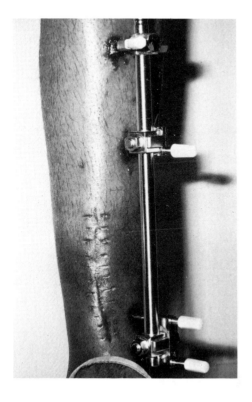

Fig. 3. Single bar unilateral frame in anteromedial position.

180

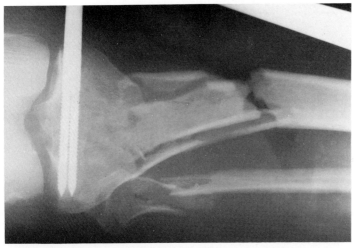

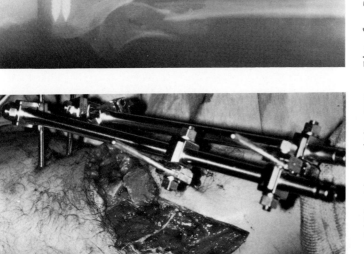

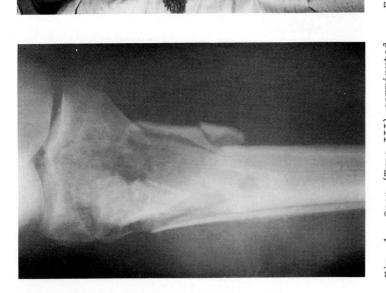

Fig. 4. Open (Type III) comminuted fracture of the tibial plateau.

Fig. 5. Immobilization with two transverse half pins proximally and two anterior half pins distally.

Fig. 6. Radiographic appearance of same injury after fixator application.

Joint motion.

Knee motion. Excluding the two knee fusions, 29 patients were assessed. The total range of motion was 125.4° on the normal, and 115.7° on the in- jured side. Using the 2-tailed T-test, the difference of 9.8° ± 26.35° was statistically not significant at the 95% level. If four patients with ipsilateral intra-articular knee injuries were omitted, the average difference in knee motion between the injured and normal leg dropped to 1.0° ± 7.8°.

Ankle motion. Considering all 31 patients, the total range of motion on the normal side was 37.0° and on the injured side 31.7°. The average difference was 5.3° ± 13.0° (p=<0.05). If four patients with permanent sciatic nerve or peroneal nerve lesions were excluded, 27 patients remain. Their average difference in ankle motion was 2.7° ± 10.0°. This again was not statistically significant (p=>0.05°).

Weight bearing

Apart from two patients, all progressed to partial weight bearing with crutches. One patient had the fixator replaced by a cast at 21 days, and the other never walked due to the sequelae of a severe head injury.

Half of the patients with open and closed fractures were changed to another method of immobilization - generally a short leg walking cast - before they were full weight bearing with the external fixator. The remainder pro- gressed to full unaided weight bearing with the fixator after an average of 56 days. All patients with nonunions or knee fusions were fully weight bearing with the external fixator after less than one month (Table I).

Table I. Weight bearing with unilateral frames

	Partial Weight Bearing		Full Weight Bearing	
	Range	Median	Range	Median
Open and closed fractures	6-98 d	40 d	15-104 d	56 d
Nonunions, knee fusions	2-12 d	7 d	11- 16 d	27 d

Complications

Compared with other series, the rate of complications was low. One patient with an infected ring sequestrum developed a local boil two months after removal of the fixator. Drainage stopped permanently after overdrilling of the pin tract (Table II).

Table II. Complications in 31 fixator applications

Complication	Number	Management
Cellulitis	3	systemic antibiotics (2) fixator removed (1)

Local allergies
    Bethadine
    Nitrofurazone
	2	discontinued drug (1)
		discontinued drug (1)

Pin infections (133 pins)	4	local skin care (3) pin replaced (1)
Draining ring sequestrum (late)	1	overdrilling (1)

Discussion

This preliminary study shows that unilateral external fixation, using rigid pins and connecting rods, can provide appropriate immobilization for a wide variety of lower extremity lesions. Compared with bilateral frame designs, several advantages were obvious.

Versatility. After an initial period of accommodation, the lack of universal joints became unimportant. The ability to insert pins independently and in different directions facilitated the construction of nonstandard frames which were optimally tailored to the clinical and mechanical demands of various injury patterns.

Wound access. No difficulties were encountered during the initial debridements and secondary soft tissue and bone procedures.

Strength. The stiffness of the principal fixator components and the absence of medial bars and pins allowed early partial or full weight bearing whenever this was desirable.

Joint motion. Full ranges of motion in knee and ankle joints were preserved in most patients who were not suffering from concomitant major nerve or intra-articular lesions.

Complications. The rate of complications was lower than that reported in most comparable series.

References

1. Adrey, J.: Le Fixateur Externe d'Hoffmann Couplé en Cadre. Editions Gead, Paris, 1970.

2. Burny, F.: Complications liées a l'utilisation de l'ostéotaxis. Acta Orthop. Belg., 41, 103, 1975.

3. McCoy, M.T., Briggs, B.T., and Chao, E.Y.: A comparative study of external skeletal fixators based on bone fracture stiffness. Orthop. Res. Soc. Trans., 5, 173, 1980.

4. Raimbeau, G., Chevalier, J.M., and Raguin, J.: Les risques vasculaires du fixateur en cadre à la jambe. Rev. Chir. Orthop. Suppl. II 65, 77, 1979.

5. Vidal, J., Buscayret, C.H., Connes, H., Paran, M., and Allieu, Y.: Traitement des fractures ouvertes de jambe par le fixateur externe en double cadre. Rev. Chir. Orthop., 62, 433, 1976.

External Fixation About the Foot and Ankle

Ch. C. Edwards

External fixation can provide a versatile and highly satisfactory means for
stabilizing the foot and ankle. The Hoffmann External Fixation System, in
particular, can be used to fix any segment or the entire foot-ankle unit.
During the past four years, we have used Hoffmann External Fixation about
the foot and ankle at the University of Maryland Hospital with generally
favorable results and few complications. In this paper, we will discuss
our management plan for major injuries, the technical principles of external
fixation, the basic frame configurations, and postoperative care, all relative to the foot and ankle.

Management of Major Injuries about the Foot and Ankle

Special anatomic features of the foot-ankle unit must be considered in
selecting the appropriate method of fixation. The foot-ankle unit is composed of multiple small bones of various shapes. They have many complex
articulations which provide the foot with flexibility and motion in all
planes. Accordingly, the foot is subject to a great variety of injuries,
making restoration of the normal anatomy difficult. Even the optimum position for aligning a disrupted foot may not be apparent initially. Thus, an
ideal fixation system for the foot must be sufficiently versatile to address
this wide range of injury patterns and must provide both intraoperative and
postoperative adjustability.

The precarious nature of foot soft tissues must also be considered in selecting a fixation system. Indeed, during the first week after injury the preservation of the foot is frequently dependent on the condition and care of
these tissues. The skin overlying the Achilles tendon and posterior calcaneus in particular has fragile vascularity. It is in a watershed area
between the posterior tibial and peroneal arterial trees and has little
subcutaneous padding; thus, the small vessels posterior to the calcaneus
are easily occluded and the skin is subject to quick breakdown from external pressure. Moreover, since the arterial supply and venous outflow of the
foot must pass through the leg, associated tibial injuries further compromise foot vascularity. For these reasons, frequent unobstructed observation
of the entire foot, the avoidance of any pressures against the skin, and
initial elevation are important factors in managing major foot trauma.

Alternatives for foot and ankle fixation

Cast fixation. Casting is a satisfactory method of fixation for most closed fractures with minimal comminuted and/or soft tissue injury. On the other hand, poor results have been obtained with plaster fixation for major open foot injuries (Omer and Pomerantz, 1972). An occlusive cast can contribute to an unrecognized compartment syndrome or pressure sores. A windowed cast does not provide sufficient access for necessary serial wound debridements. Moreover, the foot has a propensity to sweat and to retain bacteria under nails, between toes, and within thick plantar keratin. Thus, the growth of microorganisms under a damp cast may cause infection in adjacent open wounds.

Internal fixation. Because the bones of the foot are small and irregularly shaped, metal plates are generally not applicable. Staples, on the other hand, are sometimes used to maintain midfoot position following elective arthrodeses and fractures. Staples, however, frequently fail to produce sufficient stability, and once they are in place the foot position cannot be adjusted postoperatively. Kirschner wires and lag screws have proven to be the most useful types of internal fixation about the foot and ankle. Lag screws are most useful for malleolar, talar, and calcaneal fractures. Kirschner wires are effective in forefoot and midfoot displaced fractures and closed dislocations. Kirschner wire fixation alone, however, has several disadvantages in the treatment of more severe foot injuries. First, when several foot bones or joints are disrupted, anatomic reduction may be diffi- cult to obtain; Kirschner wire fixation does not permit the needed postoper- ative adjustment. Second, Kirschner fixation may not allow for subsequent compressibility; as a result, the wires may actually serve to distract fracture fragments following resorption at the fracture sites. Third, wire fixation does not provide sufficient stability to maintain length in cases of bone loss. And, fourth, Kirschner wires do not keep the foot in a neu- tral position to prevent contracture.

Skeletal traction. Traction using a Böhler frame, and when necessary over- head traction as well, overcomes most of the objections to casts or internal fixation. Properly erected traction provides circumferential skin access- ibility, is fully adjustable, and can maintain skeletal length. On the other hand, it has three great limiting factors: First, it is difficult to keep the severely injured foot in a reduced position with traction. Second, two- plane traction is tedious and places significant time demands on nursing and physician personnel. Third, traction greatly impedes patient mobility. Many patients with severe foot trauma have associated injuries to other bones and organ systems. Maximum mobilization is important for the multiple-injury patient. These patients benefit from frequent change of position to facili- tate their pulmonary management. They also must be easily transportable for diagnostic testing, serial wound debridements, and other surgical procedures.

External fixation. Although external fixation is unnecessary for simple fractures and dislocations, it fulfills all of the requirements discussed above when applied to the management of severe foot injuries. Hoffmann external fixation is sufficiently versatile to stabilize almost any injury involving the foot, ankle and/or leg. Pin groups can be placed in the metatarsals, midfoot tarsal bones, calcaneus, talus, or distal tibia. The number of these pin groups can be varied according to the degree of stability

required. Large 4 mm diameter pins can be used for the distal tibia and
calcaneus whereas smaller 3 mm pins can be used in the forefoot. Half pins
are preferable for most situations; however, transfixion pins can be used
when maximum stability is desired.

Hoffmann external fixation permits intraoperative and subsequent three-plane
adjustment. The pin clamps are attached to universal joints connected by
adjustable rods. Accordingly, if a postoperative radiograph demonstrates
unacceptable foot posture or fracture reduction, foot alignment can be easily
adjusted postoperatively. Usually, this can be accomplished in the patient's
bed without anesthesia.

External fixation of the foot provides good soft tissue access and leg
mobility. This facilitates regular inspection of skin vascularity and wound
condition, and permits repeated measurement of foot compartment pressures.
During subsequent wound debridements, skin grafting and reconstructive procedures, one side of a bilateral frame can be removed for unobstructed
access while the opposite side of the frame maintains fracture alignment.

Indications for Hoffmann external fixation

External fixation provides a useful method of fixation for many traumatic,
infectious and degenerative conditions affecting the foot and ankle. Based
on the rationale presented above and our recent clinical study of foot and
ankle external fixation at the University of Maryland (Kenzora et al, 1981),
we feel that external fixation is indicated:

- to stabilize major open fracture dislocations of the foot and ankle,

- to maintain length when bone is extensively comminuted or has been
  lost from injury or debridement,

- to prevent contracture following extensive leg or foot muscle loss
  from injury or ischemia,

- to control joint position for ankle or foot arthrodeses, and

- to provide stability with unobstructed access for soft tissue reconstruction following skin avulsion or traumatic amputation.

Treatment plan for massive trauma or extensive debridement of infection

Initial treatment includes extensive debridement, irrigation, antibiotics,
and external fixation. For extensive injuries to bone and soft tissue, a
rigid frame should be considered since fracture stabilization provides the
best milieu for soft tissue healing. In addition, the fixator provides an
ideal point of attachment for elevation of the injured foot and leg. The
suspended frame promotes venous drainage and permits circumferential observation of the soft tissues during the early critical days following injury.

During the early phase of treatment, the status of the soft tissues should
be checked regularly. Crushing of the soft tissues about the foot and more
proximal vascular injuries generally cause edema during the first few days
following injury. Accumulated edema can cause local ischemia within the

foot leading to compartment syndromes and necrosis of toes and skin flaps. If compartment syndromes are diagnosed on the basis of clinical changes or pressure measurements, fasciotomies should be performed promptly (Omer and Pomerantz, 1972). After several days, the patient with large open foot wounds should generally be taken back to the operating room for one or more repeat wound debridements. Open wounds should not be closed primarily but packed open. Contracture of skin flaps can be prevented by placing retention sutures in the flaps and tying them very loosely over gauze packed into the wound.

Despite fasciotomies, when necessary, open wound treatment, and serial debridement, proximal and local vascular compromise has led to areas of distal necrosis in 15% of our patients with severe foot and ankle region injuries. As soon as necrotic areas begin to demarcate, it is best to proceed with amputation at the lowest adjacent level compatible with acceptable foot function. In some cases, it may be necessary to adjust the distal pin group from the metatarsal to the midtarsal bones. As the injured foot recovers, it is often possible to successfully cover the end of the foot amputation stump with skin grafts or local flaps.

Within the early treatment period, most Hoffmann frame configurations permit adequate radiographic views of the foot bones. Good radiographs might indicate displaced or comminuted articular fragments. For large displaced fragments, open reduction and wire fixation might be attempted when the wounds are clean to restore articular congruity; in such cases the external fixator remains useful as a neutralization device. When subchondral plate comminution is severe, delayed primary joint fusion following soft tissue wound healing can save the patient several months of convalescence.

The first step in the reconstructive phase is to achieve skin coverage. This can usually be accomplished by delayed primary closure or with skin grafts over granulating wounds (Omer and Pomerantz, 1972). In patients with focal bone and soft tissue loss as well, we have had success with the Papineau open cancellous grafting technique. After granulation tissue covers the cancellous bone, a split thickness skin graft can be applied (Kenzora et al, 1981). More extensive grafting procedures are most successful when performed following good skin coverage.

During the consolidation phase of bone healing, less rigid fixation and increased joint motion may be desirable. If a bilateral frame was used initially, it can be converted to a single frame to produce less rigid fixation which will transfer greater load to the healing bone. When the covering soft tissues are mature, and when the injured bone has regained sufficient intrinsic stability, we generally remove the fixator and treat the injured foot in a cast. Casts should be used with great care, however, if at all, when significant portions of the foot have been covered with split thickness skin or when the injured foot has diminished sensation.

Once soft tissues have recovered and bone union is underway, we generally permit partial weight bearing ambulation with the device in place. Other authors feel that full weight bearing ambulation offers sufficient advantage to justify the addition of extra pins and more extensive frames than we

generally use (Mears, 1979). The degree of weight bearing must be highly
individualized for each case. The extent of local injuries, associated
injuries, and the patient's gait control all must be considered. For example, early partial weight bearing following ankle arthrodesis fixed with
a tibiotalar frame is probably advantageous. On the other hand, full weight
bearing ambulation in a light, flexible frame following extensive comminution or bone loss might cause collapse, nonunion, and pin loosening.

Technical Principles for External Fixation about the Foot and Ankle

Pin selection

In general, threaded, Bonnel-type pins provide the most reliable fixation.
The pins are available in two diameters. The 3 mm (C-series) pins are preferred in the forefoot and in pediatric cases. The larger 4 mm (B-series)
pins are recommended in the tibia and hindfoot of adult patients; these
pins may also be used to fix the first metatarsal in adults.

Either half pins or transfixion pins can be selected. The half pins are
designed to enter the bone from one side and penetrate several millimeters
beyond the opposite cortex. We generally prefer to use half pins about the
foot and ankle. When minimal weight bearing in the fixator is allowed,
there is much less muscle force acting on the pins in the foot-ankle region
than on pins placed in the tibia or femur. Hence, the strength imparted by
transfixion pins and double frame is generally not required. Transfixion
pins penetrate skin on either side of the bone. When placed across the
metatarsals, transfixion pins occasionally impinge on or injure the digital
neurovascular structures. In both the metatarsal and distal tibial locations, transfixion pins are prone to impale extensor tendons causing them
to scar in position and create an unwanted tenodesis. When half pins are
placed on the medial side of the tibia, calcaneus or first metatarsal, they
do not pass through neural or tendinous tissues and thus provide a more
innocuous form of fixation.

Pin placement

External fixation pins should be inserted after fracture reduction with the
foot in a neutral position. The pins should pass through an incision in
normal skin whenever possible. Since fixation in the foot can usually be
obtained from a variety of pin placement sites and from either medial or
lateral directions, an area of normal skin can usually be identified for the
pins. The standard points of insertion for foot-ankle fixation include the
proximal first phalanx, head or base of the first and second metatarsals,
midtarsal bones, calcaneus, talus, and distal tibia. Two parallel pins are
usually satisfactory for the metatarsal or midfoot locations. Three pins
are preferable for calcaneal, talar, or tibial fixation. When full weight
bearing is anticipated, additional pins are needed as detailed by Mears
(Mears, 1979 in Brooker and Edwards). As in other areas of the body, it is
important to make a sufficient skin incision before placing the Bonnel pins
to prevent injury and tenting of the surrounding skin. In cortical bone,

the pin site should be predrilled to lessen the chance of thermal necrosis
and subsequent pin loosening.

Pin group placement

In planning pin group placement sites, it is necessary to provide sufficient
pin groupings to rest the injured soft tissues, maintain length, and stabilize bone and joint reductions. On the other hand, no more groups than necessary to achieve these goals should be used to preserve micromotion for
nourishment of the articular cartilage of the foot joints (Edwards and
Chrisman, 1979), to minimize the number of pin tracts and the chances of
tissue impalement. It is also important to keep the number of rigidly immobilized joints at a minimum. To accomplish this, the pin groups should be
placed as close to the injured segment as possible, taking care not to span
more adjacent normal joints than necessary. For example, when treating an
ankle condition, consider tibiotalar fixation; for a comminuted talus, consider tibiocalcaneal fixation; for open disruption of the Lisfranc's joint,
consider metatarso-midtalar bone fixation. Saving uninjured joints from prolonged rigid immobilization may lessen residual stiffness and perhaps the
chance of late degenerative arthritis.

Frame configuration

The first step in designing a frame configuration is to decide whether to
use a single, double, or quadrilateral frame. A single frame with one rod
or adjustable rod between pin groups is satisfactory to stabilize the forefoot. A unilateral double frame can be constructed with adjustable rods
placed dorsal and plantar to the half pin groupings. A double frame is
recommended for fixation of unstable midfoot injuries and reconstructions.
A quadrilateral (bilateral double) frame consists of anterior and posterior
adjustable rods connecting two or more pin groups both medially and laterally. Quadrilateral frames are necessary in the foot-ankle region only when
there has been extensive disruption, comminution, or bone loss affecting the
distal tibia or hindfoot. In these very unstable injuries, transfixion pins
are generally used to provide maximum rigidity. Rigid fixation with transfixion pins in a quadrilateral frame is also desirable for ankle or subtalar
arthrodeses. It is often helpful to combine different frame configurations
to serve different purposes in the same extremity. For example, massive
ankle injury with bone loss might be treated with transfixion pins and a
quadrilateral tibial frame combined with a single frame extension to a half-
pin grouping in the first metatarsal to maintain normal foot posture.

It is always important to support the forefoot in a neutral position following foot trauma or major foot surgery. Severe injuries affecting the tibia
often damage the anterior compartment muscles that are responsible for foot
dorsiflexion. Relative ischemia following trauma may also impair their
action. Even without injury, there may be reflex inhibition of the dorsiflexors due to pain about the foot and ankle. As a result, the patients
generally hold their injured foot in a plantarflexed position which quickly
develops into a fixed equinus contracture. For these reasons, we agree with
Omer (Omer and Pomerantz, 1972) that it is essential to splint or fix an in-

jured foot in a neutral position promptly after surgery or injury. If return of active, painless dorsiflexion is anticipated within a couple of weeks, a splint made from orthoplast or any moldable plastic and attached to the fixator with adjustable elastic support straps is recommended. If active dorsiflexion is likely to be permanently impaired or greatly prolonged due to anterior compartment injury or extensive foot trauma, we have found it highly desirable to hold the forefoot in a neutral position using external fixation half pins in the base of the first metatarsal attached to a more proximal portion of the Hoffmann frame. Since single rod fixation between the half pins and the more proximal frame provides relative and not rigid fixation of the intervening joints, we have observed little subsequent difficulty with unwanted stiffness or painful arthritis.

Basic Frame Configurations

Tibiometatarsal frame (Fig. 1)

The tibiometatarsal frame is constructed by first placing pin groups in the base of the metatarsals and distal tibia. Half pin fixation is preferred for the metatarsal grouping. In most cases, two parallel half pins are placed in the base of the first metatarsal. A thread length is selected to anchor the pin to both the first and second metatarsal for better fixation. The proximal pin group consists of three parallel pins placed into the medial side of the distal tibia. Pin clamps are placed over the two pin groupings. These can be connected with either one or two adjustable rods. When more rigid fixation is needed, a second set of half pins can be placed in the base of the fifth metatarsal as well and transfixion rather than half pins can be used in the distal tibia. This permits attachment of both medial and lateral adjustable rods (Edwards, 1979; 1980).

The tibiometatarsal frame achieves stability of the intervening joints by means of a biologic tension-band phenomenon. With the foot held in a neutral position, the plantar fascia and Achilles tendon become tight. As the forefoot is moved into slight dorsiflexion, these structures serve as a tension band to neutralize tensile forces across the posterior and plantar aspect of the foot-ankle unit to balance the compressive forces over the dorsal aspect resulting from passive dorsiflexion. With balanced forces across both the anterior and posterior aspect of the foot-ankle unit, the intervening bones and ligaments are held in a relatively stable position.

There are three main indications for tibiometatarsal fixation:

1) *Anterior and/or lateral tibial compartment muscle loss*. This is often associated with open tibial fractures and massive foot trauma. Tibiometatarsal fixation is used to hold the foot in a neutral position to prevent equinus and cavus contractures. In case of a complete destruction of the anterior compartment muscles, tibiometatarsal fixation permits autotenodesis of the extensor tendons in a functional position. Our recent study of 33 massively traumatized feet treated with external fixation demonstrates that patients with a functional extensor tenodesis usually regain a satisfactory and painless gait (Kenzora et al, 1981). In patients with open

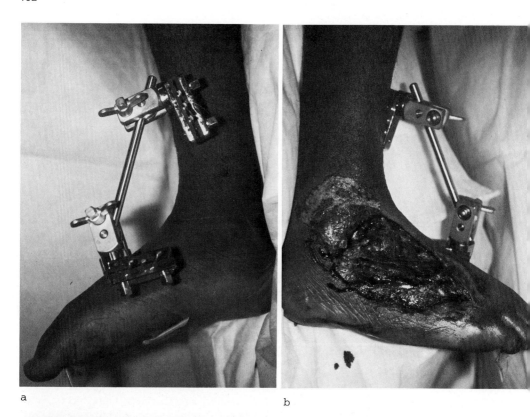

a   b

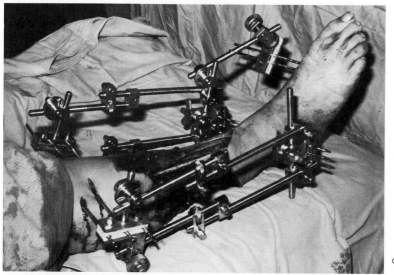

c

Fig. 1. Tibiometatarsal frame. a) and b) Simple unilateral M-T frame to stabilize lateral foot ligamentous disruption and provide access for skin coverage. c) Metatarsal extension from standard quadrilateral tibial frame to hold foot in a neutral position following traumatic disruption of anterior compartment muscles.

tibial injuries who already have a tibial frame in place, the metatarsal pin group can simply be attached to the distal end of the tibial Hoffmann frame.

2) *Stable fracture dislocations with overlying soft tissue injury.* Many ankle, subtalar or midfoot open fracture dislocations with large wounds are quite stable following reduction if the foot is held in dorsiflexion. These are ideal indications for tibiometatarsal fixation. This technique provides good access for treatment of the open wound and saves the foot from excessively rigid fixation.

3) *Extensive soft tissue loss.* Degloving injuries, heel pad avulsions, and other major soft tissue injuries can be optimally managed in a simple tibiometatarsal frame. This frame provides sufficient stability to rest the injured soft tissues and excellent access for coverage procedures.

The principal advantages of tibiometatarsal fixation are:

- excellent access to the hindfoot and midfoot for wound debridements and skin grafting - no part of the frame is in the way of the surgical procedures;
- the foot can be easily suspended from an overhead frame by attaching ropes to the anterior adjustable rods connecting the tibial and metatarsal pin groups;
- tibiometatarsal fixation provides relative stability for the foot-ankle unit with only five pins;
- since the many joints between the tibia and metatarsals remain nonfixed, a certain amount of motion is possible in each of these joints. This micromotion appears sufficient for articular cartilage nourishment, lessening the chance of late arthritic change and foot stiffness.

On the other hand, tibiometatarsal fixation is limited to injuries that are basically stable following reduction and can only be used in patients whose plantar fascia and Achilles tendon are intact. Since fixation is obtained via the biologic tension-band principle, disruption of the posterior band (plantar fascia and Achilles tendon) would jeopardize the stability of the system. Likewise, disruption of the rigid anterior bony column from either bone loss or comminution would jeopardize stability in dorsiflexion as well.

The triangular frame (Fig. 2)

The triangular frame has three points of attachment to the skeleton: a longitudinally directed pin group in the distal tibia and horizontally directed pin groups in the calcaneus and metatarsals. The calcaneal and metatarsal pin groups are connected by a simple rod. Two adjustable rods connect the tibial pin group with the rod attached to both lower pin groups to construct a unilateral triangular frame. When transfixion pins are used or double sets of half pins for the metatarsals, both medial and lateral adjustable rods are used to create a bilateral triangular frame (Connes, 1977; Edwards and Browner, 1981; Mears, 1979, in Brooker and Edwards). The bilateral triangular frame is sufficiently stable to maintain length and bony relationships for any injury involving the foot-ankle unit. Biomechanically, it should be used, when possible, to maintain bony position by traction rather than compression across all the joints of the foot. Ligaments and soft tissues around the bones are then placed under mild stretch and

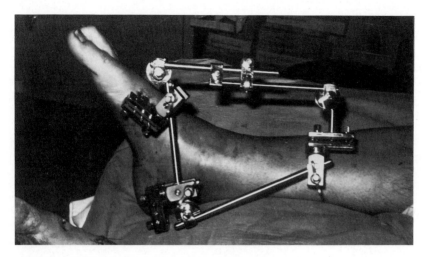

Fig. 2. Unilateral triangular frame with half pin groups in the tibia, calcaneus and metatarsals.

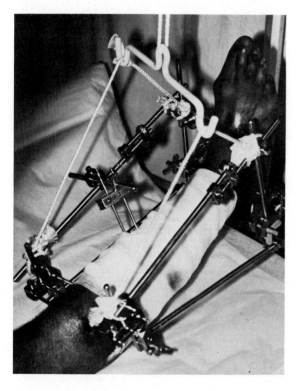

Fig. 3. Bilateral triangular frame with additional half pin group attached to adjustable rod to stabilize a segmental fragment.

hold the enveloped bones in reasonably normal position. This principle has been named "ligamentotaxis" (Vidal et al, 1979).

The triangular frame is indicated when there is:

Disruption of the plantar fascia or Achilles tendon. In such cases, the simple tibiometatarsal frame will generally not provide sufficient stability.

Comminution or loss of bone stock. Bone may be lost from trauma or from extensive debridement in the treatment of osteomyelitis.

Unstable intercollated bone segments. In severe injuries, one or more bones between the tibia and metatarsals may remain unstable or out of position following reduction of the foot to a normal posture. In such cases, a bilateral triangular frame can first be applied. A half pin group is then inserted into the unstable segment. This pin group is connected to the adjustable rods of the triangular frame to create stable fixation for the entire injured complex (Fig. 3) (Edwards and Browner, 1981).

The triangular frame produces more stability for severe foot-ankle disruptions than other frame configurations presented in this paper. It accomplishes stable reductions without the need to place metal in the open fracture wounds. The frame serves as an inboard traction system and, accordingly, helps maintain reduction of comminuted and intra-articular fractures via the ligamentotaxis principle. In addition to its intrinsic stability, the triangular frame still permits soft tissue treatment and reconstructive procedures. One side of the frame can be removed for better access while the opposite side of the frame maintains fracture reduction.

The main disadvantage of the bilateral triangular frame is that it is rigid enough to produce noticeable stiffness in the foot following prolonged use. Likewise, particularly if some of the foot joints are inadvertently held under some compression, interference with cartilage nutrition and late arthritis remain a possibility. For these reasons, lesser injuries should be treated, when possible, with more limited frames.

The tibiotalar frame (Fig. 4)

The tibiotalar frame was presented at the Seventh International Conference on Hoffmann External Fixation (Edwards, 1979). It consists of a longitudinal grouping of transfixion pins in the distal tibia and a horizontal grouping of two or three pins in the talus. The distal pin clamp is attached to a plain horizontal rod. Four adjustable rods are then connected to the proximal and distal pin clamp rods using couplings (Green, 1980).

The tibiotalar frame functions as a rigid fixation device for the ankle joint, permitting effective compression across the joint with the four adjustable rods. Because the quadrilateral frame is fully adjustable, precise control of the talar position relative to the tibia is possible. The tibiotalar frame is indicated for elective ankle fusions and, occasionally, in the initial fracture treatment when ankle articular trauma is great enough that delayed primary fusion is considered.

The advantages of tibiotalar fixation include the high degree of ankle joint control and the relatively small number of fixation pins (4-6) required. Most important, tibiotalar external fixation spares the subtalar joint. Theoretically, this is very important in the case of arthrodeses where compression is applied. Sustained compression across articular cartilage is known to cause cartilage necrosis and subsequent arthritis (Crelin and Southwick, 1960; Edwards and Chrisman, 1979). Moreover, following an ankle

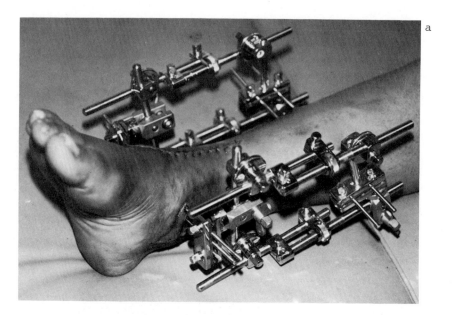

a

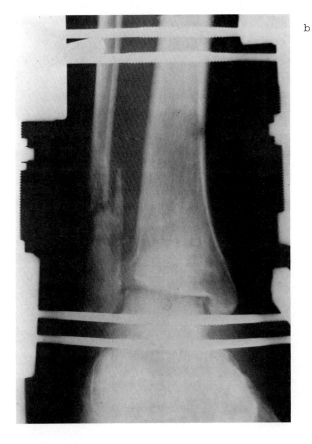

b

Fig. 4. a) and b) Tibiotalar frame used primarily for ankle arthrodesis.

fusion, normal gait depends on the development of an increased range of motion in the subtalar and midfoot joints. The inevitable stiffness that follows compression arthrodesis across the subtalar joint must limit the ultimate clinical result to some extent. On the other hand, the advantage of sparing the subtalar joint should not be overemphasized at this time since other investigators have not recorded significant problems in using tibiocalcaneal fixation for ankle arthrodeses (Mears, 1979).

The main limitation of tibiotalar fixation is the difficulty of inserting the distal pins through the talus. Because of the proximity of the posterior tibial artery to the medial surface of the talus and the small size of this bone, it is risky to attempt talar pin fixation blindly. External pin fixation of the talus is not difficult using image intensification control or when placing the pins during an arthrodesis procedure. Placement of talar pins is simplified by removal of the distal 1 cm of both malleoli. Especially good visualization of the talus is obtained in the transfibular approach to the ankle joint. Satisfactory visualization for pin placement is also possible with the standard anterior approach (Edwards, 1979).

The tibiocalcaneal frame (Fig. 5)

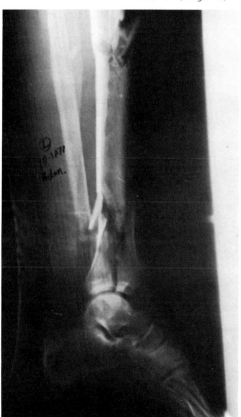
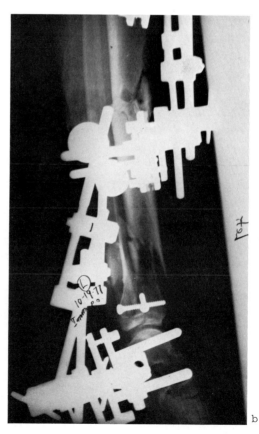

a

b

Fig. 5. a) and b) Treatment of a comminuted, segmental, intra-articular fracture using a calcaneal extension from a tibial frame for ligamentotaxis and lag screws to reduce the intra-articular fractures.

The tibiocalcaneal frame is constructed in the same manner as the tibiotalar frame except that the distal horizontal pin group is placed in the calcaneus and three or more pins are used for each of the two pin group sites (Mears, 1979). Like the triangular frame, the tibiocalcaneal frame is used in distraction to provide "inboard" traction for unstable hindfoot and subtalar injuries. It is indicated for highly comminuted fractures involving the talus or distal tibia. It is also indicated for extensive tissue loss about the ankle requiring long-term treatment for bone or soft tissue grafting procedures.

The tibiocalcaneal frame spares unnecessary mid- and forefoot fixation in patients who have good foot posture control. When additional calcaneal and tibial pins are used, partial weight bearing ambulation in adults and full weight bearing in children is possible (Mears, 1979). Tibiocalcaneal fixation often cannot be used in cases of associated calcaneal comminution. Its principal limitation is in patients who do not have good forefoot dorsiflexors. Weak dorsiflexors may be due to pain inhibition or anterolateral tibial compartment injury. To reiterate an important point, when good active control of forefoot dorsiflexors is absent, equinus contracture quickly develops if the foot is not adequately splinted or fixed in a neutral position.

The unilateral foot frame (Fig. 6)

Due to the smaller size of the forefoot and midfoot bones and the lesser forces acting upon them, 3 mm half pins are usually sufficient fixation. The foot frame consists of a half pin grouping into the distal end of the affected metatarsals or proximal phalanx and a proximal pin group into either the base of the metatarsals or midtarsal bones. Two C-series adjustable rods can then be attached to the pin clamps to stabilize the position of the fore-

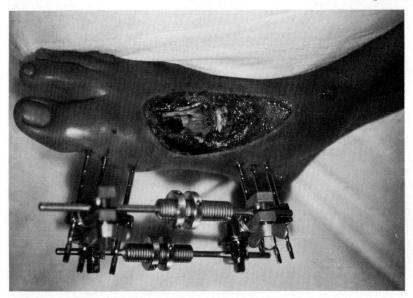

Fig. 6. Unilateral foot frame using smaller external fixation components to maintain length following shotgun obliteration of the first metatarsal shaft.

foot bones (Kenzora et al, 1981). Foot frame advantages include versatile fixation, continuous adjustability, and good wound access. This frame configuration does not fix hindfoot joints and is, in our experience, well tolerated by patients.

The forefoot frame is indicated for: treatment of metatarsal or midtarsal bone loss to preserve length; forefoot fracture-dislocations with major soft tissue wounds or skin loss; and articular comminution when delayed fusion of metatarsal-tarsal or midtarsal joints is anticipated. Although experience with elective midfoot arthrodeses is limited, the Hoffmann frame may provide more rigid fixation than staples, permit postoperative position adjustments, and provide better wound access than a cast.

Postoperative Care

Following construction of the external fixator, it is important to observe the skin for tenting about the skeletal pins. Areas of skin pressure discovered postoperatively should be released with a scalpel so that no skin margins are pressing against the pins, because any constant skin pressure will result in necrosis and predispose to pin tract infections.

After release of any skin tenting, pin site care can be divided into two stages. In the first stage, a tight gauze wrap is placed between the pin clamp and the skin after bleeding stops. This sterile occlusive dressing can often be left in place for some time. The second stage consists of removing major incrustations and regular cleaning with hydrogen peroxide or alcohol.

For several days following major surgery or injury to the foot, the foot and leg can be elevated by tying the fixator to an overhead frame. To keep the knee at about 90° of flexion a calf sling may be used. As discussed in detail under the management plan section of this paper, we advocate open treatment of major traumatic foot wounds. Patients with severe open wounds should generally be returned to the operating room several days after injury for at least one subsequent debridement. When the wound base is clean and viable, secondary closure and/or split thickness skin grafting should be performed.

After the soft tissues recover, early partial weight bearing helps prevent stiffness in the unfixed portions of the foot and promotes more normal local physiologic processes. In general, we do not advocate full weight bearing ambulation. After removal of the external fixator, the pin sites can be cleaned with alcohol and covered with a sterile dressing. Patients are advised to soak their feet in salt water twice daily until skin coverage of the pin sites occurs.

Results

Based on our experience using foot-ankle Hoffmann external fixation in the treatment of over 50 traumatized feet, we find this technique of great value in managing fracture dislocations with major open wounds, bone loss, or comminution. External fixation helps prevent traction deformities, stabilizes injured soft tissues, and facilitates subsequent reconstruction. It achieves good control and rigidity for fusions about the foot and ankle as well. On the other hand, external fixation is not necessary for the majority of closed injuries to the foot. For less severe injuries, we advocate conventional casting for simple fracture dislocations, use of lag screws for major fragment fixation of hindfoot and ankle, and Kirschner wires for such unstable forefoot disruptions as the Lisfranc dislocation.

Our recent study of 33 cases of major foot trauma suggested that external fixation made possible the salvage of many feet which would otherwise have been lost using other conventional methods. The external fixation technique facilitated close observation of the injured soft tissues, elevation, serial wound debridements and subsequent soft tissue reconstructive procedures. Of the 33 cases studied, 85% of the severely injured feet treated with external fixation achieved normal position and painless ambulation; however, some degree of stiffness and cosmetic deformity was present in all cases. Even when the entire foot could not be salvaged, the management plan discussed above permitted a lower level of amputation in several cases than would have otherwise occurred. Likewise, external fixation was useful in elective arthrodeses about the foot and ankle. In all cases, excellent bone position was maintained.

Complications using the external fixation frames as described above have been few. Pin tract drainage developed in only 11% of our patients. In only one patient was any procedure other than removal of the draining pin necessary. This one patient had a curettage to remove a ring sequestrum. In fact, pin tract problems were much less common about the foot and ankle in our experience than with the tibia, femur, or pelvis. This is probably because there is very little compressible soft tissue between the skin and bone about the foot and ankle. The incidence of pin tract drainage appears to correlate with thickness and mobility of the skin at the pin bone interface. Pin tract difficulties in our series may have also been minimized by restricting all but partial weight bearing ambulation. Impalement of extensor tendons and digital nerves occurred in several of our patients; however, none suffered functional deficits. Impalement of tendons can be eliminated when medial half pin groupings are used rather than transfixion pins.

In summary, external fixation about the foot and ankle is a simple technique to master. External fixation is sufficiently versatile to stabilize almost any injury complex about the foot and ankle. Following major trauma or surgery, most major complications can be prevented or minimized with the continuous observation of soft tissues made possible by the application of external fixation to this region. We have found the external frames described above sufficiently adjustable to maintain good bony position and stability as well as functional foot posture regardless of the magnitude of the injury. Consequently, even when massive soft tissue injury and muscle loss have occurred, autotenodesis leaves the foot in a functional position, usually permitting painless ambulation.

If pin placement and frame configuration is planned with care, the complications of external fixation about the foot and ankle are possibly fewer than at any other anatomic site. If, nevertheless, external fixation cannot be continued, it does not preclude other subsequent treatment modalities.

Finally, it is important to emphasize that external fixation for foot-ankle injuries or reconstructions is but one stage of the reconstructive program. In certain cases, internal fixation techniques may be indicated in addition to external fixation. In others, after soft tissue healing, the fixator can be removed and adequate stabilization accomplished with casts or orthoses.

References

1. Connes, H.: Hoffmann's External Anchorage Techniques, Indications and Results. Edition Gead, 4th Ed. 1977, pp 164.

2. Crelin, E.S., and Southwick, W.O.: Mitosis of chondrocytes induced in the knee joint articular cartilage in rabbits. Yale J. Biol. Med. $\underline{33}$, 243, 1960.

3. Edwards, C.C.: New directions in Hoffmann external fixation: The Maryland experience with major trauma. Proc. 7th Int. Conf. on Hoffmann External Fixation. Ed., J. Vidal, S.A. Diffinco, Geneva, Switzerland 1979, pp 51-59.

4. Edwards, C.C.: Management of multisegment injuries in the polytrauma patient. In, Advances in External Fixation. Ed., R.M. Johnston, Symposium Specialists, Inc., Chicago, 1980. pp 43-60

5. Edwards, C.C. and Browner, B.D.: The Application of Hoffmann External Fixation. Zimmer USA, Inc., Warsaw, 1981. p 28.

6. Edwards, C.C. and Chrisman, D.D.: Articular cartilage. In, The Scientific Basis of Orthopaedics. Eds. J.A. Albright and R.A. Brand, Appleton-Century-Crafts, New York, 1979, pp 313-347.

7. Green, S.A.: Arthrodesis. In, Advances in External Fixation. Ed., R.M. Johnston, Symposium Specialists, Inc., Chicago, 1980, pp 134-154.

8. Kenzora, J.E., Edwards, C.C., Browner, B.D., Gamble, J.G., and DeSilva, J.B.: Management of acute major trauma involving the foot and ankle with Hoffmann external fixation. Foot and Ankle, 1981. In press.

9. Mears, D.C.: Percutaneous pin fixation. In, Materials and Orthopaedic Surgery. Ed., D.C. Mears. Williams and Wilkins Co., Baltimore, 1979. pp 404-479.

10. Mears, D.C.: The use of external fixation in arthrodesis. In, External Fixation: The Current State of the Art. Eds., A.F. Brooker and C.C. Edwards. The Williams and Wilkins Co., Baltimore, 1979, pp 241-275.

11. Omer, G.E., and Pomerantz, G.M.: Initial management of severe open injuries and traumatic amputations of the foot. Arch. Surg., $\underline{105}$, 696, 1972.

12. Vidal, J., Buscayret, C., and Connes, H.: Treatment of articular fractures by "ligamentotaxis" with external fixation. In, External Fixation, The Current State of the Art. Eds., A.F. Brooker and C.C. Edwards. Williams and Wilkins Co., Baltimore, 1979, pp 75-82.

Anatomic Considerations in the Placement of Percutaneous Pins

A. Giachino

There is no region of the femur which innocuously accepts percutaneous pin fixation. Transfixation of soft tissues has predictable complications. Obviously, any structure present in the thigh can be transfixed, resulting in total or partial loss of function. Damage to a major nerve or vessel must be avoided at all costs. Avoidance of joint cavity invasion assumes secondary importance, followed by considerations of muscle belly transfixation and nursing care.

Nerves

The femoral nerve branches into a cauda equina anterior to the hip joint and lateral to the femoral artery, and thus is partially protected by its division into smaller parts. Additional protection to the distal medial branches results from their relationship to the femoral artery in the adductor canal and the avoidance of this area when inserting pins.

The sciatic nerve enters the thigh posteromedial to the head of the femur and runs most of its course posterior to the shaft of the femur. Pins entering the femur posterior, or those exiting posterior, create such difficult nursing care problems that this area is never considered in clinical practice.

Vessels

The superficial femoral artery travels with its accompanying veins through the femoral triangle and adductor canal on the medial aspect of the thigh.

The exact relationship of the artery to bone, in the coronal plane, was sought in 20 cadaveric limbs. With the patella facing anterior, the adductor canal was dissected and the points where the artery lay midway between, and definitely posterior, to the anterior and posterior cortices were recorded. The proximal pole of the patella and the anterosuperior iliac spine (ASIS) were used as bony reference points (Fig. 1). On average, the artery was posterior to the femur 19.2% of the distance from patella to ASIS (Fig. 2), and bisected the femur at 49.2% (range 40.8% to 58.7%) (Fig. 3). In theory, therefore, any pin inserted in the coronal plane bisecting the femur, and not more proximal than 40.8% of the distance from proximal pole of patella to ASIS, should avoid contact with the femoral artery. The level of absolute safety must be taken as 12.7% (Fig. 2). This relationship of femoral artery to femur illustrates why pins in the coronal

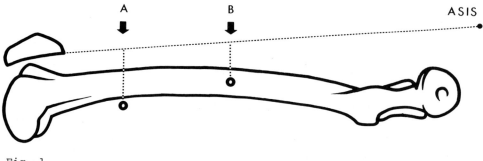

Fig. 1.

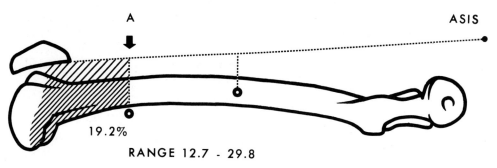

19.2%

RANGE 12.7 - 29.8

Fig. 2.

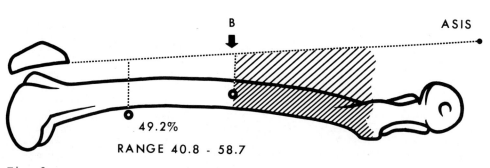

49.2%

RANGE 40.8 - 58.7

Fig. 3.

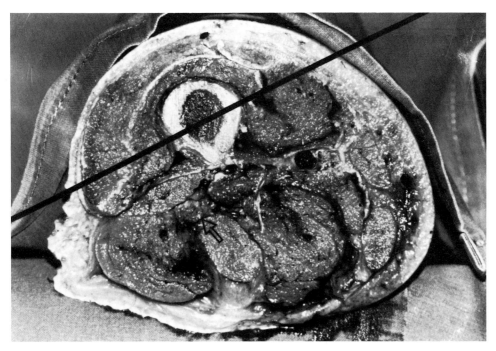

Fig. 4. Right thigh. External rotation of the plane of the pin provides increased safety. Light arrow shows sciatic nerve.

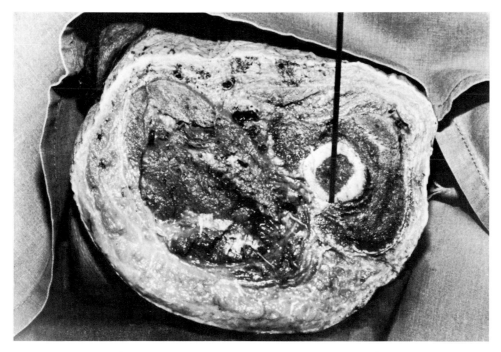

Fig. 5. Left thigh. Anterior half-pin fixation of proximal femur. Note the femoral vessels medially.

plane are less safe as one proceeds proximally. Externally rotating the
plane of the pin 30° can increase the degree of safety and yet not endanger
the sciatic nerve (Fig. 4). The alternative solution is to use half pins,
entering laterally in the area of concern, or to perform an open placement
of the pins.

Anterior and lateral half pins in the proximal diaphysis of the femur avoid
the femoral artery and sciatic nerve and do not impede nursing care (Fig. 5).

Joints

Pins in the head and neck of the femur are obviously in the hip joint.

The knee joint's domain is larger than that of the hip. The suprapatellar
pouch reaches an average of 6.3 cm proximal to the proximal pole of the
patella, or 1.3 times the length of the patella proximally (Fig. 6).

Pins entering the joint cavity may give rise to joint sepsis or adhesions
and must be avoided.

Muscles

Pins transfixing muscles limit their excursion and thus affect proximal and
distal joints. Anterior femoral pins will affect motion of the knee to a
greater extent than pins placed in the coronal plane. On an average, the
patella moves 6 cm distally when the knee flexes from 0° to 90° in an adult.
An anterodistal femoral pin must be a half pin to avoid the sciatic nerve
and femoral-popliteal vessels. It will limit knee motion and be associated
with skin inflammation, and is best used when movement of the knee is not
required (eg, knee arthrodesis).

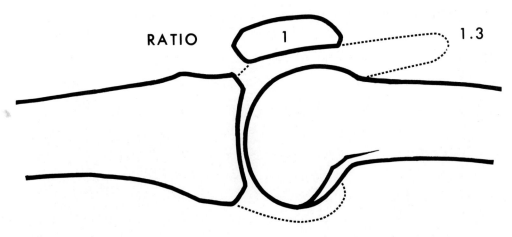

Fig. 6.

Use of the External Fixator in Thigh Fractures

K. W. Klemm

Indications

Evaluation of the advantages and disadvantages of external fixation as a
method of stabilizing fractures and nonunions - particularly in cases of
fractures and nonunions of the femur - is directly related to the general
attitude in different countries of how such conditions should be treated:
by conservative measures with traction and plaster cast, or by surgical
stabilization by means of compression plates and intramedullary rods.

Compared with conservative treatment, the external fixator achieves better
stabilization and better alignment of the fragments than does immobilization by means of traction and plaster cast. It is also more convenient
for the patients. They can move around and be discharged from hospital at
an early date.

In the past 40 years, the techniques of surgical stabilization of fractures
by means of compression plates, intramedullary rods, and other devices have
been highly perfected. There is no doubt, however, that the risk of postoperative wound infection is present in any bone surgery, particularly in
the surgical treatment of open fractures, and that such infections may
result in delayed healing and serious adverse effects. In comparison with
internal fixation of fractures, the fixateur externe generally allows good
alignment of the fragments as well as correction of the axis if required.
Furthermore, early physiotherapy after surgical stabilization of fractures
is possible, although to a somewhat limited degree because the bone pins
may hinder muscle movement.

In the case of closed fractures, external fixation has an intermediate
position between conservative and surgical treatment. In the case of open
fractures, however, particularly those in which extensive additional damage
to the soft tissues must be treated, external fixation is superior to all
other methods of treatment.

Taking these factors into consideration, the following indications are proposed for the use of external fixation:

1. Third degree open fractures, in which conservative treatment is difficult or practically impossible because of soft tissue damage or in
   which surgical stabilization cannot be attempted because of the risk
   of infection.

2. Closed fractures with soft tissue damage, as in burns (for the same
   reasons mentioned above).

3.   Closed fractures in patients in poor general condition, to avoid
     immobilization and the risk of extended surgery.

External fixation is particularly valuable in emergency situations where
a number of injured persons must be treated as soon as possible under
unsatisfactory conditions and requiring immediate transportation (war
casualties, for example). For these reasons, the fixateur externe has
become standard equipment for many military medical units since it can
be applied quickly and without risk. More important, however, is that
necessary alignments of the fragments can be effectively made later on
under better conditions. This applies particularly to the fixateur
externe of Raoul Hoffmann.

Contraindications

There are no contraindications for the use of external fixation of thigh
fractures, in general. In fractures with involvement of the adjacent
joints, however, good alignment of fragments can only be achieved by open
reduction. In addition, satisfactory stabilization of the fracture
affords bridging of the joint by the fixateur externe.

The Fixateur Externe of Raoul Hoffmann

Many external fixation systems are available. Following is a description
of the technique of application of the Hoffmann fixateur externe. This
particular system is unique for its versatility of application, allowing
simultaneous correction of the axis in all three planes, and for its
relatively uncomplicated technique.

The basic components include six different parts for the outer frame and
two different forms of bone pins for anchorage of the bone to the frame.
With these components, all required mountings for the femur are possible.

The bone pins are affixed in sets in the clamps of the universal ball joints
with or without rod. The almost unlimited radius of motion of the universal
ball joints together with the articulating couplings allow by means of the
connecting rods a rigid mounting of the pin sets in all directions. This
enables simultaneous axis alignment on three planes, which is the main
advantage of this system.

The anatomical situation of the thigh requires the use of two types of bone
pins: half pins with threading at one end for the two proximal sets of pins
and transfixing pins with central thread for the distal set. Both types of
pins are available in different total lengths and different thread lengths
(Fig. 1). All pins are self-drilling and self-tapping.

The instrumentation includes a drill brace for manual insertion of the pins,
a pin guide for parallel insertion of three or more pins on a single plane
to be connected to the clamps, and pilot grips for easier adjustment of the
fracture. These pilot grips are particularly useful if an image intensifier is used to keep the surgeon's hands out of the field of direct
radiation.

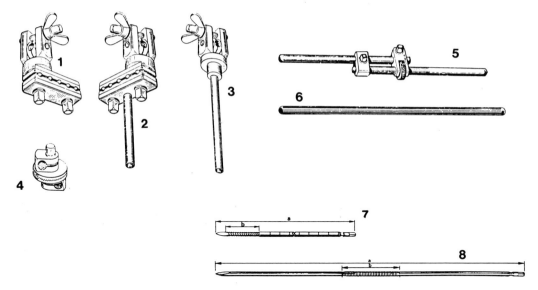

Fig. 1. Components of Hoffmann's fixateur externe. 1) Universal ball joint; 2) universal ball joint and rod; 3) reversed universal ball joint; 4) articulation coupling; 5) adjustable connecting rod; 6) connecting rod; 7) half pin threaded at one end; 8) transfixing pin with central threading.

Technique

The application of the fixateur externe can be done on a conventional operating table or on a fracture table. The use of the latter facilitates the operation since the fracture can be set and held in place before application of the frame. Under these conditions, the pins are inserted at the correct location in accordance with the underlying bone. When the fracture is set after the insertion of the bone pins, too much tension on the soft tissue usually results.

For application of the fixateur externe for the femur, the patient is placed in supine position on the fracture table. Reduction of the fracture with correction of the axis is carried out under control of the image intensifier. Open reduction is rarely necessary; if necessary, however, reduction a minima under sterile conditions should be performed.

The dihedral frame for the femur combines two sets of proximal half pins at 90° to each other and one distal set of transfixing pins.

For the insertion of the first proximal pin on the lateral side, the central axis of the femur is localized by the use of either probe pins or an image intensifier. If optimal anchoring is to be achieved, the pins must pass through both corteces.

The tip of the pin is inserted through a stab incision. Manual drilling of the pins is strongly recommended to avoid thermal necrosis of the bone. If the drilling becomes difficult, the pin tip is probably clogged with bone

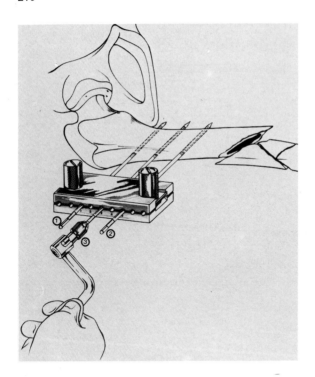

Fig. 2. Insertion of the lateral proximal set of pins with the drill brace and the pin guide.

meal. It is advisable to remove the pin, clean the tip, and reuse the hole that has already been made.

Whereas the first pin is positioned without the use of the pin guide, the subsequent two pins are positioned with the help of this instrument in order 1, 2, 3 (Fig. 2). It is always better to insert the two outer pins first, leaving the middle pin to the last, as this is the best way to assure that all the bone pins are securely anchored in the bone and that none has merely perforated the soft tissues.

The distal set of transfixing pins should be inserted before the second set of proximal half pins when good alignment of the fragments, and some stability of the frame by mounting of the first connecting rod, has already been achieved (Fig. 3). If the distal set pins with central threading are used, they are inserted in the same way.

The application of the frame follows by sliding two universal ball joints with rod on the lateral ends of the bone pins, one universal ball joint without rod on the medial ends of the distal transfixing pins, and then tightening them. By affixing one or two pilot grips, it is now possible to align the axis and to maintain the desired result by means of the first connecting rod (Fig. 4).

The second set of proximal pins is inserted at a 90° angle, paying careful attention to spacing of vertical and horizontal pins to avoid blocking inside the bone. For higher stability, the outer frame is then completed by affixing a second connecting rod over two articulation couplings (Fig. 5).

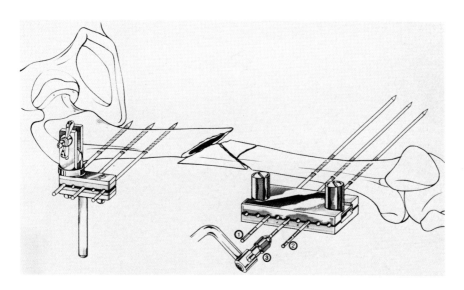

Fig. 3. Insertion of the distal set of transfixing pins with the drill brace and the pin guide

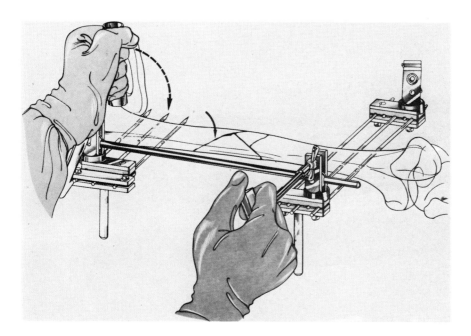

Fig. 4. Mounting of two universal ball joints with rod on the lateral sets of pins and one universal ball joint on the medial ends of the distal transfixing pins. Reduction by means of a pilot grip and application of the first connecting rod.

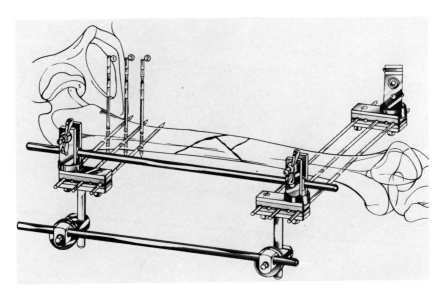

Fig. 5. Insertion of the ventral set of proximal pins; completion of the outer frame by means of a second connecting rod; and two articulation couplings.

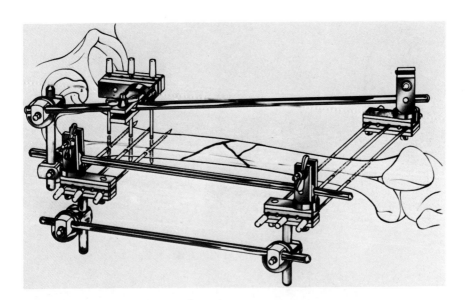

Fig. 6. Mounting of a universal ball joint on the ventral set of proximal pins; connecting this proximal set of pins with the distal set exiting medially. Note two connecting rods and two articulation couplings connecting the lateral proximal set with the ventral proximal set.

One connecting rod between the ventral proximal set of pins and the medial
distal set, and a second connecting rod between the ventral connecting rod
and the first lateral rod affixed by means of two articulation couplings,
form the inner half of the frame (Fig. 6).

In the case of comminuted fractures, only simple connecting rods are used
since compression cannot be applied. When dealing with a transverse or a
short oblique fracture, adjustable connecting rods allowing compression
are recommended. Screw No. 1 (Fig. 7) is tightened and compression then
applied by turning the knurled head screw towards the negative. Distraction is achieved by turning it towards the positive. To prevent unwanted
movement at the knurled head screw and loss of correction, screw No. 2
must be tightened.

In the operating room and within a few days after the operation, roentgenograms should be taken to control the axis. Whereas compression and distraction and minor varus and valgus deformities can be adjusted by means
of the connecting rods, adjustment of rotational deviation and gross varus
and valgus deformity can only be accomplished by loosening of the frame at
the universal ball joints and the articulation couplings. Several days
after the operation, it is possible to correct deviation of the axis at
the patient's bedside without anesthesia.

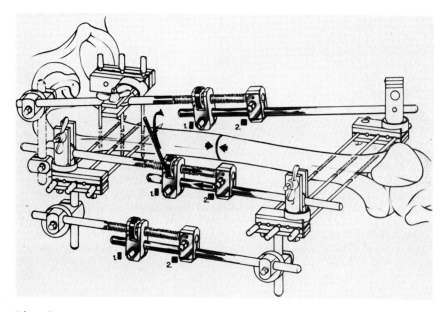

Fig. 7. Application of adjustable connecting rods for compression.

Follow-up Care

To avoid pin track infection, it is essential that skin tension at the site
of the pins be avoided. Even when adequate incisions have been made during
the operation, skin necrosis may result due to postoperative swelling. In

this case, the incision is enlarged under local anesthesia to release the tension on the skin.

The skin in the area of the bone pins must be carefully cleaned each day and any crust removed. The patient should be asked to assume responsibility for the care of the fixateur externe.

The excellent stabilization of the fracture by the fixateur externe and freedom from pain allows the patient to get out of bed after one or two days. At this time, physiotherapy can begin, although in the case of external fixation of the femur this may cause some difficulty since the distal transfixing pins can inhibit muscle movement, thus permitting only limited knee bending. The patient can return home as soon as the skin lesions have healed. It is sometimes amazing how ingenious patients are in solving the problem of dressing by use of zippers or means of enlarging pantlegs to enable them to go out and lead a normal social life.

Control roentgenograms should be taken at three to four week intervals and weight bearing allowed when the radiologic findings show sufficient bone consolidation.

According to the type of fracture and the age of the patient, fracture healing will occur within three to six months. If bone regeneration is slow and inadequate, the healing process can be speeded up by cancellous bone grafting. For easy access to the site of operation, the connecting rods can be removed and reapplied thereafter.

In cases of delayed bone consolidation, it is advisable to remove the frame in two stages to avoid fatigue fractures. The connecting rods as shown in Fig. 5 are left for another month or two, with the ventral proximal set of pins already removed.

Complications

Pin track infection is the only typical complication of this method of treatment. In mild infections, orally administered antibiotics will control the infection until bone consolidation permits removal of the pins. In severe infections, with loosening of the pin in the bone, either this particular pin or the whole set of pins have to be removed. The pin tracks are thoroughly curetted and rinsed with saline solution. Gentamicin inserts are temporarily implanted and will control the infection without additional systemic antibiotic therapy. A new set of pins is then inserted more proximally or distally.

Conclusion

Stabilization of closed fractures by external fixation takes an intermediate position between conservative and surgical treatments, but is superior to all other methods of treatment in fractures with extensive soft tissue damage. The fixateur externe provides excellent stability with a low risk of infection and is much more comfortable for the patient than traction and plaster cast, particularly in cases of thigh fractures.

The External Fixator for the Prevention and Treatment of Infections

S. Weller

In recent years, the external fixator has increasingly proved its value
and effectiveness in the prevention of infections after open fractures,
and in the treatment of postoperative infections and infected pseudarthroses. Apart from numerous impressive animal experiments, clinical practice
and experience have demonstrated that immobility in the area of the fracture, ie, the stability of osteosynthesis, must be achieved before initi-
ating therapy. It is equally important in the prevention of infection.
Obviously, other important measures have to be taken to prevent or control
infections of bones and joints. Nevertheless, stable fixation of the
fracture is imperative.

Local blood supply to soft tissue covering the bone and an intact vascular
system supplying the bone also play an important role in preventing infections and maintaining the vitality of the bone.

Extensive additional damage may be caused while treating surgically a
fracture or pseudarthrosis or while performing an osteotomy. Here, internal stabilization using plates, screws, wires, pins and nails are not
only harmful but may even damage tissues locally. Moreover, these procedures might impair the healing process.

Less damage is done with the external fixator which serves as a stabilizing device for bones and joints, thus preventing and controlling infections
(Fig. 1, 2). The use of an external fixator avoids implantation of large
foreign bodies into the immediate area at risk. Moreover, stabilization
through an external fixator away from an open fracture or an osteotomy
reduces possible damage to soft tissues, does not impede blood supply, and
permits mobilization. These are important factors in the prevention and
control of infection and in the speed of healing.

While fixation must not necessarily be stable for bone healing to occur in
cases of noninfected fractures, in the presence of infection only external
tighteners and clamps, precisely fitted as a three-dimensional device to
the limbs, will assure optimum stability.

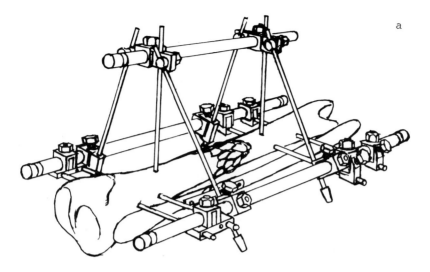

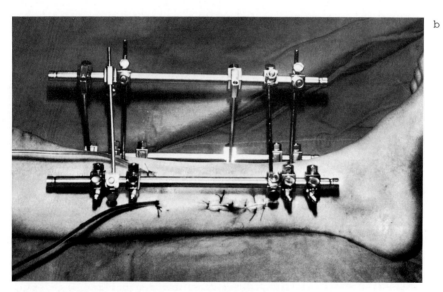

Fig. 1. The AO 3-dimensional external fixation offers
high stability: a) model; b) clinical application in
a postoperative infection with suction-irrigation
drainage.

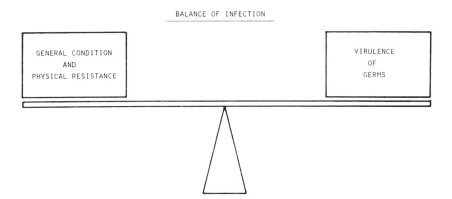

Fig. 2. The balance of infections. The scale should tip to
the left side.

Clinical experience and experimental investigations have impressively demonstrated the importance of stability in the successful treatment of osseous
or articular infections.

Generally, post-traumatic and postoperative therapy aims to

- limit and control infections

- transform an acute into a subacute infection to assist spontaneous bone
  healing; and, if required, stimulate in the healing process by appropriate measures such as cancellous bone grafting or other similar methods.

Acute infections should be classified according to degree and site:

- infected hematoma (superficial infection) (Fig. 3);

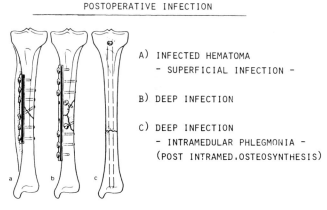

POSTOPERATIVE INFECTION

A) INFECTED HEMATOMA
   - SUPERFICIAL INFECTION -

B) DEEP INFECTION

C) DEEP INFECTION
   - INTRAMEDULAR PHLEGMONIA -
   (POST INTRAMED.OSTEOSYNTHESIS)

Fig. 3. Three stages of postoperative infection
after internal fixation.

- deep infections, reaching or starting from the bone;
- deep infection of the medullary canal with the so-called medullary canal phlegmonia (such as following medullary nailing).

During the early stage of an infection, it is extremely dangerous to confine therapy to the administration of systemic antibiotics, immobilization by plaster cast and local antiseptic dressings. Also, topical spraying of a surgical or traumatic wound is an insufficient precaution and cannot prevent the infection from progressing to deeper layers or prevent externally induced superinfection and, consequently, loosening of implants.

The diagnosis of a post-traumatic or postoperative wound infection must be followed by immediate surgical intervention. The following points should be observed:

- Draining of an infected hematoma or abscess
- Direct culturing and sensitivity testing
- Removal of necrotic tissue (soft tissue and bone) - debridement
- Thorough wound lavage
- Determine whether fixation is stable; if necessary, change to external fixator or proceed with adequate internal fixation method
- Closed or open suction irrigation
- If necessary, and especially in cases where cavities are formed, insert PMMA-gentamicin beads as chains
- Wound closure with stay sutures or, preferably, open wound treatment with temporary wound dressing or skin grafts and secondary closure
- Postoperative elevation of the extremity
- Initially, high parenteral doses of broad-spectrum antibiotics; then changeover to a specific antibiotic depending on the result of culture and sensitivity tests
- Daily inspection of the wound
- General supportive measures to improve resistance (eg, blood transfusion, infusion, high caloric diet)
- Investigation and treatment of concomitant diseases (such as diabetes, circulatory disorders, gastrointestinal diseases)

Local infection and purulent secretions will subside as treatment progresses. The erythrocyte sedimentation rates should be determined frequently.

Once infection is controlled, the following additional surgical measures may be initiated:

- Secondary wound closure after open wound treatment:

    temporary skin cover and conditioning of wound base by synthetic skin substitute (Epigard);

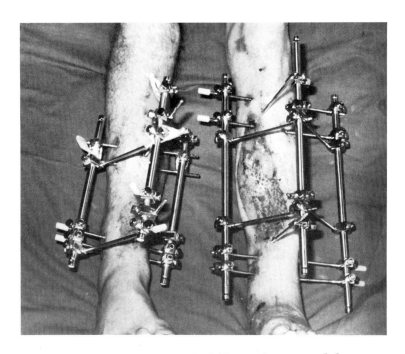

Fig. 4. External fixator in bilateral compound lower
leg fracture.

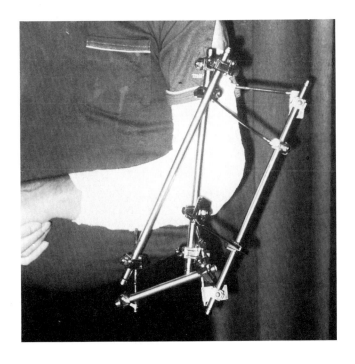

Fig. 5. Severe compound
fracture of the elbow
joint with secondary in-
fection treated by ex-
ternal fixation with
temporary immobilization
of the joint.

    skin transplantation - meshgraft;

    delayed closure

- Autologous cancellous bone graft (when wound conditions are favorable)
- In the last stage, possible change of plate fixation ↔ external fixator, medullary pin ↔ external fixator (Fig. 4, 5).

Although postoperative infection constitutes a serious complication after internal fixation of closed and open fractures, application of proven techniques permits a favorable prognosis. Regular monitoring of the wound, and of the stability of fixation (preferably achieved with external fixation), suction-irrigation-drainage, local application of PMMA-gentamicin bead chains and high dosages of systemic antibiotics, on a short-term basis, after sensitivity testing, are important steps to assure a high success rate.

Septic Nonunion

S. A. Green

General Considerations

This paper deals with the application of external skeletal fixation to one of the most serious complications of musculoskeletal trauma: septic nonunion of long bone. The fixator serves as an adjunct to therapy in several ways: 1) limb length can be maintained after resection of cortical bone; 2) the fixator allows access to the wound for dressing changes and serial debridement; 3) the fixator, by stabilizing osseous tissue, promotes healing of the septic process.

It must be appreciated that the application of an external fixator constitutes only one aspect of the management of these problems. In some situations, a draining fracture will stop discharging purulent material within a few days of fixator application. Unfortunately, if osseous union is not obtained while the fixator is in place, the septic process will flare up again as soon as the fixator is removed. Needless to say, such an occurrence is very discouraging to both patient and physician. To make matters worse, the external skeletal fixator, by reducing physiologic fracture motion, retards external callus formation. Likewise, primary bone healing is retarded because the external fixator rarely will achieve the rigid fixation and interfragmentary compression obtainable with internal fixation. Thus, the biologic processes of fracture repair are inhibited by the fixation system, suggesting that bone healing must be supplemented with fresh autogenous bone graft.

Bone grafting in the face of sepsis is an established procedure with a high likelihood of success provided that certain precautions are followed: only cancellous bone should be used for the grafting procedure, and free drainage from the septic focus must be provided. Cancellous bone seems to be quite tolerant toward pus if free drainage is permitted. Cortical bone graft, on the other hand, may form sequestra, thereby becoming a source of persistent wound sepsis. It is important when applying a cancellous bone graft to use fresh autogenous bone harvested from an appropriate site. The anterior or posterior ilac crests can be utilized as well as the greater trochanters and the proximal tibial metaphyses. Additional donor sites include the proximal ulna and distal radius.

Efforts should be made to maintain the viability of the transplanted bone tissue. Bassett (1972) has demonstrated that although the osteocytes die shortly after removal of the cancellous graft, some of the osteoblasts lining trabecular surfaces survive the ordeal of transplantation.

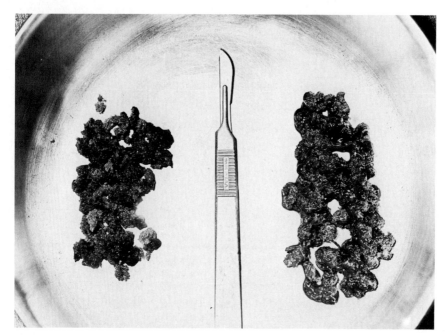

Fig. 1. Fresh autogenous cancellous bone graft, curretted from the greater trochanter of the femur (left) and the iliac crest (right). This is the only type of bone graft recommended if there is any risk of graft sepsis.

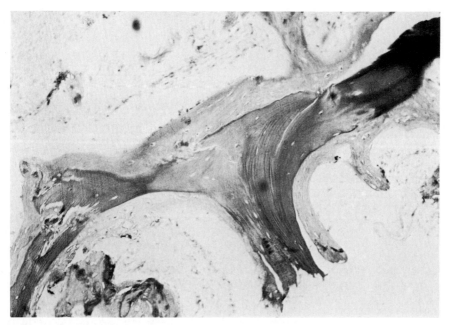

Fig. 2. Fresh autogenous cancellous bone graft six weeks after transplant. Note new bone formation directly on the dead bone trabecular. (From Green, S.A.: Complications of External Skeletal Fixation. Thomas, Springfield, 1981, by permission.)

The graft should be kept in a physiologic irrigating solution (such as Ringers or Normosol) until the tissue is placed into the recipient bed. To reduce the danger of contamination of the donor site by microorganisms from the recipient area, it is wise to obtain the bone graft before surgical procedure.

An important consideration when contemplating bone grafting is the quality of the recipient graft bed. Bone grafts seem to take better when placed into a healthy well vascularized bed of soft tissue. Bone grafts fare poorly indeed when inserted into dense collagenous scar tissue (Edwards et al, 1979).

These considerations suggest that the bone graft should be placed in healthy tissue, away from the area of drainage. Certain surgical approaches to the limbs are preferred for bone grafting. For the tibia, the posterolateral approach (Harmon, 1945) avoids the scarred and poor quality tissue which is usually present anteriorly. This approach also allows the creation of a tibiofibular synostosis.

Several pitfalls are associated with the posterolateral approach. For example, a fracture deformity involving both the tibia and fibula also involves distortion or damage of the interosseous membrane (which usually forms the floor of the recipient graft bed). A tear of the interosseous membrane makes the approach especially dangerous, because the anterior tibial artery and deep peroneal nerve may be inadvertently damaged. Furthermore, the interosseous membrane, being attached to the anterior edge of the fibula, is somewhat difficult to locate during surgical dissection. One must carefully elevate the tibialis posterior muscle from the medial surface of the fibula and the interosseous membrane. The dissection is simplified by starting distally where the tibialis posterior muscle becomes tendinous. Proximalward dissection will usually find the correct plane.

Another consideration when planning a posterolateral bone graft is the prospect of injury to the posterior tibial artery, or more commonly, to the veins associated with it. If there is any question about the integrity of all the vessels of a limb before surgery, an arteriogram will usually clarify the nature of the problem. Generally speaking, such a study is not necessary if a dorsalis pedis pulse and a posterior tibial pulse are present before surgical intervention.

Equally important is the viability of the muscles which will serve to nourish and support revascularization of the bone graft. Muscle of poor vascularity will not sustain a bone graft placed upon its surface. (This problem is most apparent when a bone graft is applied to a limb that has suffered the effects of a compartment syndrome.) A cancellous bone graft applied to the surface of a nonviable muscle will become a necrotic cheesy mass within a few weeks.

Septic Nonunions

Two basic strategies of surgical treatment can be applied to a septic nonunion. One plan of attack calls for completely eliminating the septic process, thereby creating an uninfected nonunion. Bone reconstruction then follows in an effort to obtain skeletal stability. The alternative strategy is to attempt osseous union while the fracture is still draining in the hope that union of the fracture will result in spontaneous resolution of the infection. The decision which of these approaches to select is based on a simple question: Is a sequestrum present?

In some cases, the sequestrum may prove to be a loose fragment of bone, devoid of soft tissue attachment, floating in soft infected granulation tissue. Such a fragment should be removed. Unfortunately, not all sequestra are so easily defined. Commonly, the necrotic bone is in continuity with viable osseous tissue. Usually, this occurs when the outer millimeter or two of bone is exposed to air and dries. An advancing front of granulation tissue has the capacity to dissolve this dried necrotic bone and adhere to the underlying viable cortex. If, on the other hand, the cortical necrosis is full thickness (rather than only on the surface), granulation tissue will not adhere to it. The granulation tissue will heap up instead and grow across the bone without actually adhering to it. This unfortunate situation results in the development of an abscess space between the contaminated necrotic bone and the granulation tissue, leading to persistent drainage.

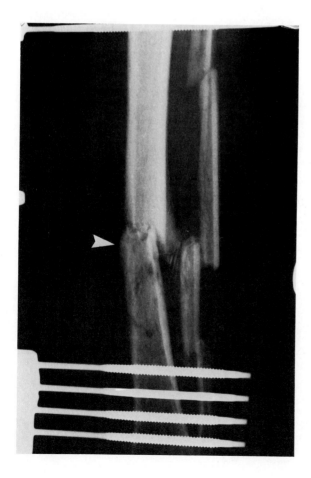

Fig. 3. Characteristic appearance of a septic nonunion with necrotic bone on one side of the fracture line. Note that all reactive changes occur at the end of the viable fragment.

It is difficult to determine whether or not the bone necrosis is full thickness or only surface deep from the outward appearance of the bone itself.
Roentgenograms, however, are extremely helpful because they will usually
reveal a characteristic relative radiodensity of the necrotic fragment when
compared with the surrounding radiolucency associated with disuse of the
limb.

Contaminated exposed bone should not be covered with skin flaps (Edwards
et al, 1979; Vidal et al, 1979). Such a strategy will result in the development of a deep abscess which may compromise further treatment. Exposed bone
can be safely covered if the superficial necrotic surface is shaved off
(down to bleeding bone) and if adequate drainage of contaminated fluids is
allowed. If there is any doubt about the viability of the bone, one should
not proceed with soft tissue coverage.

Different types of infected nonunions require different strategies of management. A hypertrophic nonunion without evidence of sequestra formation responds extremely well to external skeletal fixation alone. If the nonunion
is transverse, a rigid frame with compression across the fracture site usu-

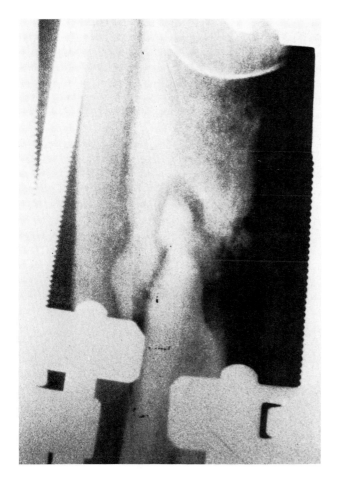

Fig. 4. Another example
of septic nonunion while
in a fixator. The non-
viable (distal) fragment
produces motion-related
bone resorption of the
viable proximal fragment.

ally results in resolution of the nonunion in ten to 12 weeks. When dealing with a tibial hypertrophic nonunion (transverse type), a fibial osteotomy may be necessary to ensure adequate contact of the fracture site. When bone union appears to be present radiographically, the external frame can be removed but the pins left in place for an additional week. This permits the union to be tested, yet allows the reapplication of the frame without reinsertion of pins.

As the site of nonunion becomes more oblique, compression is less desirable since there is a tendency for the fracture fragments to slide past each other. In this situation, the stability offered by the external fixator is usually sufficient to promote union without compression, although a supplementary cancellous bone graft may be necessary.

With hypertrophic nonunions, sepsis may be present but will usually resolve when union is complete. The infected process can be considered a consequence of motion of the bone ends and can be expected to resolve when the fracture is stabilized. It is important to realize that this therapeutic plan applies only to septic nonunions not associated with the presence of a segment of necrotic bone.

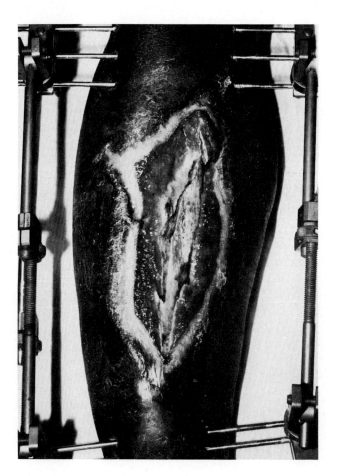

Fig. 5. Sequestration of a large segment of cortical bone requiring extensive debridement. The debridement should proceed in layers until viable osseous tissue is encountered. In this case, the limb was salvaged because function and sensibility of the foot were normal.

When a draining fracture shows no progress towards union and displays roent-genographic and clinical features that indicate the presence of a necrotic bone segment, debridement should be carried out. If, after debridement, a transverse defect of the bone diaphysis remains, it is reasonable to shorten the limb in the external fixator if the total resultant loss of limb length is one inch or less. This procedure greatly simplifies patient management because it eliminates the need for reconstruction of a diaphyseal defect. If, on the other hand, the defect proves to be greater than one inch, recon-struction with bone graft will be necessary.

In most patients, following debridement, contact between the bone ends will be present at one point but a saucerized crater-like defect will be present at the fracture site. The most appropriate surgical treatment here is to bone graft the defect as soon as the recipient soft tissues will support such a graft. If the cancellous bone graft matures slowly, one or more supplemental bone grafting procedures may be necessary.

As indicated earlier in this paper, a viable bone graft requires a well vas-cularized recipient bed. Since many complex Type III open fractures are frequently associated with skin and soft tissue loss, reconstruction of the soft tissues is usually desirable before application of the bone graft. This treatment protocol requires aggressive soft tissue management. Fre-quent debridement of necrotic bone and soft tissue should be followed by early skin and soft tissue coverage. Where exposed muscle is present, split thickness skin grafts can be applied. If the defect involves loss of skin, soft tissue and underlying muscle, a soft tissue flap should be planned.

Many tissue flaps have been described. For transposition flaps one uses local tissue (Ger, 1970), while for cross leg flaps and free flaps one employs tissue from distant sites. Free flaps (Daniel and May, 1978), where the transferred tissue is supplied by blood vessels which are attached to the recipient vascular supply with microsurgical technique, have lately gained popularity. It is technically exacting and requires the diligent efforts of a team well trained in microvascular technique (Derman and Schenck, 1977). As indicated earlier, such flaps should not be applied if there is any doubt about the viability of bone being covered.

A simpler method of obtaining soft tissue cover is to use local muscle or musculocutaneous flaps (Ger, 1970). In the lower leg, the gastrocnemius muscle or soleus muscle serve this function well. The gastrocnemius may be transferred with its overlying subcutaneous tissue and skin. If the soleus muscle (a deep structure) is used, the exposed muscle belly must be covered with a split thickness skin graft. Because of the danger of a partial slough of the distal end of such a transposition, it is worthwhile waiting five days before covering the exposed soleus muscle belly with skin. In this manner, the viability of the transposed muscle can be ascertained. There are certain disadvantages with transposition flaps and free flaps. For example, the transferred muscle is no longer able to function in its original capacity. Furthermore, there is always the danger of slough of some or all of the flap, leading to additional surgery.

Once soft tissue cover has been obtained and there is no evidence of deep sepsis, a close corticocancellous bone graft should be applied. The free edge of the transposed muscle can be elevated and the graft placed beneath it. Alternatively, the graft may be inserted through intact skin elsewhere on the limb.

Papineau (1973) and Roy-Camille (1976) have advocated the use of the open bone graft. Such a graft is applied directly to the exposed but clean granulating tissue and viable muscle belly, and the wound is permitted to heal by second intention. Vascularized granulation tissue will grow into and around the graft and nourish it. The cancellous graft material incorporates within the granulation tissue and begins to form new bone. When the graft is completely covered by granulation tissue, a split thickness skin graft may be applied. (Alternatively, healing and epithelialization by secondary intention can be allowed to occur.)

Unfortunately, cortical bone cannot be used in this situation because the graft material is contaminated while it is exposed, becoming the focus of chronic sepsis. Cancellous bone, as indicated earlier, appears to be tolerant toward such contamination provided free drainage is present.

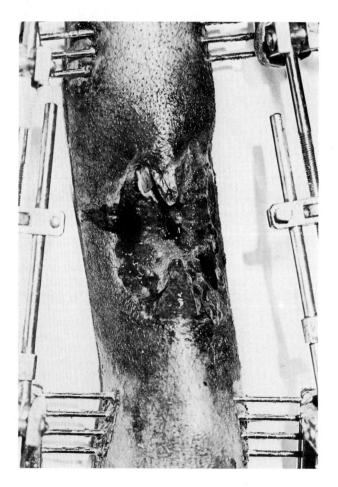

Fig. 6. Septic non-union with a large segmental defect requiring additional debridement. Extensive reconstruction is required to salvage such a limb. The patient's foot was anesthetic and without motor power. For these reasons, the limb was amputated.

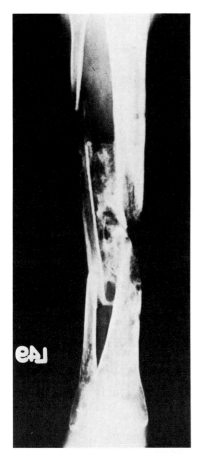

Fig. 7. A well placed tibio-fibular synostosis, applied through the posterolateral approach.

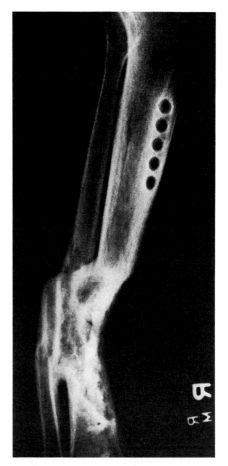

Fig. 8. An open cancellous bone graft which incorporates the fibula into the graft mass.

The technique of open cancellous bone grafting is associated with several serious problems. The center of the graft usually becomes necrotic because it is far from its source of nourishment. In general, the degree of central necrosis appears to be dependent on the nutritional status of the patient and the quality of the recipient bed. The problem can be overcome - but not completely eliminated - by keeping the graft wet until completely covered by granulation tissue. Furthermore, elevation of the patient's limb with continued bedrest for approximately one week after the grafting procedure seems to ensure an adequate graft take.

Pseudarthrosis of the graft mass is another problem that occurs when a large segment of diaphysis is reconstructed with cancellous bone (Green, 1970). I believe the pseudarthrosis occurs because of micromotion of the graft mass. To eliminate this problem, it is imperative to employ a fixator frame con-

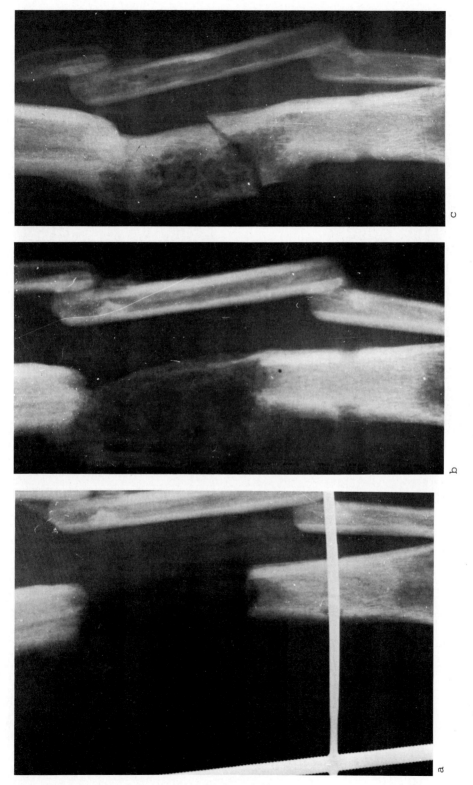

Fig. 9. a) Segmental defect created by resection of necrotic infected bone. b) Open (Papineau) cancellous bone graft. c) Transverse fracture of the graft mass. A synostosis to the fibula would have prevented this complication.

figuration that is extremely rigid. The standard Vidal-Adrey quadrilateral frame configuration should be supplemented with an additional anterior bar and half pins in an oblique plane (Vidal et al, 1979). Other configurations will be necessary for other fixator systems.

Graft fractures (Green, in press) also have been seen with cancellous reconstruction of diaphyseal bone. The fracture can occur with minimal trauma, and has a radiographic appearance similar to that which is seen in Pagetoid bone. Two basic·principles should be followed to avoid such problems:

1) Wherever possible, the graft mass should be stabilized by synostosis to an intact bone, such as the fibula in the lower leg; and 2) prolonged ambulation in a fracture orthosis is important because it allows proper maturation and corticalization of the cancellous bone graft. The brace will be necessary for at least three years if a major diaphyseal reconstruction is accomplished.

In view of the problems associated with open cancellous bone grafting, it is recommended that closed bone grafting be used whenever possible (Sudman, 1979). With this in mind, consultation with a surgeon knowledgeable in plastic and reconstructive techniques is desirable early in the course of patient management whenever one is faced with a draining ununited fracture associated with necrotic bone and deficient soft tissues.

New Developments - Comment

Several recent developments have been introduced to deal with the problem of septic nonunion. These include: a) the use of gentamicin PMMA beads; b) the use of electrical stimulation for bone healing. These two modalities, while not mutually exclusive, approach the problem of septic nonunion from the two alternative directions described at the beginning of this paper. The goal of treatment with gentamicin-PMMA beads is to eliminate the septic focus, permitting treatment of an uninfected nonunion by the usual methods suitable to such a problem. With electrical stimulation of bone healing, on the other hand, one attempts to gain union in the hope that sepsis will subside spontaneously.

The gentamicin-PMMA beads (Jenny et al, 1977; Klemm and Jenny, 1979) have the appearance of small white pearls strung on a wire. They are placed into an abscess cavity which is sutured closed. Gentamicin in high concentrations leaches from the surface of the beads into the local tissues. Extremely high local concentrations of this antibiotic have been reported while the systemic levels are negligible. Adequate antimicrobial concentrations of the gentamicin persist for several weeks. At the end of this time, the beads are removed through a small incision, and the abscess cavity can be filled with bone graft. This product is not yet available in North America, but it deserves consideration when it is released for use by the orthopedic community.

Electrical stimulation of bone healing has been shown to be effective in resolving the septic process when bone union occurs. Of the three systems of electrical stimulation currently available, the external (noninvasive) pulsating electromagnetic field offers the most benefit to the patient with septic nonunion. (The percutaneous method developed by Carl Brighton may stimulate a quiescent septic process.)

Our preliminary experience with the electromagnetic system has been very encouraging. Further clinical research is needed to define the role of electrical stimulation in conjunction with external fixation in the management of septic nonunion of long bone.

References

1. Bassett, C.A.L.: Clinical implications of cell function in bone grafting. Clin. Orthop. 87, 49, 1972.

2. Burri, C.: Post-Traumatic Osteomyelitis. Huber, Bern, 1975.

3. Chao, E.Y.S., Briggs, B.T., and McCoy, M.T.: Theoretical and experimental analysis of Hoffmann-Vidal external fixation system. In, External Fixation, The Current State of the Art. Eds, Brooker, A.F., Jr., and Edwards, C.C. Williams and Wilkins, Baltimore, 1979.

4. Connes, H.: Hoffmann's Double Frame External Anchorage - Methods, Applications and Results in 160 Observations. GEAD, Paris, 1973.

5. Daniel, R.K. and May, J.W., Jr.: Free flaps: An overview. Clin. Orthop. 133, 122, 1978.

6. Derman, G.H., and Schenck, R.R.: Microsurgical technique - Fundamentals of the microsurgical laboratory. Orthop. Clin. North Am. 8, 229, 1977.

7. Edwards, C.C., Jaworski, M., Solana, J., and Aronson, B.: Management of compound tibia fractures in the multiply injured patient using external fixation. Am. Surg., 45, 190, 1979.

8. Ger, R.: The management of open fracture of the tibia with skin loss. J. Trauma, 10, 112, 1970.

9. Green, S.A.: Complications of External Skeletal Fixation. Thomas, Springfield, Ill., 1981.

10. Green, S.A.: Placement of the double frame. In, Proc. 7th Internat. Conf. on Hoffmann External Fixation, Ed., Vidal, J.; Diffinco, Geneva, 1979.

11. Green, S.A., and Bergdorff, T.: External fixation in chronic bone and joint infections: The Rancho experience. Orthop. Trans. (in press).

12. Harmon, P.H.: A simplified surgical approach to the posterior tibia for bone grafting and fibular transference, J. Bone Jt. Surg., 27, 496, 1945.

13. Hoffmann, R.: L'ostéotaxis, ostéosynthèse par fiches transcutànées et rotules. Helv. Chir. Acta, 18, 282, 1951.

14. Jenny, G., Kempf, I., Jaeger, J.H., and Konsbruck, R.: Utilisation de billes de ciment acrylique à la gentamicine dans le traitement de l'infection osseuse. Rev. Chir. Orthop. 63, 491, 1977.

15. Karlstrom, G., and Olerud, S.: Percutaneous pin fixation of open tibial fractures. Double-frame anchorage using the Vidal-Adrey method. J. Bone Jt. Surg. 57A, 915, 1975.

16. Klemm, K., and Jenny, G.: Traitement des pseudarthroses infectées par fixateur externe et gentabilles. In, Proc. 7th Internat. Conf. Hoffmann External Fixation, Ed: Vidal, J., Diffinco, Geneva, 1979.

17. Krempen, J.F., Silver, R.A., and Sotelo, A.: The use of the Vidal-Adrey external fixation system, Part 2: The treatment of infected and previously infected pseudarthrosis. Clin. Orthop. 140, 122, 1979.

18. Nicoll, E.A.: Fractures of the tibial shaft. A survey of 705 cases. J. Bone Jt. Surg. 46B, 373, 1964

19. Olerud, S.: Treatment of fractures by the Vidal-Adrey method. Acta Orthop. Scand. 44, 516, 1973.

20. Papineau, L-J.: L'excision-greffe avec ferméture retardée deliberée dans l'ostéomyelitis chronique. Nouv. Presse Med. 2, 2753, 1973.

21. Perren, S.M.: Physical and biological aspects of fracture healing with special reference to internal fixation. Clin. Orthop. 138, 175, 1979.

22. Roy-Camille, R., Reignier, B., Saillant, G., and Berteaux, D.: Résultats de l'intervention de Papineau. A propos de 46 cas. Rev. Cir. Orthop. 62, 347, 1976.

23. Shaar, C.M., and Kreuz, F.P.: Manual of Fractures. Treatment by External Skeletal Fixation. Saunders, Philadelphia, 1943.

24. Sudman, E.: Treatment of chronic osteomyelitis by free grafts of cancellous autologous bone tissue. Acta Orthop. Scand. 50, 145, 1979.

25. Vidal, J., Connes, H., Buscayret, C., and Trouillas, J.: Treatment of infected non-union by external fixation. In, External Fixation, The Current State of the Art., Eds., Brooker, A.F., Jr., and Edwards, C.C.; Williams and Wilkins, Baltimore, 1979.

26. Vidal J., Pous, J.G., Allieu, Y., Adrey, J., and Goaland, C.: Notre expérience de l'irrigation continuée dans le traitement des suppurations et des fracas de membres. Montpellier Chir., 16, 481, 1970.

Therapy of Post-Traumatic Osteomyelitis

K. H. Müller

The absolute number of patients with post-traumatic osteomyelitis has risen due to an increasing incidence of open fractures and to the extended indication for surgery of the bone (Böhm and Hörster, 1979; Müller, 1981; Müller and Rehn, 1978). The consequences of osteomyelitis are not limited to the affected bone or surrounding tissue. Lengthy illness, uncertain healing results, and the disruption of family and social ties lead to psychologic behavioral disorders and social conflicts. In addition, the direct costs and financial consequences of osteomyelitis represent problems. Post-traumatic osteomyelitis, however, is preventable. Aside from prophylactic measures, this catastrophy can almost certainly be avoided with expert clinical assessment and optimal, preferably early therapy (Fig. 3, 5, 7, 8) (Müller and Rehn, 1978).

The treatment of post-traumatic osteomyelitis includes four main aspects (Müller, 1981):

- thorough debridement of necrotic tissue (Fig. 2)

- stabilization of infected fragments (Fig. 1, 2, 3, 4, 5, 8)

- autologous cancellous bone grafting and osteogenic stimulation (Fig. 1, 2, 4, 5, 8)

- local and systemic chemotherapy (Fig. 6, 7, 8).

These four measures are interdependent and are not replacable by other measures. In each case, the duration of the infection, the extent of the defect, its anatomic location, the condition of the tissue, and the age of the patient determine the therapeutic procedures. Such procedures cannot be schematized. The fifth therapeutic step, skin closure (with meshed split skin and a flap), is usually held up until the bone consolidates (Fig. 7). In the final analysis, however, tissue conditions capable of withstanding stress are an indication of lasting therapeutic success (Fig. 8).

1. Debridement

Debridement includes the removal of all necrotic tissue. Excision and freshening of inflamed vital structures should be done sparingly and cautiously. Sufficient drainage of the wound bed is mandatory (Fig. 1, 2, 6). Compared with debridement of the bone, debridement of soft tissue (fistulae, abscesses, infected scar tissue) can be more radical. Nevertheless, in chronic osteomyelitis, especially in the femur and pelvic area, extirpation of widely branching fistulae not connected to bone can cause difficulties (Müller, 1981). Skin closure without tension should be endeavored, but it should not be a limiting factor in thorough soft tissue debridement.

Bone debridement requires a great deal of experience, if sufficiently vital bone at the fracture ends is to be exposed without causing unnecessary tissue loss (Fig. 2, 3, 5). Due to the difficulty of performing a radical excision while preserving tissue, the degree of visible and microscopic bone vitality following debridement varies. It also depends on the extent of the osteomyelitis. Total debridement is thus a goal which cannot be attained either surgically or microbiologically (Müller and Decker, 1980). Bone debridement leaves a surgically clean cavity (Fig. 1, 2), frequently causing loss of all fragment contact (Fig. 3, 4, 5, 6, 7, 8). During bone revision, periosteal reactive edges must be treated with care since, in addition to cancellous bone grafts, they represent an important source for bridging defects (Fig. 4a, 4b). Incomplete debridement and stability are incompatible since dead tissue harbours the infection, and continued infection in turn leads to a loosening of fixation (Burri, 1979; Müller, 1981).

Naturally, debridement includes removal of implants which have loosened since they no longer serve their purpose; to the contrary, they support the infection (Fig. 1, 2, 4b). On the other hand, our clinical experience and histologic observations show that the rule of maintaining stabilizing internal implants should be modified (Fig. 3, 8). In daily practice, the decision to replace internal implants with an external fixator is most difficult. It is not unusual to find that a fracture, although internally stabilized, nevertheless fails to heal, and that removal of the plate reveals that sequestration of the cortical bone in contact with the metal is the cause (Fig. 3a, 3b). Contrary to a totally separated sequestrum surrounded by pus, we have here a case of irreversible bone devitalization caused by the osteomyelitis in which a firm union with adjacent vital bone is retained. Being dead hard tissue, necrotic cortical surfaces which are not dislocated and only microscopically separated still maintain a macroscopically stable internal fixation for a long time (Fig. 3a, 3b). Bone healing, however, should not be expected since revitalization of such necrotic cortices is impossible (Fig. 8b). Internal implants should, thus, only be left in place if they stabilize vital or revitalizable bone. On the other hand, early infection should not lead to early removal of the internal implant, especially when the fractures are para-articular and intra-articular. External fixation at these sites may be difficult; moreover, healing in the metaphyseal area generally tends to be more rapid.

2. Stabilization

Healing of an infected fracture is hindered by mechanical instability as well as inflammatory osteolysis. Primary treatment must include, in addition to debridement, interfragmentary stabilization through fixation. Furthermore, to fix the unstable infected bone mechanically, it is essential that every surgical procedure be also a measure to control the infection. This requirement is difficult to achieve because an osteosynthesis in the presence of an infection confronts the surgeon with a number of adverse mechanical and biologic factors (Fig. 1):

Mechanical factors

- reduction or loss of interfragmentary friction due to inadequate or absent contact between the fragments (Fig. 4)
- inadequate anchorage of the implant due to poor bone stock (osteoporosis) (Fig. 2)
- few or no implants in the area of infection (Fig. 1, 7, 8)

Biologic factors

- loss of physiologic properties of bones, soft tissues, and other functional tissues (Fig. 2)
- impaired vascularization of the site of infection due to necrosis, osteolysis, and general dystrophy of the surrounding area (Fig. 4)
- disrupted local and general endogenous defence mechanisms

Especially in the presence of an accumulation of these adverse conditions an external fixator must be the basic principle for stabilizing these infected fragments (Fig. 1, 2, 3, 4, 5, 6, 8). The advantages are as follows:

- sufficient stabilization of fragments away from the site of infection without immobilizing a joint (Fig. 4)
- even when close to the site of infection, the pins do not act as biologically or mechanically irritating foreign bodies; disrupted vascularization is not further compromised, and an optimal secondary intervention is feasible (Fig. 7).

The various anatomic locations, however, require an appropriate choice between the available forms of external fixators.

The advantages of the external fixation device for post-traumatic osteomyelitis in the *tibia shaft*, where infection occurs most often, are evident (Burri, 1979). Using the possibilities offered by external fixation in a three-dimensional application, external fixation has been experimentally and clinically perfected to a point where it can also be used in the presence of extensive bone and tissue defects. Alternatives for stabilization are no longer even debatable (Fig. 2, 4, 8).

When the infection is in the *femoral shaft*, however, there are anatomic and biomechanical limits to the stabilizing and surgical possibilities with the external fixator. For this reason, we prefer plate fixation for the treatment of post-traumatic osteomyelitis of the femur, even in the presence of larger defect areas in the bone (Fig. 5). We discourage plate osteosynthesis as the first choice of treatment only when the anchorage is unreliable, when there is no skin closure possible, and when the infection could not be brought under control. The unsatisfactory mechanical characteristics of the lateral bracket fixator in respect to knee function can also be improved in the femur by external fixation in a three-dimensional application (Müller, 1981). We might mention, for example, the good results achieved with the external fixator for hip arthrodesis when pyogenic coxitis is present and for the stabilization of infected unstable fractures of the *pelvic girdle* (Müller, 1981).

Bone defects of the *humerus*, since shortening is functionally insignificant, should be treated by compression osteosynthesis with a plate. In the presence of widespread soft tissue damage, secondary to infection, in particular when nerve dissection is risky, external stabilization of the humerus is a successful procedure due to the reduced biomechanical load.

The complex topography and the various functions of the *forearm* require protection of the soft tissue; therefore, internal plate osteosynthesis is indicated (Rehn and Müller, 1978). Only the application of the external fixator on the muscle-free edge of the ulna is without risk. When the radius is infected, the fixator is only indicated when plate osteosynthesis has been unsuccessful. In the presence of osteomyelitis of bones close to or in communication with a joint, eradication of the infection and restoration of satisfactory function can often only be achieved by radical resection arthrodesis with an external fixator (Fig. 2). On the other hand, in the initial phase of para-articular osteomyelitis immobilization with an external fixator which bridges the joint is also indicated if the joint is to be saved.

3. Cancellous Bone Grafting

Probably the most effective step in osteomyelitis therapy is autologous cancellous bone grafting. As a biologic building material and catalyst, autologous cancellous bone grafts are essential for appropriate surgical management. Furthermore, based on biologic principles, such grafts often guarantee long-term control of bone infection (Fig. 1, 3c, 4, 5c, 5d, 7, 8c). The transplanted autologous cancellous bone is incorporated despite bone infection, provided the bed is vital and stable and the infection is not extensive (Decker and Müller, 1980; Müller and Decker, 1979; Schweiberer, 1976). Evidently, an optimal preparation of the graft bed is an essential requirement.

In summary, one can state that autologous cancellous bone grafts for cases of post-traumatic osteomyelitis fulfill four tasks (Fig. 4):

- As soon as vascularization begins, local endogenous defence mechanisms are activated.

- Bone is built up through the bone's own osteogenesis, and osteogenic activity is stimulated in the osseous bed.

- The osteosynthesis becomes more stable after the cancellous bone has been surrounded by vital tissue, and bone strength is increased following the bridging of fragments.

- Optimal biologic filling material is used for the bone defect.

In general, a sleeve-type cancellous bone graft should be used to speed bone consolidation and to control the infection even when there is contact between the main fragments. Tibia defects can be bridged in three ways:

239

- by open, anterior, direct autologous cancellous bone grafts (Fig. 1, 2f, 3d, 4a, 7, 8c)

- by closed, lateral, direct or bridge-type autologous cancellous bone grafts (Fig. 4b)

- by the formation of lateral fibulotibial synostosis (Fig. 4c).

The latter bridging method, using a so-called fibula-protibia graft, is only indicated when direct access is contraindicated and when the defect is very large. In the femur and humerus, only autologous cancellous bone is used to directly bridge a defect (Fig. 5). Due to the well vascularized surrounding muscles, even large diaphyseal defects can be built up and transformed into bone capable of bearing weight. Bone defects of the lower arm are bridged by interposing a corticocancellous bone splint which is integrated into the internal compression osteosynthesis. The whole osteomyelitis therapy is reflected in the optimal preparation of the graft bed. Failure to graft successfully autologous cancellous bone has the following consequences:

- local conditions deteriorate

- time is lost, thus increasing the danger that the osteosynthesis will loosen

- valuable autologous cancellous bone tissue is lost.

4. Antibiotic Therapy

Antibiotic therapy must be based on identification of organisms and their sensitivity (Hierholzer and Lob, 1978). In cases of post-traumatic osteomyelitis, antibiotic therapy is only indicated combined with surgical measures. When the identity of an infectious microorganism is not available following the acute onset of an infection, the nonspecific use of a broad-spectrum bactericidal antibiotic is indicated which is also effective against the specific hospital microbial environment. Thereafter, susceptibility testing will determine which specific antibiotic is indicated. High dosages of a parenteral antibiotic are required shortly before and after surgery in cases of osteomyelitis associated with septicemia.

Our clinical, histologic and experimental investigations have confirmed the effectiveness of local antibiotic therapy in the form of gentamicin-PMMA chains (Septopal®)(Fig. 8). From the time the first tests were performed more than four years ago until March 1981, we have been able to treat 521 patients with gentamicin-PMMA chains. Even in the absence of local blood flow or interstitial fluid exchange, the antibiotic is continuously released from the synthetic material (polymethylmetacrylate) at the site of the infection in bactericidal concentrations (Klemm et al, 1979). The prerequisite for the effectiveness of this method is the sensitivity of the causative pathogens to gentamicin. With the rapid formation of granulation tissue with little or no inflammation, the infection subsides (Fig. 3, 5b, 6, 8c)(Klemm et al, 1979; Müller and Biebrach, 1979). For basic surgical reasons, we use suction drainage to drain an osteomyelitic defect cavity which has been filled with chains and closed (Fig. 6)(Müller and Biebrach, 1979). It is possible that some gentamicin is lost due to the suction

Treatment of Posttraumatic Osteomyelitis

① Debridement

② Stabilisation

③ Autologous cancellous - bone grafting

④ Antibiotics ⎾ systemic
                ⎿ local

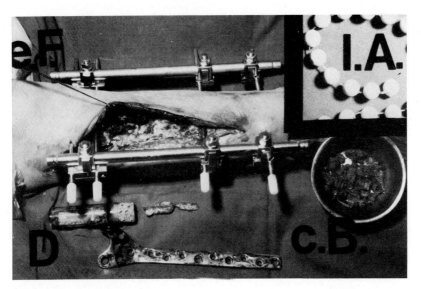

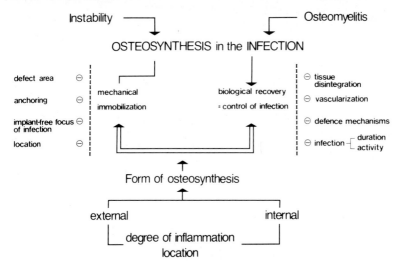

Fig. 1. Main elements in the therapy of post-traumatic osteomyelitis; schema of factors associated with stable osteosynthesis in the infection which affect each other.

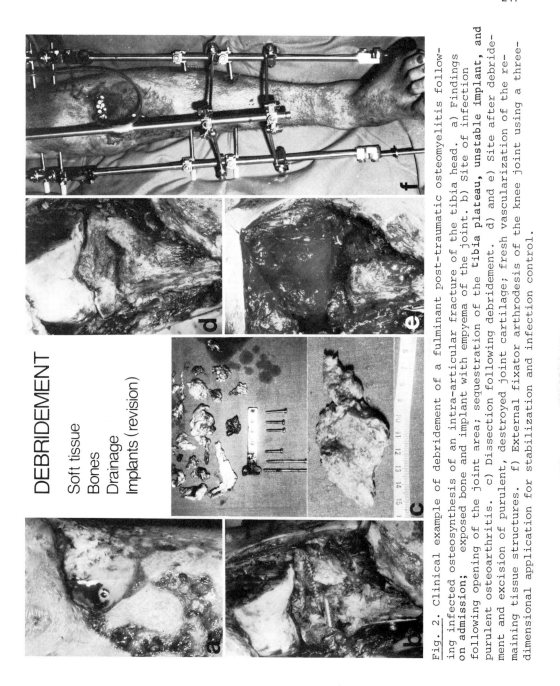

DEBRIDEMENT

Soft tissue
Bones
Drainage
Implants (revision)

Fig. 2. Clinical example of debridement of a fulminant post-traumatic osteomyelitis following infected osteosynthesis of an intra-articular fracture of the tibia head. a) Findings
on admission; exposed bone and implant with empyema of the joint. b) Site of infection
following opening of the joint area; sequestration of the tibia plateau, unstable implant, and
purulent osteoarthritis. c) Dissection following debridement. d) and e) Site after debridement and excision of purulent, destroyed joint cartilage; fresh vascularization of the remaining tissue structures. f) External fixator arthrodesis of the knee joint using a three-
dimensional application for stabilization and infection control.

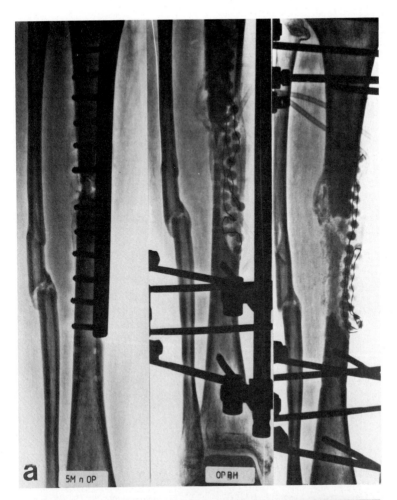

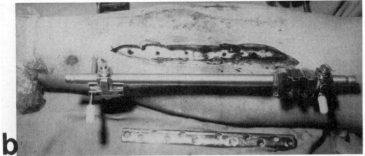

Fig. 3. Clinical example of an infected pseudarthrosis
in the tibia when plate osteosynthesis appears stable.
a) Series of roentgenograms showing the bone defect
after debridement and the removal of the implant.
b) Nondislocated sequestrum of the tibia corticalis adjacent to the plate.

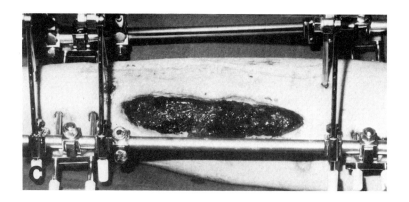

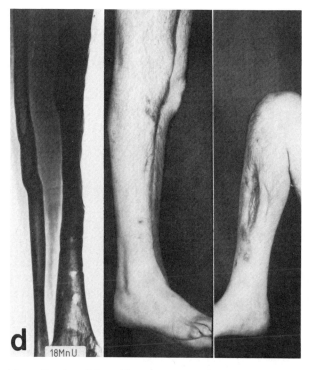

Fig. 3. (continued)
c) Open, secondary cancellous bone grafting and external fixation. d) Roentgenogram and clinical healing.

244

Open direct autologous cancellous bone graft

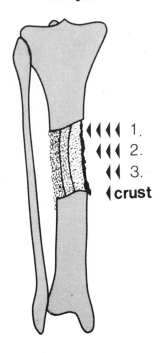

1.
2.
3.
crust

a

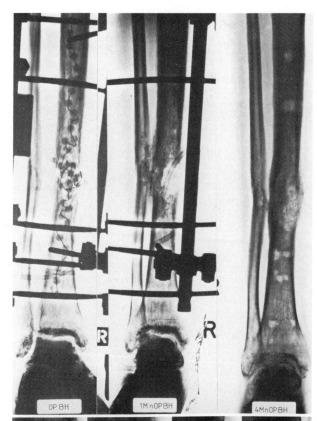

OP BH   1Mn0PBH   4Mn0PBH

Closed lateral autologous cancellous bone graft

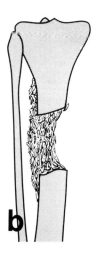 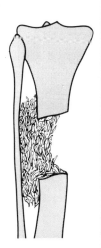

b

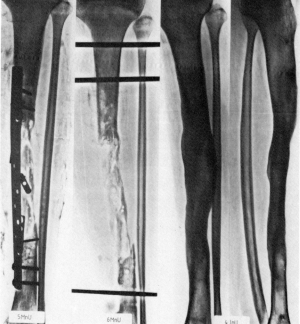

5MnU   6MnU   4 Inll

Fig. 4. (See next page for description)

Modifikations of fibulo-tibial Synostosis

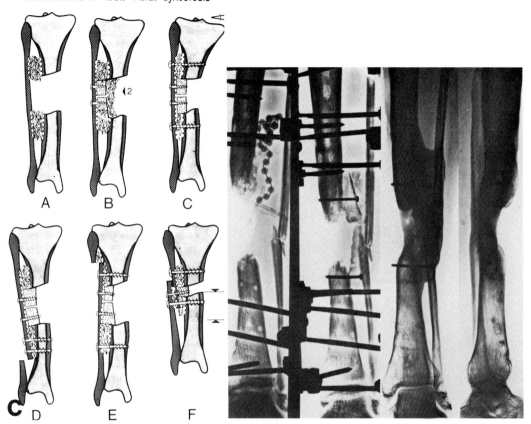

Fig. 4. Schematic presentation and a series of roentgenograms showing the
forms of autologous cancellous bone grafting when infected tibia defects are
present. (a and b on previous page). a) Open, direct cancellous bone grafting; the defect cavity is progressively filled in onionskin-like layers.
b) Closed, lateral, direct or bridge-type cancellous bone grafting of the
main tibia fragments. c) Fibulotibial bridging with a variety of surgical
modifications (fibula-pro-tibia-grafting).

246

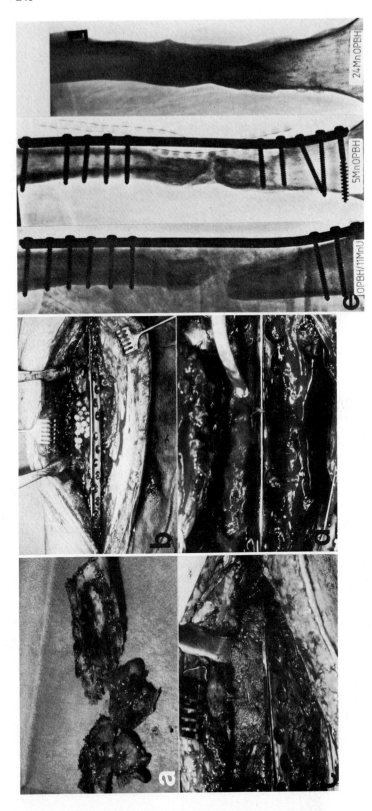

Fig. 5. Clinical example and roentgenogram series showing the build-up of an infected defect pseudarthrosis in the femur following autologous cancellous bone grafting. a) Dissection of the sequestrum. b) Infection control by means of stable plate osteosynthesis and intermediary insertion of gentamicin-PMMA chains. c) Secondary autologous cancellous bone grafting. d) Vital, strongly vascularized, still soft bridging of the defect by an autologous cancellous bone graft which has taken. e) Roentgenogram series.

Suction Drainage Coupled with Gentamycin-PMMA-Chains

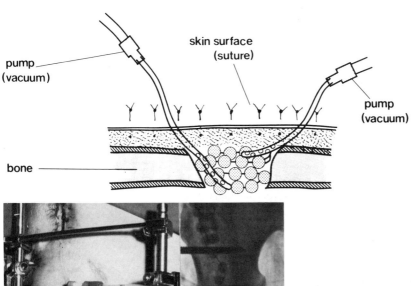

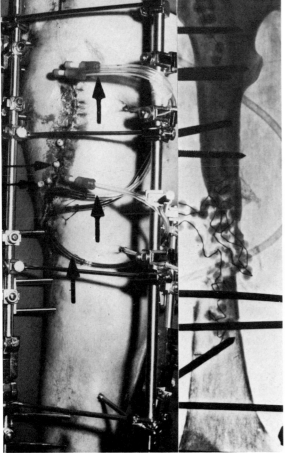

Fig. 6. Schematic and clinical example of the technique of local antibiotic therapy using gentamicin-PMMA chains; primary skin closure of the osteomyelitic defect cavitiy, which has been filled with chains, and suction drainage.

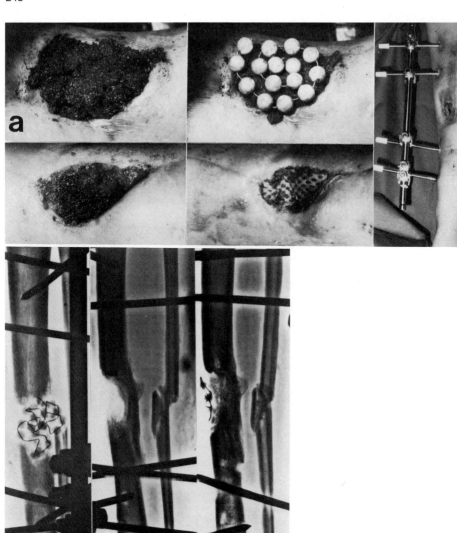

Fig. 7. Clinical representation of the course of a direct autologous cancellous bone graft; an infected tibia defect is shown which is locally protected
by gentamicin-PMMA chains. a) Fresh, secondary, open autologous cancellous
bone grafting; a gentamicin-PMMA chain is placed on the wound in a spiral
form (daily replacement of the dressing using moist gauze strips); after the
grafted cancellous bone has taken, meshed split skin is used for skin coverage. b) Roentgenogram series showing the three consecutive bone grafts.

drainage. Our tests have shown, however, that the concentrations reached in the granulation tissue and in the cancellous bone are many times higher, and in the cortical bone (with few exceptions) at least as high, as the tissue levels obtainable with parenteral administration of gentamicin (Müller and Dingeldein, 1981). When appropriate, we also combine autologous cancellous bone grafting with this form of local antibiotic therapy (Fig. 7)(Müller and Decker, 1980).

The first 171 patients treated from December 1976 to May 1978 were carefully documented (Müller and Biebrach, 1979). Histologic examinations of this group of patients showed that the condition of chronic post-traumatic osteo-myelitis is considerably improved when gentamicin-PMMA chains are used (Böhm and Hörster, 1979). As a preliminary long-term study, 145 patients in this group were reexamined on an average of 31 months after completion of therapy. In 94% of the patients, the infection had abated; of these, 60% showed primary and 34% secondary control of the infection (Fig. 8). In 19% of patients, osteomyelitic reactivation (ie, when fistulae, abscesses, and sequestra with general signs of infection recur) was observed. Due to the advantages of local antibiotic infection control - low risk for secondary interventions, reduced hospitalization, and favorable long-term results - it has supplanted irrigation-suction-drainage in our clinic in most cases. It does not replace or diminish the priority of surgical measures (debridement and stabilization), but effectively augments them.

References (continued after figures)

1. Böhm, E., and Hörster, G.: Histologische Verlaufsuntersuchungen bei der lokalen mit Gentamycin behandelten chronischen Osteomyelitis. In, Burri, C., and Rüter, A.(Ed.): Lokalbehandlung chirurgischer Infektionen. Huber, Bern-Stuttgart-Wien, 1979.

2. Burri, C.: Posttraumatische Ostcitis, 2nd Ed. Huber, Bern-Stuttgart-Wien, 1979.

3. Decker, S., and Müller, K.H.: Morphologisch-experimentelle Untersuchungen über die vom Lager ausgehende Vascularisation autologer Spongiosatrans-plantate. In, Hierholzer, G., and Zilch, H. (Ed.): Transplantatlager und Implantatlager bei verschiendenen Operationsverfahren. Springer, Berlin - Heidelberg - New York, 1980.

4. Hierholzer, G., and Lob, G.: Antibioticatherapie in der Unfallchirurgie. Unfallheilkunde 81, 64, 1978.

5. Klemm, W., Contzen, H., and Lennert, K.H.: Gentamycin-PMMA-Kugeln bei Knochen- und Weichteilinfektionen - Ergebnisse aus der Berufsgenossen-schaftlichen Unfallklinik Frankfurt/Main. In, Burri, C., and Rüter, A. (Ed.): Lokalbehandlung chirurgischer Infektionen. Huber, Bern-Stuttgart-Wien, 1979.

6. Müller, K.H. Exogene Osteomyelitis von Becken und unteren Gliedmassen. Springer, Berlin-Heidelberg-New York, 1981

7. Müller, K.H., and Rehn, J.: On prophylaxis, early recognition and early treatment of infected osteosyntheses. Arch. Orthop. Traumat. Surg. 92, 127, 1978.

ADVANTAGES of Gentamycin-PMMA-Chains

① Infection control ↗

② Risk of secondary interventions ↘

③ Functional therapy ↗

④ Duration of hospitalization ↘

⑤ Long-term results ↗ ?

⑥ Dynamic concept of treatment

Gentamycin-PMMA-Chains

Follow-up examination of the 1st group of patients (n=145)

∅ 31 months following completion of treatment

94% infection controlled ⎧ primary   60%
                         ⎩ secondary   34%

19% osteomyelitic reactivation

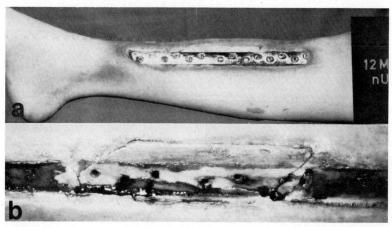

Fig. 8. Advantages of local antibiotic therapy using gentamicin-PMMA chains and the results of a preliminary long-term study of 145 treated patients. Clinical and roentgenographs summarizing the therapeutic steps in the treatment of post-traumatic osteomyelitis. a) Clinical picture of an infected pseudarthorsis of the tibia at the beginning of treatment, 12 months after a simple fracture. b) Sequestration of the middle-third of the tibia for a distance of 13 cm.

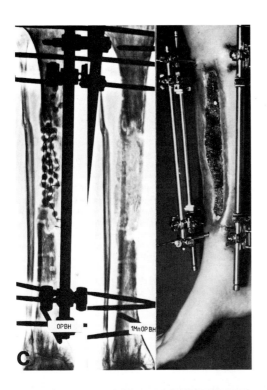

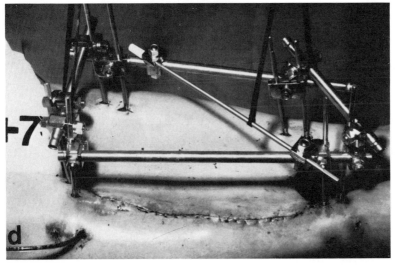

Fig. 8 (continued)
c) Roentgenogram series showing osteoplastic reconstruction
of the defect, three-dimensional external stabilization, and
local antibiotic therapy. d) Complete skin coverage using
cross-leg grafting and immobilization with an external
fixator.

252

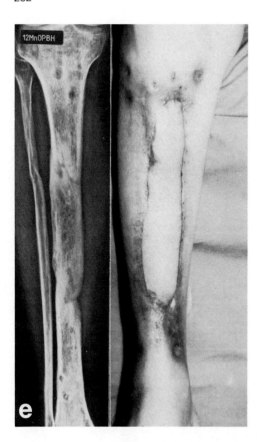

Fig. 8. (continued)
e) Healing result one year after treatment.

References (continued)

8. Müller, K.H., and Biebrach, M.: Die lokale Antibiotikatherapie von
    Knochen- und Weichteilinfektionen mit Gentamycin-Kunststoffketten -
    Ergebnisse und Erfahrungen am "Bergmannsheil" in Bochum. In, Burri, C.,
    and Rüter, A. (Ed.): Lokalbehandlung chirurgischer Infektionen. Huber,
    Bern-Stuttgart-Wien, 1979.

9. Müller, K.H., and Decker, S.: Zur Vorbereitung des Transplantatlagers
    und Vorgehen zur Verpflanzung autologer Spongiosa bei der Osteomyelitis.
    In, Hierholzer, G., and Zilch, H. (Ed.): Transplantatlager und Implantatlager bei verschiendenen Operationsverfahren. Springer, Berlin-Heidelberg
    New York, 1980.

10. Müller, K.H., Dingeldein, E., and Müller, K.: Untersuchungen der Gentamycinkonzentration in verschiendenen Geweben und Sekreten nach lokaler
    antibiotischer Therapie mit Gentamycin-PMMA-Ketten (in preparation, 1981).

11. Rehn, J., and Müller, K.H.: Die posttraumatische Osteomyelitis des
    Unterarms. Unfallheilkunde 81, 353, 1978.

12. Schweiberer, L.: Theoretisch-experimentalle Grundlagen der autologen
    Spongiosatransplantation im Infekt. Unfallheilkunde 79, 135, 1976.

Treatment of Infected Fractures and Pseudarthroses with External Fixation and Gentamicin-PMMA Beads

K. Klemm

In most patients with infected pseudarthroses the causes derive from two sources:

1) first to third degree open fractures with subsequent development of chronic osteomyelitis due to highly contaminated and severely traumatized soft tissues and bone;

2) surgically-treated fractures with implantation of rods and plates complicated by deep postoperative infection.

At the Post-traumatic Osteomyelitis Service of the Frankfurt Accident Clinic about 25% of the total number of 53 beds are occupied by adolescents and young men between 16 and 25 years of age who were in a motorcycle accident and had suffered open fractures, mostly of the lower leg. There is general agreement today that these fractures should primarily be stabilized by external fixation; yet, quite a number of patients are transferred to our clinic from other hospitals where such fractures were treated by fixation with plates and rods.

Infected pseudarthrosis is the dreaded dual complication of chronic osteomyelitis with sequestration of bone and persisting instability at the fracture site. Bone consolidation is hindered by sequestrated fragments and/or instability. Classic treatment consists of radical removal of all sequestrated bone and alloplastic implants followed by irrigation-suction drainage and combined with systemic or local antibiotic therapy. Restabilization is achieved by application of an external fixation. Subsequent bone grafting is performed if necessary.

A new approach in local antibiotic therapy consists of temporary implantation of gentamicin-containing plastic beads. These beads have a diameter of 7 mm and contain 4.5 mg gentamicin base and 20 mg zirconium dioxide as radiologic contrast medium. The broad-spectrum antibiotic is slowly released in high doses from the plastic material, polymethyl methacrylate. As was shown in *in vitro* studies by Wahlig and Dingeldein, initially 400 to 500 µg gentamicin base per day is released from one single bead. Around the 10th day, 120 µg, and at the 20th day, 50 µg is detectable. On the 80th day, 10 µg gentamicin base is still present.

These *in vitro* studies were confirmed by determination of gentamicin concentrations in wound secretions following implantation of the beads. The concentrations exceed about 10 to 100-fold the minimal inhibitory concentrations for the most common organisms. Moreover, they exceed by far serum and tissue levels obtainable with the same antibiotic administered systemically.

Pharmacokinetic studies in patients indicate that only traces of gentamicin can be measured in the serum a few days after implantation of the beads.

In the urine, however, gentamicin can still be measured several months after bead implantation; concentrations were always under 10 µg/mL. Any fear of toxic side effects is therefore groundless, and additional parenteral administration of gentamicin or other antibiotics at the usual dosage can be prescribed if this should be necessary.

Gentamicin-PMMA beads are on the market in most of the European countries as single beads of 10, 30 or 60 beads on a braided wire in the form of chains. For the temporary implantation of these beads, in cases of infected pseudarthroses, gentamicin-PMMA chains are advantageous.

The following surgical technique is recommended. The patient with an infected pseudarthrosis of the femur or tibia is placed on the traction table. Using the traction table instead of the normal operating table has many advantages. After removal of the sequestrated bone fragments and implants, such as rods and plates, the alignment of the major fragments is kept without danger of axis deviation and shortening. There is easy access for the image intensifier to check the position of the pins, particularly important for the insertion of pins at the femur.

We prefer to do the sequestrectomy under vital staining with disulphine blue, which is especially helpful for early identification of devitalized bone fragments. In an adult with normal weight about 30 mL of the dye are injected intravenously one hour before the operation. All tissue with blood supply show more or less intensive staining while tissue without blood supply, such as teeth, retain their natural color. This applies to sequestrated bone as well. Some authors have expressed the viewpoint that sequestrectomy under vital staining may result in larger defects than necessary. Our experience, however, with patients referred to us from other hospitals, indicates that in most infected pseudarthroses sequestrectomy was not done radically enough resulting in new sinus formation. Sequestrectomy under vital staining has to be performed in a bloodless field by application of a tourniquet; otherwise impeded vision by the stained blood in the operative field will result in false interpretation of the findings. Furthermore, the uselessness of any antibiotic treatment in chronic osteomyelitis without surgical intervention can be demonstrated by vital staining.

Following removal of sequestrated fragments and alloplastic implants, one or more gentamicin-PMMA chains, depending on the size of the cavity, are placed into the wound. A Redon drainage tube is inserted as well and the wound closed tightly as in aseptic operations. The drainage tube is connected to a secretion bag serving only as an overflow drainage to avoid tension to the wound closure (Fig. 1).

In our opinion, by carrying out this procedure the gentamicin is slowly released into the hematoma, and the gentamicin-enriched hematoma carries the antibiotic in the opposite direction of the stream of secretion.

The external fixator is then applied. We prefer the external fixator of Raoul Hoffmann because of its almost unlimited versatility due to the universal ball joints. Once a surgeon has become acquainted with the Hoffmann

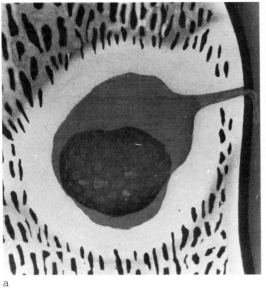

a

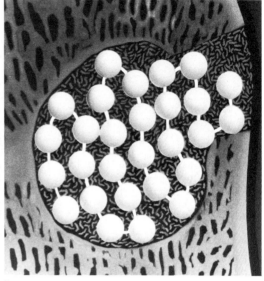

b

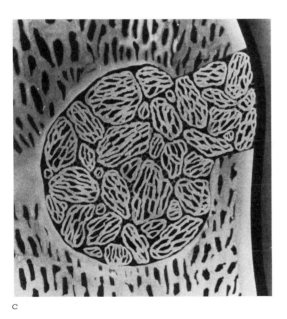

c

Fig. 1.
a) Sequestrating osteomyelitis.
b) Implantation of gentamicin-PMMA chain.
c) Cancellous bone grafting.

apparatus, its application is easy. The system can be adapted to the topographic situation in each individual case, and corrections can be made at any time thereafter without changing the pins. Positioning of the bone pins proximally and distally to the pseudarthrosis can be done at any level and direction without consideration of the frame's mounting.

Following implantation of gentamicin-PMMA chains, wound healing, as under aseptic conditions, can generally be expected. Contrary to irrigation-suction drainage, this method of treatment gives the patient the freedom to leave his bed the day after the operation. He can be discharged when wound healing is completed. There is no reason to keep a patient with an external fixator at the hospital. He will be readmitted either for bone grafting or final removal of the fixator. The patients are very clever in arranging their clothes to accommodate the mounting of the frame.

Additional systemic antibiotic therapy combined with the local implantation of gentamicin-PMMA chains is not necessary for the treatment of chronic osteomyelitis around the infected pseudarthrosis; but with the removal of sequestrated bone and application of the external fixator in the course of one operation, there is always the danger of pin tract infection. We therefore give the patients oral cephalosporins prophylactically during the first two weeks after the operation.

At the second operation for bone grafting, the wound is reopened and the gentamicin-PMMA chain removed. Depending on the length of time the chain has been implanted, the beads are more or less encapsulated in granulation tissue. At this point the infection-free cavity is firmly filled with can- cellous bone. There is no doubt that autologous cancellous bone is the best for bone transplantation; but in quite a number of cases the donor sites at the iliac crests and tibial heads are devoid of spongy bone or of insufficient quantity or poor quality, so that deep frozen homologous bone grafts are a good substitute. The homologous cancellous bone is taken from femoral heads, deep frozen down to $-75°$ C.

If the skin and soft tissue at the anterior aspect is so scarred that tension-free wound closure over the bone graft is endangered or impossible, the dorsomedial approach is recommended for bone grafting.

At the tibia, the final outcome always depends on the condition of the soft tissue and not so much on the extent of the bone defect. Cross leg flaps or muscle transposition flaps are good means to improve the situation.

The patient is discharged again, and readmitted to hospital either for a second bone transplantation, if necessary, or the final removal of the external fixator.

Pin tract infection and refracture are threatened complications in the course of treatment and after. In severe pin tract infection with loosen- ing of the pins, the pins have to be removed and replaced somewhere else. In mild pin tract infection with little purulent discharge and no loosen- ing of the pins, the original mounting can be kept until sufficient bone consolidation has taken place. Following removal of the pins, the pin tracts are curetted and rinsed thoroughly. Gentamicin-PMMA sticks are inserted into the pin tracts for about a week. As gentamicin-PMMA chains cannot be used in the narrow pin tracts, these sticks of gentamicin-PMMA around K-wires, currently handmade, are a good solution to the problem of pin tract infection.

In cases of infected pseudarthroses where a more or less extensive bone defect had to be reconstructed, the newly formed bone is of poor quality, lacking the normal structure. It is a bone slab instead of a tube of much higher bending strength. Refracture without new trauma is not a rare complication. To avoid this complication and to give the bone enough time to regain normal strength under protection, patients with healed pseudarthrosis of the tibia are equipped with an orthotic device.

If a refracture occurs, the patient as well as the surgeon face the threat that the whole problem and prolonged treatment may start all over again. According to our experience, refracture may be a desired complication. As there is almost never a displacement of the fracture, restabilization in a rather simple mounting without opening the fracture site is sufficient. We observed in our cases periosteal callus formation of surprisingly good quality, adding new stability which was not achieved by all the previous measures. We have never seen refracturing happen after bone consolidation of a former refracture.

Two case histories may illustrate the point (Fig. 2, 3).

A 19-year old man was admitted with an infected pseudarthrosis of the right femur eight months after angulated plate osteosynthesis of a supracondylar fracture. Sequestrated bone fragments were removed and the remaining defect filled with gentamicin-PMMA chains. Because of the short distal fragment and the stiffness of the knee joint, an external fixator with extension below the knee joint was applied. Cancellous bone grafting was performed twice. The external fixator was removed 12 months later (Fig. 2).

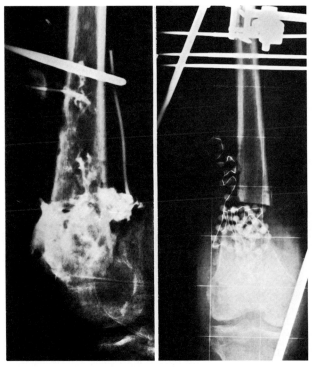

Fig. 2. a) Infected pseudarthrosis of the femur. b) Implantation of gentamicin-PMMA chains following radical sequestrectomy of an external fixator.

a   b

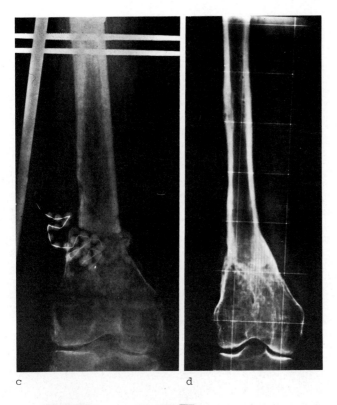

c   d

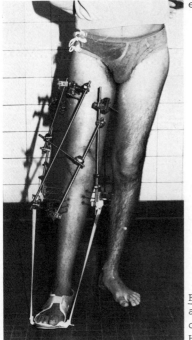

e

Fig. 2. c) Partical bone consolidation after first bone grafting. d) Complete bone consolidation within 12 months. e) External Hoffmann fixator.

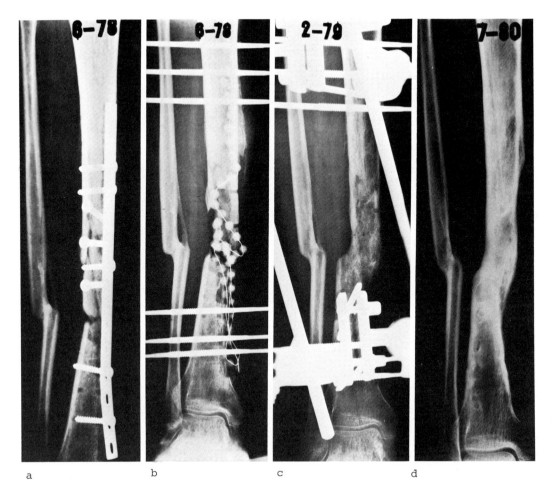

Fig. 3. a) Infected pseudarthrosis of the tibia. b) Implantation of gentamicin-PMMA chains following radical sequestrectomy and application of an external fixator. c) Partial bone consolidation following bone grafting, triangulation added to the external fixator. d) Complete bone consolidation within
2 years.

Another case history concerns a 17-year old boy who was admitted because of
infected pseudarthrosis of the left tibia. The plate and sequestrated bone
were removed and the defect filled with gentamicin-PMMA chains. Cancellous
bone grafting was performed twice and the third dimension added to the external fixator for more stability. He was carrying an orthopedic splint
apparatus for about one year after removal of the external fixator (Fig. 3).

From 1976 to 1979, 131 patients with infected pseudarthroses were treated
in this way at the Accident Clinic at Frankfurt (Dr. Klemm), Strasbourg
(Dr. Jenny) and Vienna (Dr. Vecsei). Eight were located at the humerus,
seven at the forearm, 40 at the femur and 76 at the tibia. Table I shows
the results of the 76 patients with infected pseudarthroses of the tibia.

Twenty-one resulted from closed fractures, 27 from open fractures Type I or II, and 28 from third degree open fractures. Fifty-three patients were primarily treated with plate osteosynthesis, 11 with intramedullary nails and 12 by other means. The average time between accident and the combined treatment was 11 months.

There can be no doubt that in a high percentage of the 55 patients with open fractures the development of infected pseudarthrosis could have been avoided if they had primarily been treated by external fixation.

Table I. Results in 76 patients with infected pseudarthrosis of the tibia treated with external fixation and gentamicin-PMMA chains (Klemm and Jenny, 1979).

n = 76			
Sex		**Age**	
♂ = 64 ♀ = 12		Ø 35 years	

Type of Accident			Type of Fracture	
Traffic	Pedestrian	15	Closed	21
	Cyclist	18	Open I - II°	27
	By car	11	Open III°	28
No traffic		32		

Time between injury and E.F.+ gentamicin-PMMA-treatment	Primary treatment of fractures	
Ø 11 months	Plates	53
	Intramedullary nail	11
	Another	12

Results	n	%
Pseudarthrosis consolidated, infection subsided	64	84.2
Pseudarthrosis persisted, infection subsided	2	2.6
Pseudarthrosis consolidated, infection persisted	5	6.6
Pseudarthrosis persisted, infection persisted	5	6.6
Amputation	5	

Complications		
Pin tract infection	10	
Refracture after removal of E.F.	2	

References

1. Klemm, K., Jenny, G.: Traitement des pseudarthroses infectées par fixateur externe et Gentabilles - A propos d'une serie de 127 cas. Compte rendu des 7èmes journées internationales du fixateur externe d'Hoffmann. Montpellier/Avignon, France, janvier 1980. Diffinco Sa Geneva/Suisse, 1979.

2. Wahlig, H., E. Dingeldein, R. Bergmann, K. Reuss: The release of gentamicin from polymethylmethacrylate beads. J. Bone Jt. Surg. 60B, 270, 1978.

External Fixation as a Secondary Procedure

A. K. Hedley and M. L. Bernstein

Introduction

Primary use of external fixation devices is commonplace wherever major trauma is encountered. Application of these devices is primarily restricted to compound fractures, both of the upper and lower limb of Type II and Type III magnitude. Use of these devices allows access to the associated soft-tissue injuries, facilitating adequate nursing care and eventual soft tissue procedures (Brooker, 1978; Connes, 1973; Jackson, 1978; Karlstrom, 1975; Krempen, 1979; Lawyer, 1980; Stone, 1981). The use of external fixation as a secondary procedure after failure of primary treatment has not yet been extensively reviewed in the literature. Krempen, Silver, and Sotello (1978) presented their results in the treatment of 23 pseudarthroses using the Hoffmann device. All infections were eradicated and only two cases failed to unite, with a mean healing time of ten months. Vidal and Connes (1978) reported on 100 cases of infected nonunions treated with the external fixator. An 80% rate of control of infection was reported with healing times ranging from seven to ten months.

We would like to report on a series of patients who have had external fixation devices applied after failure of primary treatment. The majority of these patients were infected or had a history of infection associated with their injury in the recent past. The external fixator was selected as the treatment of choice in these cases due to the presence of infection or to the situation of the fracture which rendered it difficult to treat by more conventional methods.

All but one of these patients have been successfully treated both in terms of the infection and of delayed union. Angular deformities have been virtually minimal and residual shortenings have all been within acceptable limits.

Materials and Methods

Our series of 22 patients consists of 18 men and four women (Table I). Average age was 30 years. Eighteen suffered from high velocity injuries in motor vehicle accidents. The patients had an average of two other significant orthopedic problems.

TABLE I

CASE	AGE	INJURY	INFECTION	LOCAL PROBLEMS	TIME SINCE INJURY	TIME ON	OTHER PROCEDURES	WEIGHT BEARING	PIN PROBLEMS	TIME TO HEALING
R.M.	27	Open Tibia, Delayed Union	No	Skin necrosis	4 Mo.	24 Wk.	None	T.D.W.B.	Multiple pin drainage, device off	10 Mo.
A.M.	43	Open Tibia, Delayed Union	No	100% anterior displacement	3.5 Mo.	10 Wk.	None	N.W.B.	None	8 Mo.
B.S.	23	Open Radius with Carpal Dislocation, Delayed Union	No	None	3 Mo.	8 Wk.	None	----	None	2.5 Mo.
A.F.	24	Closed Tibia, Non-union	No	None	7 Mo.	11 Wk.	Iliac crest graft	T.D.W.B.	None	5 Mo.
D.P.	25	Open Tibia, Non-union	No	None	6 Mo.	11 Wk.	None	N.W.B.	None	7 Mo.
T.H.	28	Open Tibia, Non-union	No	None	21 Mo.	12 Wk.	Fibular osteotomy	N.W.B.	Single pin out for drainage	8 Mo.
C.M.	34	Open Tibia, Non-union	No	None	42 Mo.	16 Wk.	Iliac crest graft	T.D.W.B.	None	10 Mo.
G.D.	30	Open Tibia, Non-union	Yes	Draining	8 Mo.	10 Wk.	Debridement	Unrestricted	Single pin out for drainage	8 Mo.
R.K.	34	Open Tibia, Non-union	Yes	Draining	6 Mo.	13 Wk.	Debridement	T.D.W.B.	None	6 Mo.
L.J.	32	Open Tibia, Non-union	Yes	30° Valgus	36 Mo.	12 Wk.	Debridement, Iliac crest graft	T.D.W.B.	None	6 Mo.
D.G.	26	Open Tibia, Non-union	Yes	30° Valgus	6 Mo.	30 Wk.	Debridement, Iliac crest graft	Unrestricted	Loosened after fall	10 Mo.
J.M.	24	Open Tibia, Non-union	Yes	Draining, Skin loss	7 Mo.	12 Wk.	Debridement, Iliac crest graft	Unrestricted	Single pin out for drainage	7 Mo.

TABLE I (CONTINUED)

CASE	AGE	INJURY	INFECTION	LOCAL PROBLEMS	TIME SINCE INJURY	TIME ON	OTHER PROCEDURES	WEIGHT BEARING	PIN PROBLEMS	TIME TO HEALING
R.S.	25	Open Tibia, Non-union	Yes	Draining, multiple sinuses	30 Mo.	28 Wk.	Debridement, Iliac crest graft	T.D.W.B.	None	10 Mo.
C.G.	22	Open Tibia, Non-union	Yes	Failed Lotte's nail	36 Mo.	10 Wk.	Debridement, Iliac crest graft	Unrestricted	Superficial pin infection	6 Mo.
R.F.	47	Open Tibia, Non-union	Yes	Poor skin	33 Mo.	32 Wk.	Debridement, Iliac crest graft	T.D.W.B.	None	10 Mo.
B.G.	20	Closed Tibia, Non-union	Yes (2° to prior treatment)	Drainage, deformity	7 Mo.	10 Wk.	Debridement, Iliac crest graft	T.D.W.B.	None	4 Mo.
J.E.	33	Open Humerus, Non-union	Yes	25° Varus	24 Mo.	20 Wk.	Debridement, Iliac crest graft	----	Superficial pin infection	6 Mo.
C.A.	24	Open Humerus, Non-union	Yes	Draining	14 Mo.	38 Wk.	Debridement, compression	----	None	10 Mo.
A.K.	32	Open forearm, segmental Ulna, Non-union	Yes	Draining	60 Mo.	10 Wk.	Debridement, Iliac crest graft	----	None	4 Mo.
D.T.	25	Open, Segmental Femur	No	Extruded fragment	2 Mo.	11 Wk.	Sterilized segment plus Iliac crest graft	N.W.B.	Multiple pin drainage, device off	13 Mo.
A.S.	48	Open, Segmental Femur	Yes	Drainage	6 Mo.	22 Wk.	Debridement, Iliac crest plus fibular graft	T.D.W.B.	None	13 Mo.
D.F.	25	Open, Segmental Femur	Yes	Drainage	27 Mo.	10 Wk.	Vascularized fibular graft	N.W.B.	Loosening, drainage	Not Healed

Injuries treated included three delayed unions, four noninfected nonunions, 12 infected or previously infected nonunions, and three open femoral injuries with segmental bone loss. Four upper extremity cases, three femurs, and 15 tibias were treated in this series.

Average duration from injury to our application of external fixation was 17 months, with a range of $2\frac{1}{2}$ to 60 months. The patients had undergone an average of three previous procedures, with one patient having undergone seven previous procedures.

For the purpose of this review, a nonunion is defined as clinical instability persisting at six months after injury, without roentgenographic evidence of union. Time to union is defined as the time from application of the fixator to unprotected use of the extremity.

Management

1. External fixators were applied in conjunction with thorough debridement in infected cases or bone grafting in noninfected cases. Grafting with cancellous or corticocancellous bone was performed two to four weeks after debridement in infected cases. Pins were inserted percutaneously with the hand brace, avoiding tension in the skin and soft tissues.

2. All patients with positive preoperative and/or intraoperative cultures were treated with intravenous antibiotics for six weeks. The choice of antibiotic was based on sensitivity studies and consultation with the Infectious Disease Service.

3. Compression was applied whenever bone apposition was possible due to the configuration of the fracture; shortening of one centimeter or less was accepted to obtain compressible surfaces. Patients were followed at one to two-week intervals with the adjustment of compression at these visits. In patients in whom the fixator was initially applied as a neutralization or distraction device, compression was gradually applied as callus was seen radiologically.

4. Pin cleansing was performed with hydrogen peroxide followed by providone-iodine paint three times per day. Erythematous, tense skin was incised at follow up visits. Superficial erythema or infection was treated with elevation and oral antibiotics. Pin loosening accompanied by drainage was treated by removal of the involved pins.

5. After device removal, all patients were protected with a cast or orthosis for a minimum of four to six weeks before unrestricted use of the extremity was allowed.

Results

Overall, 22 of 23 fractures (96%) united with this treatment and 13 of 14 infected cases (93%) were free from drainage at last follow-up.

Delayed Unions

External fixation was selected for these patients because of skin problems or fracture configurations which made treatment difficult with conventional methods. These three fractures united without grafting on an average of 6.8 months. Average duration of fixation was 14 weeks.

Noninfected nonunions

These patients were treated with external fixation for an average of 12.5 weeks with bone union at 7.5 months. Two patients had iliac crest bone grafting at the time of application of the device. The other two patients had transverse fractures which were successfully treated by compression without grafting.

Infected nonunions

Seven of the 12 patients in this category had frank drainage at the time of admission. The remaining five had previously documented but inadequately treated infections. Initial treatment consisted of debridement and application of the fixator, plus appropriate intravenous antibiotic therapy.

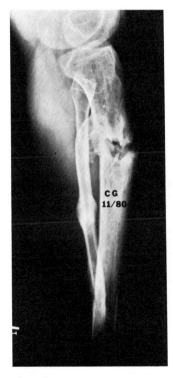
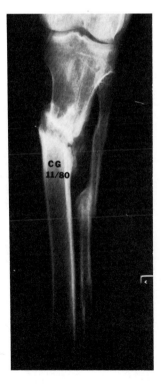
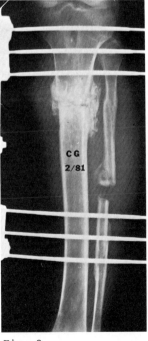

Fig. 2.

Fig. 1.

268

Nine patients were subsequently grafted with iliac crest bone. The other three patients healed with debridement and compression without graft. The external fixator was applied for an average of 18.8 weeks. Functional union was achieved on an average of 7.3 months. No significant difference in healing times between grafted and ungrafted fractures was observed. All infection were eradicated, and none has recurred to date (Fig. 1-5).

Segmental femur fractures

One patient was treated with replacement of a sterilized, freeze-dried extruded segment of his own femur. Another had fibular plus iliac crest grafting (Fig. 6) while the third was treated with a vascularized free fibular graft anastomosed to a branch of the profunda femoris artery. The first two patients healed in approximately 13 months; the third patient is in the eighth month after a vascularized graft and the fracture has not united. The Hoffmann device loosened at ten weeks and he was placed in a spica cast. He also has persistent wound drainage.

Complications

Nine patients (41%) experienced pin tract problems, of whom two had multiple pin loosening requiring device removal. One was in a severely osteoporotic patient, while the other occurred in a patient who fell with the device in

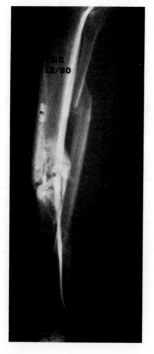 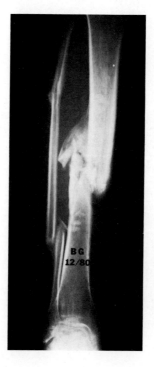 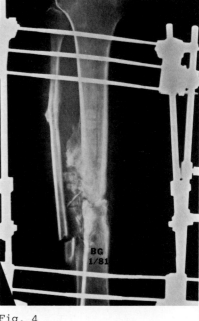

Fig. 4

Fig. 3.

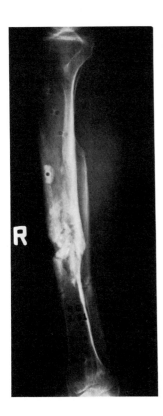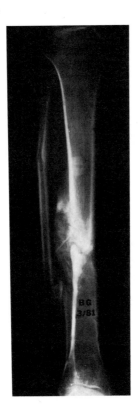

Fig. 5.

situ 30 weeks after its application; his fracture was clinically stable at that time.

Pin tract drainage occurred in seven cases: Two patients had multiple pin drainage requiring removal of the entire device. A single loose pin was found in three patients and was removed, followed by continued use of the fixator. Loose pins tended to be in metaphyseal rather than diaphyseal positions. Two patients with superficial drainage responded to incision of tight skin, elevation, and oral antibiotics.

No cases with drainage went on to persistent pin tract infection or have required treatment other than pin removal.

No patients had neurologic or vascular injury resulting from the use of external fixation in this series. No refractures occurred after discontinuance of protection of the extremity.

Weight bearing

In patients allowed unrestricted weight bearing, 75% experienced single or multiple pin loosening and drainage. This contrasts with pin tract problems in only 12% of patients restricted to touch-down gait with crutches.

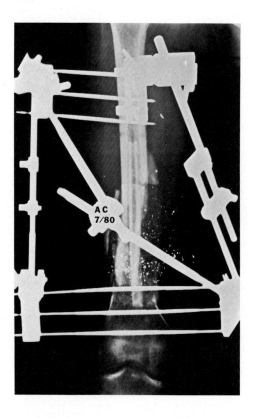

Fig. 6.

Discussion

Delayed and nonunions have historically been challenging orthopedic problems.
An overall rate of union of 96% with resolution of infection in 93% of infected cases was achieved in this series. This compares favorably with
results of other treatments reported in the literature (Meyer, 1975; Müller,
1979).

The external fixator offers clear advantages over other forms of treatment
in allowing ready access for skin and wound care, permitting frequent dressing changes and whirlpool therapy in patients for whom this is desirable.
The rigid fixation and maintenance of near-anatomic alignment offered by the
device also improves the soft tissue environment and promotes granulation.
We found that skin defects up to approximately 5 cm frequently granulated and
epithelialized or required only split thickness skin grafts; full thickness
flap coverage was more frequently necessary with other forms of treatment in
the past. Other authors have had similar results (Lawyer, 1980; Vidal, 1978).

Infected fractures or nonunions appear to be effectively treated by this combination of rigid immobilization, adequate debridement, maximal antibiotic
therapy, and secondary bone grafting when the wound is clean.

The fixators also allow interfragmentary compression where internal fixation
cannot be prudently employed. Stone and Mears (1981) propose that the frame

be gradually made more flexible, and other forms of treatment employed as union proceeds. Our protocol has been somewhat different, maintaining rigid fixation and gradually applying and augmenting compression until clinical stability is achieved. Several established nonunions were treated in this series with compression without grafting and went on to successful union without prolonged healing time compared with grafted fractures. Transverse fractures compressed without graft were observed to heal with minimal callus, attesting to the rigidity of the fixation that can be established. This has also been observed by Lawyer (1980).

Use of these devices requires frequent physician supervision, with inspection of the device and pin tracts at one- to two-week intervals. Pin problems have constantly hampered the use of external fixation and have been largely responsible in the past for the lack of acceptance of this form of treatment. Certain principles of pin care have emerged from our experience:

1. Pins must always be inserted with the hand brace. Use of power equipment will result in wide rings of thermal necrosis with subsequent pin loosening and sometimes persistent pin tract infection (see Fig. 3).

2. Loosened pins cause persistent drainage and must be removed.

3. Conversely, superficial erythema or drainage with a secure pin frequently responds to elevation, restriction of activity, and short courses of oral antibiotics.

4. Skin under tension around pins will undergo necrosis and superficial infection will result. Tight skin must be sharply released at clinic visits.

5. Unrestricted weight bearing leads to loosening. Touch-down weight bearing does not appear to increase the frequency of pin tract problems in lower extremities.

6. Compression should be frequently adjusted, but sufficient overcompression to significantly deform the pins probably contributes to loosening.

7. Protected use of the extremity for a minimum of four to six weeks after discontinuance of the fixator is essential due to the multiple stress risers provided by the pin tracts. While the pin tracts are visible on the roentgenograph long after treatment, the "stress riser" effect is decreased by locally increased trabeculae about the tracts.

External fixation is an effective and desirable secondary treatment for injuries that have failed to unite with primary treatment. Rigid immobilization enhances soft tissue healing while compression of bone fragments further increases stability and augments union. External fixation requires considerable physician involvement and especially close attention to details of pin management.

References

1. Brooker, A., and Edwards, C. (Eds.): External Fixation: Current State of the Art. Williams and Wilkins, Baltimore, 1978.

2. Connes, H: Hoffmann's Double Frame External Anchorage, GEAD, Paris, 1973.

272

3. Jackson, R.P., Jacobs, R.R., and Neff, J.R.: External skeletal fixation in severe limb trauma. J. Trauma 18, 201, 1978.

4. Karlstrom, G., and Olerud, S.: Percutaneous pin fixation of open tibial fractures: Double frame anchorage using the Vidal-Adrey method. J. Bone Jt. Surg. 57A, 915, 1975.

5. Krempen, J.F., Silver, R.A., and Sotello, A.: The use of the Vidal-Adrey external fixation system. Cl. Orthop. 140, 111, 1979.

6. Lawyer, R.B., Jr., and Lubbers, L.M.: Use of the Hoffmann apparatus in the treatment of unstable tibial fractures. J. Bone Jt. Surg. 62A, 1264, 1980

7. Meyer, S., Weiland, A.J., and Willenegger, H.: The treatment of infected nonunions of fractures of the long bones. J. Bone Jt. Surg. 57A, 836, 1975.

8. Müller, M., and Thomas, R.: Treatment of non-unions in fractures of the long bones. Clin. Orthop. 138, 141, 1979.

9. Olerud, S.: Treatment of fractures by the Vidal-Adrey method. Acta Orthop. Scand., 44, 515, 1973.

10. Stone, J.P., and Mears, D.C.: External fixation of open tibial fractures Contemp. Orthop. 3, 310, 1981.

11. Vidal, J., Connes, H., Buscayret, C., and Trovillas, J.: Treatment of infected non-unions by external fixation. In, External Fixation: Current State of the Art. Eds., Brooker and Edwards., Williams and Wilkins, Baltimore, 1978.

12. Vidal, J., Buscayret, C., Connes, H., and Melka, J.: Treatment of open fractures with a loss of osseous substance: Examples from clinical cases. In, External Fixation: Current State of the Art. Eds., Brooker and Edwards; Williams and Wilkins, Baltimore, 1978.

External Fixation of Pelvic Fractures.
Principles of the Trapezoid Compression Frame

P. Slätis, E. O. Karaharju, J.-P. Kaukonen, and A.-L. Kairento

External fixation of the pelvis may be regarded as a routine procedure in all injuries affecting the posterior weight-bearing arch, ie, fractures of the sacrum, the sacroiliac joint, and the massive posterior part of the iliac bones. Accurately applied, external fixators give considerable stability to the fractured pelvis, enabling the patient to use crutches within a few weeks after the accident. The end results are gratifying (Brooker and Edwards, 1979; Karaharju and Slätis, 1978; Muller et al, 1978; Slätis and Karaharju, 1980; Tile and Pennal, 1980). Several mountings have been suggested, in most of which the frame is attached to the iliac wings with one or more crossbars connecting the two sides. Carabalona et al (1973) used single or double transverse crossbars to connect the iliac crests. Mears et al (1980) suggested four ventral compression bars or, in unstable cases, an external frame encircling the entire pelvic girdle and taking hold of the iliac bones with bars introduced through the iliac wings. Boltze et al (1976), of the AO school, mounted their tubular external fixator as a quadrilateral frame attached to the iliac crests. In 1975, we suggested the use of a trapezoid compression frame mounting for the treatment of unstable pelvic fractures (Slätis and Karaharju, 1975).

Surgical Anatomy

The posterior part of the pelvic ring is made up of the sacrum, the sacroiliac joints, and the massive side pillars of the iliac bones. Together, these structures form an arch with the imposts resting on the acetabular roof on either side. Anteriorly, the pelvis consists of the pubic rami which meet in the midline to form the symphysis (Fig. 1a).

In the erect subject, the weight load of the trunk is transmitted along the posterior part of the pelvic ring, the anterior part carrying a negligible load. The weakest areas of the arch are the sacroiliac joints and the juxta-articular cancellous bone. The sacrum is wedged between the iliac bones, the inferior part of the bone being broader than the superior part; hence, unless firmly held, the bone tends to slip forward and downward. The stability of the structure depends on the intricate ligamentous support provided by the dorsal sacroiliac ligaments. It is by these ligaments that the sacrum is suspended. As the weight load increases, the strain on the ligaments forces the sacroiliac joint surfaces closer to each other. It should be noted, however, that the suspension system is firm, movement in the joint normally being negligible. In the sagittal plane, the pelvic girdle is stabilized by the sacrospinous and sacrotuberous ligaments. These attachments prevent the sacrum from descending under the weight of the trunk

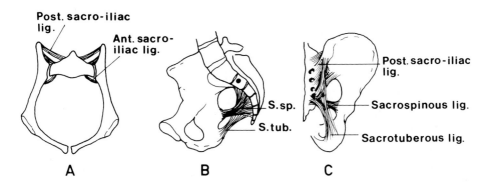

Fig. 1. The ligamentous support of the pelvic girdle in the standing position. A) The sacrum acts as an inverted keystone between the strong weight-bearing pillars of the iliac bones. In this floating position, the sacrum is suspended by strong posterior ligaments. B) Body weight tends to rotate the pelvic girdle around a transverse axis running through the sacroiliac joints (black dot). Pivoting around the axis and undue strain on the sacroiliac joints is prevented by the sacrospinous (s.sp.) and sacrotuberous (s.tub.) ligaments. C) Posterior aspect of the right sacroiliac joint. Note the attachment of the posterior ligaments: a fracture through the longitudinal foramina of the sacrum leaves the stability of the sacroiliac joint largely intact, whereas dislocation of the joint leads to severance of the ligamentous support.

and stabilize the normal inclination of the pelvis towards the axis of the body (Fig. 1b).

Fractures through the sacrum (Figs. 1c, 4a) leave the main ligamentous attachments intact, whereas dislocations of the sacroiliac joint tear the sacroiliac ligaments.

The Trapezoid Compression Frame

With the patient lying on his back, the trapezoid compression frame consists of two vertical bars connected by an upper horizontal bar and a lower compression bar (Fig. 2a).

The upper horizontal bar acts as a fulcrum for the compression force. When the screw on the compression bar is turned to decrease the span between the lower ends of the vertical bars, compression is transmitted to the pelvic girdle. Provided the joints in the connector blocks are firmly locked, the compression effect is conveyed to the sacroiliac joints and the sacrum.

When the patient is standing, the correct inclination of the trapezoid frame is 20° above the horizontal plane (Fig. 2b). With the frame mounted in this

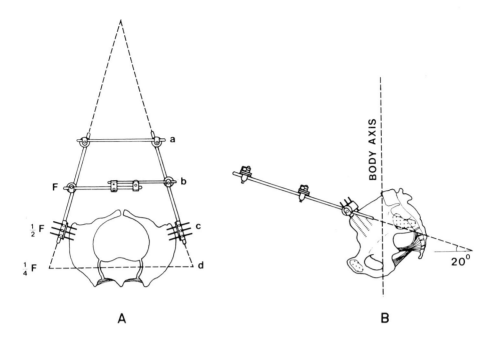

Fig. 2. Force (F) exerted by the trapezoid compression frame. A) The frame is attached to the iliac crests with pins. Compression applied to the frame at level b conveys compression through the iliac wings (level c) to the posterior part of the pelvis (level d). Cf. Table I. B) The correct inclination of the frame is 20° above the horizontal plane in the standing position. With such a mounting, the forces are transmitted through the sacroiliac joints. Note that the sacrospinous and sacrotuberous ligaments act as tension bands below the level of the sacroiliac joints and augment the compressive effect of the frame on these joints.

way, the main force is exerted on the sacroiliac joint, and only a minor force affects the symphysis (Table I). It should be noted that the compression force reaching the posterior part of the pelvis is only about one-fourth the force exerted on the compression bar of the frame.

Reduction of the Fracture

In 20-25% of unstable fractures of the pelvis, gross displacement occurs. The detached hemipelvis is often rotated slightly outward by the weight of the ipsilateral limb, and displaced cephalad by the pull of the trunk muscles. Reduction of the fracture under general anesthesia as soon as possible after admission to hospital is advocated, either in addition to other surgical interventions or as the sole procedure. A television image intensifier, a straight universal operating table, and radiographic equipment are needed.

Table I. Compression forces of a pelvic specimen measured in the compression bar of the trapezoid frame, the sacro-iliac joint and the symphysis. The right hemipelvis had been detached by complete transection of the sacroiliac joint and the symphysis, and subsequently realigned and secured with the external frame, as shown in Fig. 2 and 3.

Compression bar of the frame kp	Sacroiliac joint kp/cm^2	Symphysis kp/cm^2
1.4	0.6	0.42
3.4	1.32	0.72
5.4	1.92	0.96
7.4	2.4	1.08
9.2	3.0	1.32
12.6	3.84	1.5
14.6	4.2	1.62

Displacement of the hemipelvis is reduced in the following way: traction is applied to the ipsilateral limb and the movements of the pelvic fragments are assessed on the television monitor. In severe displacement, the fragments may often be realigned by gentle movements; undue force should be avoided during the first attempts at reduction. Once the posterior arch has been successfully reduced, the reduction is locked by slight internal rotation of the limb. Persistent dorsal displacement of the hemipelvis should now be ruled out by careful palpation of the posterior iliac spines; the patient should not be turned. Any dorsal shift of the hemipelvis is corrected by manual pressure on the dorsal iliac spine in a ventral direction; the lower limb may simultaneously be rotated outward to slacken the posterior soft tissue hinge until realignment of the posterior arch is fully satisfactory.

The pins are inserted percutaneously in the iliac crests. At a preselected point, 2 cm dorsally of the anterior iliac spine, the first of the pins is introduced into the center of the crest with a bit brace. Parallel to the first pin, the other two pins are inserted in a straight line along the crest. Care should be taken to insert the pins between the outer and the inner lamina of the iliac bone. The inclination of the iliac wing can be palpated, or ascertained with the aid of pins inserted subperiosteally, or by open exposure of the iliac crest. We have not encountered intra-abdominal lesions caused by percutaneous introduction of the pins. We have, however, frequently observed pins deviating outward into the gluteal muscles and causing irritation.

The connector blocks are slid down the pins and secured. The lower edge should be about 1 cm above the skin, and at the upper edge the pins should protrude only a few millimeters to prevent obstructing the vertical bars of the frame. The vertical bars are attached to the blocks, the joints

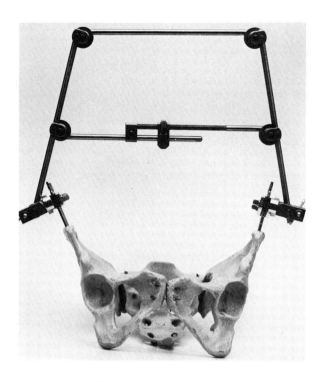

Fig. 3. The trapezoid compression frame mounted on a pelvic specimen. The connector block should be positioned close to the iliac crest, and the pins inserted deep enough in the bone to protrude only a few millimeters above the connector block. The joint in the connector block should be firmly locked before compression is applied to the frame.

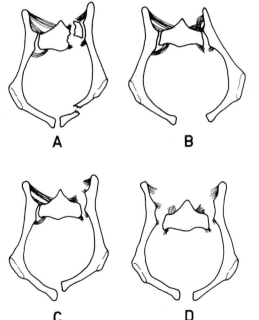

A   B

C   D

Fig. 4. Double vertical lesions to the pelvic girdle suitable for treatment with external frames. A) The commonest lesion: a longitudinal fracture through the sacral foramina with simultaneous fractures of the pubic rami. Reduction is usually simple and the trapezoid frame provides good stability until fracture union is completed. B) The open book lesion: rupture of the symphysis indicates ligamentous injury to the posterior joint. Part of the posterior ligaments here acts as a hinge, which makes realignment easy. The lesion is quite stable after reduction and fixation with a frame. C) The detached hemipelvis: simultaneous complete rupture of the symphysis and the sacroiliac joints. There is always some malalignment of the posterior arch, although the displacement may be slight. Careful reduction and external fixation usually result in good alignment and good stability. D) The dislodged sacrum: a rare lesion with bilateral ruptures of the sacroiliac joints. Reduction is difficult and the external frame merely keeps the unstable iliac wings in position.

slid down the vertical bars, and the upper ends connected with the top horizontal bar. The compression bar is finally mounted midway between the upper
horizontal bar and the connector blocks (Fig. 3).

The alignment of the fracture is checked, with the iliac wings firmly engaged
on the sacrum, the inclination of the iliac wings carefully assessed, and the
joints of the connector blocks firmly locked with the T-driver. The compression screw on the compression bar is then turned in such a way that compression is applied and turning of the screws is continued until the vertical
bars bend. All nuts are then tightened and the fracture position analyzed.
If reduction is adequate, a radiograph is taken. If alignment is unsatisfactory, the frame is removed, the repositioning maneuver repeated as needed,
and the reduction once more secured with the external frame. Fractures of
the sacrum and ilium are usually easy to stabilize with the trapezoid frame.
Dislocations of the sacroiliac joint, on the other hand, may need repeated
efforts at reduction.

The mounting of the frame needs more than one pair of hands and some dexter-
ity. Recently, we have developed a ready mounted frame with glide bearings
in the joints of both horizontal and compression bars. The advantage of
this frame is the ease with which it can be mounted and the good compression
effect obtained with the smooth bearings. Postoperatively, the patient is
transferred to an ordinary bed. Turning is allowed. The pin area is cleaned
daily and covered with dressings.

Radiographs are taken in the operating room, on the second day after the
operations, and 3, 6 and 12 weeks after mounting the frame.

Patients with unilateral fracture dislocations are allowed out of bed three
weeks after the operation and encouraged to move on crutches. The frame is
removed six weeks after the injury. In bilateral injuries to the pelvic
girdle, verticalization of the patient is postponed to eight weeks after
external fixation.

Discussion

The stability achieved with the trapezoid compression frame in the treatment
of unstable pelvic fractures is good in unilateral and satisfactory in bilateral lesions. In laboratory experiments, Gunterberg et al (1978) have
shown that pelvic specimens with unilateral dislocation of the sacroiliac
joint and secured with the frame resisted vertical loads averaging 1,390 N.
When similarly tested, unilateral fractures withstood vertical loads averaging 2,163 N. In bilateral lesions, however, the mean acceptance of load
was only 247 N. The data suggest that unilateral hemipelvic dislocations,
when stabilized with the external frame, tolerate vertical loads exceeding
the normal demands in the standing position. In case of a bilateral hemipelvic displacement, however, the frame will maintain the reduced position,
but the pelvic girdle is not usually stable enough for early weight bearing.
Vecsei et al (1979) stabilized pelvic specimens with three mountings: the
quadrilateral frame of Carabalona, the double ventral compression frame of
the AO tubular fixator system, and the trapezoid compression frame. The
figures obtained revealed that the trapezoid frame exerted three times as
much lateral compression as the quadrilateral frame and the AO tubular

frame. Similarly, the trapezoid frame yielded more rotational stability than the two other frames. The data available on external frames require critical appraisal. External fixation is not a panacea for the treatment of pelvic injuries. Two limitations should be pointed out. Firstly, the problem of the floating sacrum (Fig. 4d) remains largely unsolved. External frames attached to the iliac bones do not get a grip on the dislodged keystone of the weight-bearing arch in this lesion. The sacrum ought to be pushed dorsally and secured to the iliac bones in such a way that forward slipping is prevented. Mears (1980) has pointed out that the bone stock in the sacroiliac area is sufficient for internal fixation; perhaps a combination of internal fixation dorsally and external fixation of the iliac wings will provide stability in these rare lesions. Secondly, external frames are not always applied properly. Uncritical use of compression in unstable pelvic lesions may increase the displacement of the fragments and cause narrowing of the pelvic outlet. Careful assessment of each fracture is needed, reduction and alignment of the fragments are essential, and the effect of the compression frame should be properly understood. When the frame is accurately applied, external fixation of pelvic fractures affords gratifying results and may be used routinely in unilateral lesions. More experience is needed, however, before the merits of different mountings can be evaluated in detail.

Summary

External fixation of the fractured unstable pelvis is advocated as a routine procedure whether or not there is displacement. The frame should exert its stabilizing effect mainly on the posterior weight-bearing part of the pelvis, and should be firm enough to permit early weight bearing. The principles of the trapezoid compression frame are outlined. In clinical practice, the fractured pelvis should be reduced and secured with the frame as soon as possible after the accident.

References

1. Bolze, W.H., Fernandez, D.L., Schatzker, J.: The external fixator. AO Bulletin 62, 1976.

2. Brooker, A.F., and Edwards, C.C.: External Fixation: The Current State of the Art. Williams and Wilkins, Baltimore, 1979.

3. Carabalona, P., Rabichong, P., Bonnel, F., et al: Apports du fixateur externe dans les disjonctions du pubis et de l'articulation sacro-iliaque. Montpellier Chir. 19, 62, 1973.

4. Gunterberg, B., Goldie, I. and Slätis, P.: Fixation of pelvic fractures and dislocations. An experimental study on the loading of pelvic fractures and sacro-iliac dislocations after external compression fixation. Acta Orthop.Scand. 49, 278, 1978

5. Karaharju, E., and Slätis, P.: External fixation of double vertical pelvic fractures with a trapezoid compression frame. Injury 10, 142, 1978.

6. Mears, D.C., and Fu, F.H.: Modern concepts of external skeletal fixation of the pelvis. Clin. Orthop. 151, 65, 1980.

7. Muller, J., Bachmann, B., and Berg, H.: Malgaigne fracture of the pelvis: treatment with percutaneous pin fixation. J.Bone Joint Surg. 60A, 992, 1978.

8. Slätis, P., and Karaharju, E.: External fixation of the pelvic girdle with a trapezoid compression frame. Injury 7, 53, 1975.

9. Slätis, P., and Karaharju, E.: External fixation of unstable pelvic fractures. Experiences in 22 patients treated with a trapezoid compression frame. Clin. Orthop. 151, 73, 1980.

10. Tile, M. and Pennal, G.F.: Pelvic disruption: principles of management Clin. Orthop. 151, 56, 1980.

11. Vecsei, V. and Kuderna, H.: Therapie und Ergebnisse bei Beckenfrakturen unter Verwendung des Fixateur Externe. Hefte Unfallheilk. 140, 129, 1979.

External Fixation of Pelvic Ring Fractures

D. C. Mears

In the past, the management of the patient with an unstable pelvic ring fracture has been an enigma for most orthopedic surgeons. Especially when such a patient, who usually has other serious and potentially life-threatening injuries, is brought to a community hospital, limitations of available treatment methods and the enormous imposition on the resources of such a hospital give rise to a high incidence of morbidity and mortality.

Recently, techniques of external fixation have evolved for the application to the unstable pelvic ring which immensely decrease the magnitude of blood loss. Moreover, external fixation provides effective alleviation of pelvic pain, permits early mobilization with bed to chair transfers, markedly diminishes the risk of severe post-traumatic pulmonary complications, and greatly lessens a costly period of hospitalization.

The unstable pelvic ring fractures were classified by Pennal (1961), Tile et al., (1969), Whiston (1953), and Wilson (1971). One type of an unstable pelvic ring fracture is illustrated in Fig.1.

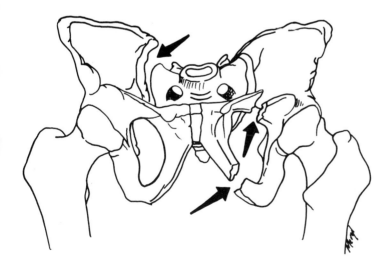

Fig. 1. A schematic diagram showing one type of unstable pelvic ring fracture in which a sacroiliac joint and the contralateral rami have been violated.

An anteroposterior compressive force provokes a disruption of the symphysis pubis with a wide diastasis or multiple fractures of the rami. A lateral compressive force, the most frequently encountered type of unstable pelvic ring fracture, may present one of several patterns of displacement. The anterior disruption may constitute a fracture of one or more pelvic rami or a dislocation of the symphysis pubis, or it may violate both structures. The posterior disruption may violate the ipsilateral or contralateral ilium, sacroiliac joint or the sacrum. Occasionally, multiple posterior disruptions may occur.

A third type of injury, the vertical shear disruption, generally follows the application of the most violent extraneous forces. Usually, the disruptive force is transmitted through a lower extremity via the hip joint and into the pelvic ring. Radiologic evidence of a vertical shear fracture includes an avulsion fracture of the ischial spine with superior migration of the entire hemipelvis. One or more branches of the lumbosacral plexus, especially the L-5 root segment, frequently are injured (Patterson and Morton, 1973). Unless multiple roentgenographic views are taken, the pelvic instability may be overlooked for it may not be evident in the conventional anteroposterior pelvic view. Ancillary roentgenograms, including pelvic inlet and outlet projections, should be obtained. Computerized axial tomography is a valuable ancillary technique which reveals the pattern and degree of disruption of a severe pelvic ring fracture.

The typical patient with an unstable pelvic ring fracture usually shows evidence of other serious injuries to the intra-abdominal organs, intrathoracic structures, central nervous system or to the limbs. Massive hemorrhage and the associated need for urgent fluid replacement should be anticipated. In the past, during the early traumatic period when urgent resuscitative measures were initiated, or during the attempts by general and thoracic surgeons to insert chest tubes and undertake laparotomy, the stabilization of the pelvic ring fracture by the orthopedist was usually deferred. Generally, the pelvic ring fracture was managed by bed rest, a pelvic sling, skeletal traction, a hip spica cast or, rarely, by internal fixation. The nonoperative methods did not provide effective cessation of osseous bleeding from the fracture site nor did they permit early mobilization of the patient. In the presence of prolonged bed rest, Trunkey et al (1974) have documented a high incidence of serious pulmonary, urinary, and psychologic problems. The delayed mortality, secondary to pulmonary complications, has ranged between 10 and 30% in several series. In the few reports where internal fixation of the pelvic ring fracture was undertaken within the first two days after injury, unacceptably high mortality rates have been reported which were attributable to surgical hemorrhage. The nonoperative modalities of treatment, also, have been associated with a high incidence of serious chronic disabilities, such as a significant leg length discrepancy, severe low back pain, sacroiliac pain, markedly displaced nonunions, and, in women, obstetric problems. During the past twenty years, sporadic attempts to employ external skeletal fixation for the immobilization of an unstable pelvic ring fracture have been reported by several American and European centres (Brooker and Edwards, 1979; Carabalona and Bonnel, 1973; Connes, 1973; Gunterberg et al, 1978; Mears, 1979; Muller et al, 1978; Riska et al, 1979). By the use of a simple anterior frame, marked diminution in the severity of fracture pain was observed although most of these early attempts were accompanied by a late loss of reduction of the fracture unless the patient was maintained at bed rest for at least a few weeks.

Nevertheless, these observations stimulated the author to undertake biomechanical and clinical studies on the use of external fixation for markedly
unstable pelvic ring fractures (Brown, personal communication). A series
of fresh cadaveric specimens obtained from young individuals were used to
assess the rigidity of a variety of previously employed frames and of
various novel designs. Combinations of internal and external fixation as
well as novel types of internal fixation were investigated. These results
will be published elsewhere (Mears et al, in press). From this study it
was evident that the previous designs of anterior frames, such as those
devised by Slätis and Carabalona, failed to provide adequate fixation to
permit early bed to chair transfers or ambulation. Two novel designs of
external fixation improvised by myself provided adequate rigidity so that
immediate bed to chair transfers could be implemented. One technique is
a modification of the Slätis design of an anterior frame in which the
rigidity of the frame is augmented (Fig. 2).

The other method involves the erection of a more sophisticated frame
(anteroposterior type) for the treatment of a markedly comminuted pelvic
ring fracture or one which is accompanied by a central acetabular or a
femoral fracture. The second method mentioned is technically challenging;
the anteroposterior frame hampers the nursing care. As a result, such a
method is reserved for very special cases. The optimal stability, however,
is obtained when an anterior frame is augmented by the use of posterior
internal or external fixation. Our clinical experience favors the use of
posterior internal fixation.

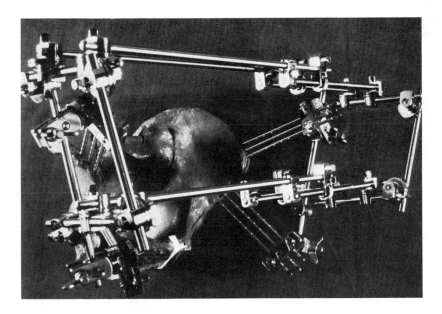

Fig. 2. A photograph presenting the modified anterior pelvic fixation frame with half pins inserted
into the anterosuperior and anteroinferior
iliac crests.

Table I. Management algorithm for the control of hemorrhage
in the patient with an unstable pelvic ring fracture

I. During the transfer to the hospital by helicopter or ambulance

   a. Administer IV fluids
   b. Apply MAST suit

II. In the Emergency Room, assess the stability of the cardiovascular system

   A. Unstable, hypovolemic patient

      1. Blood and IV fluid replacement
      2. Paracentesis or minilaparotomy; if positive, undertake laparotomy.
      3. Apply rigid external pelvic fixation.
      4. If still unstable cardiovascular system with shock, undertake selective arteriography with a balloon catheter or embolization.
      5. Upon failure of (4) explore the site of the bleeding intrapelvic vessel.

   B. Stable patient

      Undertake primary internal or external fixation of the posterior and anterior sites of pelvic disruption.

From the clinical studies undertaken at the University of Pittsburgh, and from comparable documentation reported by Edwards at the Maryland Shock Trauma Center in Baltimore, the use of external skeletal fixation has been observed to provide several benefits. The foremost is the control of hemorrhage provoked by the pelvic fracture. The protocol employed at the University of Pittsburgh for the control of hemorrhage in a patient with a pelvic ring fracture is presented in Table I above.

On the day after the application of external pelvic fixation, the patient with an unstable pelvic fracture is encouraged to logroll in bed and to undertake independent transfers from bed to chair. With this increased activity and upright posture, the patient has a marked lessening of risk in the incidence of serious pulmonary complications such as infection and pulmonary emboli. Within a few days after surgery, and provided that the management of other injuries permits, an attempt is made to discharge the patient to his home with a bed to chair existence. This technique greatly facilitates nursing care of open pelvic or appendicular wounds and prevents the problems associated with prolonged bed rest and recumbency. During the operative procedure, a closed reduction of the fracture is undertaken. When postoperative roentgenograms have been scrutinized, an adjustment of the reduction may be undertaken whenever required. Whatever reduction is accepted can be maintained until the fracture has united.

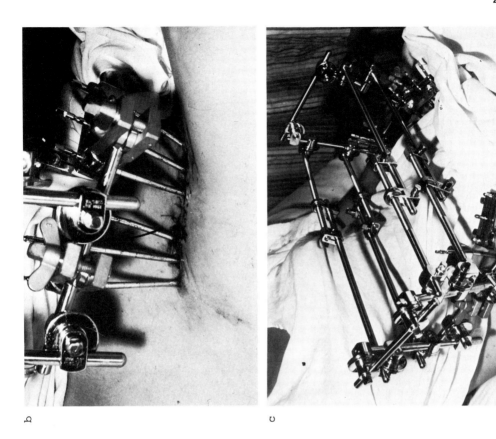

a

b

c

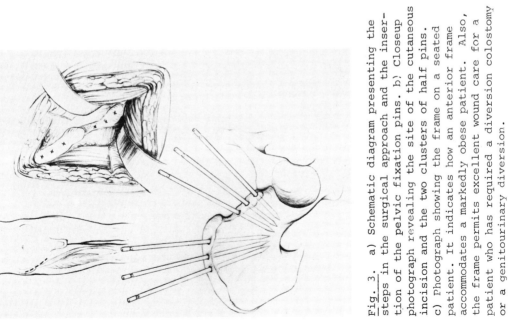

Fig. 3. a) Schematic diagram presenting the
steps in the surgical approach and the insertion of the pelvic fixation pins. b) Closeup
photograph revealing the site of the cutaneous
incision and the two clusters of half pins.
c) Photograph showing the frame on a seated
patient. It indicates how an anterior frame
accomodates a markedly obese patient. Also,
the frame permits excellent wound care for a
patient who has required a diversion colostomy
or a genitourinary diversion.

Technique

After a general anesthetic has been administered, the patient is placed in a supine position. The upper half of a Smith-Petersen incision is made along each anterior iliac crest (Fig. 3a). A subperiosteal plane is developed along the superficial and deep surfaces of the crest. The sartorius and the direct head of rectus femoris are sharply incised from the pelvis. Retractors are placed along the inner and outer tables of the iliac crest so that the bone can be visualized during the insertion of the fixation pins. With the use of a hand brace, three half pins are inserted into each anterosuperior and anteroinferior iliac crest with a space of about 1 cm between each pin (Fig. 3b). The two ipsilateral clusters of pins exit from the bone with an angle of about 45° between them. A ball joint is attached to each cluster, and a straight rod is used to bridge the two ipsilateral ball joints. Two articulation couplings are added to each of the straight rods. Another straight rod is attached to each of the four articulation couplings and directed perpendicular to the long axis of the patient. The straight rods attached to each hemipelvis are forcefully approximated to one another to reduce a diastasis. To reduce a superior migration of a hemipelvis, traction can be applied to a lower extremity, preferably by the use of a fracture table. Rotational deformity, also, can be corrected under roentgenogram control by manipulation of the straight rods which serve as lever arms and, thereby, facilitate the reduction. Two Vidal-type quadrilateral frames are assembled and attached to the four vertically aligned straight rods (Fig. 3c). A final straight rod is applied to the tips of the vertical, straight rods mounted to each hemipelvis. The wounds are irrigated and closed loosely around each cluster of pins.

On the day after external fixation, the patient is encouraged to move from his bed into a chair. Supplementary roentgenograms are taken to reveal the reduction of the fracture fragments. Adjustments in alignment are undertaken, as necessary, with the patient in bed, without general anesthesia. All fixation nuts are tightened on the first and third postoperative days, and subsequently at weekly intervals. Routine pin track care is initiated on the day after surgery. The patient and the family are shown how to clean each pin site by swabbing it with a cotton applicator soaked in hydrogen peroxide.

The patient is discharged to his home when the condition is stable and when patient and family can look after the external frame. Six to 10 weeks later, the patient is readmitted for the removal of the external frame. Under ketamine hydrochloride anesthesia, the external frame is disassembled. The union of the fracture is confirmed by clinical and radiologic assessment. Then, the half pins are removed and the pin tracks are irrigated with Betadine solution. The anterior frame is extremely useful for reduction and stabilization of the symphysis pubis. The application of the anterior frame is technically easy and can be performed quite quickly in case of massive bleeding. For the construction of more sophisticated frames that employ transfixing pins in the iliac crests, the reader is referred to previous publications (Mears, 1979; 1980).

Complex Pelvic Fractures

Certain complex pelvic ring fractures may in some cases be managed by the use of external fixation. An open pelvic fracture is particularly suited to this form of treatment. Most of the open fractures are Grade III injuries with extensive soft tissue damage and contamination. By the application of external fixation, the soft tissue injuries may be readily examined, debrided, and cleaned on the ward. In the presence of an open pelvic fracture with an open wound in the perineum, even in the presence of an intact anal sphincter, a diversion colostomy is mandatory. Otherwise, feculent material passes from the rectum into the open wounds causing a severe intrapelvic infection that usually culminates in a fatal outcome.

Materials and Results

Over the last 3 1/2 years, 20 patients with unstable pelvic fractures were treated with these methods. Most of the patients were polytraumatized and required a team approach to their management. There were 10 men and 10 women with an age range from 17 to 70 years. Most of them were involved in vehicular accidents. There were 12 Malgaigne fractures, four wide diastases of the symphysis pubis, and three complex comminuted fractures that also involved multiple pelvic rami. Four patients also had central acetabular fractures. Six of the fractures were open so that an early diversion colostomy was required. The results indicate that 14 of the patients obtained marked pain relief within a day after application. Fourteen patients were out of bed within a week after surgery, and three of the patients who were managed with an anteroposterior frame were able to ambulate. There was one postoperative loss of reduction and no non-unions. Four deaths occurred from unrelated injuries. One obese patient died from a massive pulmonary embolism one day after application of the frame. Nine of the patients were able to resume normal activities within four months after their injuries.

Discussion

While previous use of pelvic external fixation devices applied to pelvic fractures provided substantial pain relief for the patient, they did not stabilize an unstable pelvic ring fracture sufficiently to prevent late loss of reduction, nor permit early active transfers from bed to chair or independent partial weight-bearing gait. With the two configurations of external fixation devices assembled from the Hoffmann apparatus described here, we have realized these surgical objectives with minimal morbidity associated with the device and an acceptable incidence of complications. Nevertheless, the pelvic frames are cumbersome and require daily nursing care of the pin tracks and the external frame itself.

During the past two years, we have studied alternative types of external fixation devices of superior design which will be described elsewhere. Furthermore, we have undertaken biomechanical and anatomical laboratory investigations on methods to obtain stable internal fixation of comparable pelvic ring fractures. Most previous attempts at internal fixation have used wires or screws which provided inadequate stability or they have

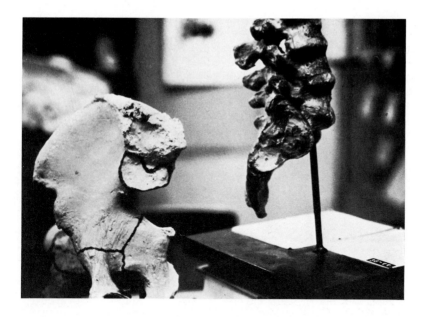

Fig. 4. Photograph showing a cadaveric pelvis in which
the thick bone stock available on either side of the
sacroiliac joint is evident.

focused on stabilization of the anterior segment of the pelvic ring where
the available bone stock does not lend itself to rigid fixation (Jenkins
and Young, 1978; Trunkey et al, 1974; Whiston, 1953; Wilson et al, 1971).
Few previous efforts have been directed towards fixation of the posterior
violation of the disrupted pelvic ring. While, at first glance, the
posterior ilium and adjacent portion of the sacrum seem to possess
irregular surfaces, unfavorably shaped for the application of internal
fixation devices, upon closer scrutiny a different impression emerges.
In fact, the vicinity of the sacroiliac joint provides a highly satisfactory source of bone stock (Fig. 4). The site is readily approached
by a longitudinal incision superficial to the sacroiliac joint. The most
superior origin of the gluteus maximus is reflected sharply in an inferior
and lateral direction. A subluxation or dislocation of the sacroiliac
joint, or of the adjacent portion of the posterior ilium, is reduced by
the application of a bone-holding forceps applied to a projecting cancellous lag screw that is deeply embedded into each of the fracture fragments. Three or four cancellous lag screws are applied in a longitudinal
array which traverse the fracture from the ilium to the ala of the sacrum.
Alternatively, the screws may be applied through an appropriately contoured
bone plate situated on the principal iliac fracture fragment parallel to
the sacroiliac joint where the plate functions as an enlarged washer. An
example is shown in Fig. 5.

After surgery, the patient is permitted to undertake active independent
movements and to walk with a partial weight-bearing gait. Generally, at
about six weeks after surgery, a full weight-bearing gait is restored.

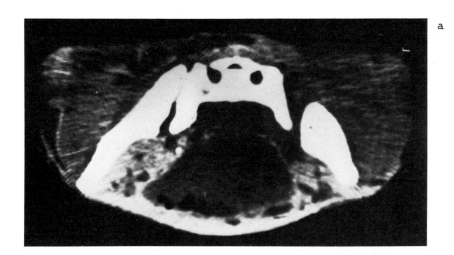

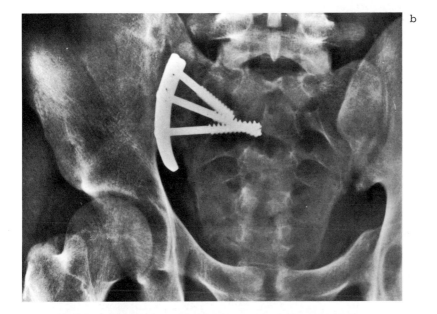

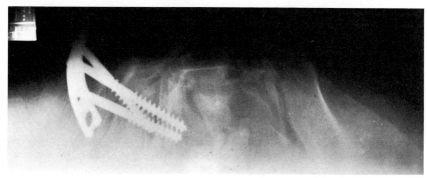

Fig 5.
(for legend
see next
page)

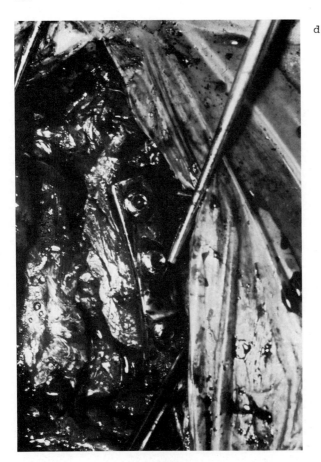

d

Fig. 5. a) A computerized axial tomogram illustrating the sacroiliac joint of a young man with a lateral compression injury causing a dislocation of the right sacroiliac joint and fractures of the left rami. As seen in subsequent anteroposterior and oblique radiographs (b and c), open reduction and internal fixation of the sacroiliac joint was performed in which three cancellous lag screws were applied across the joint. d) An intraoperative photograph revealing the plate applied to the superficial surface of the ilium adjacent to the sacroiliac joint, which serves as a large "washer".

Where the posterior fracture involves the sacrum rather than the sacroiliac joint or the adjacent posterior ilium, stable internal fixation is difficult to realize. Currently, we are studying the possible application of long plates that extend transversely from one to the other posterior ilium. When the pelvic ring is wholly unstable, such posterior fixation is combined with the application of an anterior plate on the disrupted symphysis pubis. Alternatively, a smaller anterior external frame, similar to that described by Slätis, is applied for the stabilization of the disrupted symphysis or of the adjacent rami fractures.

Summary

The management of unstable pelvic fractures remains a major challenge to the orthopedic surgeon. The principal goals should include provision for immediate reduction and stabilization of the fracture to minimize pain, hemorrhage, late pulmonary complications, and various chronic musculo-skeletal disabilities frequently associated with these massive traumas. Of all currently available treatment modalities, external skeletal fixation appears to be the most effective method.

The anterior fixation frame is simple to apply; it provides adequate stability for the patient to move independently from bed to a chair. It does not provide adequate posterior stability to resist the forces encountered in independent ambulation which, therefore, should be deferred.

A more sophisticated external frame which employs multiple transfixing pins in either ilium provides a greater degree of stability so that early ambulation can be encouraged. Special instruments, however, are required. The elaborate surgical technique necessitates appropriate expertise and familiarity by the surgical team. Currently, a variety of superior methods to obtain rigid posterior stabilization of the pelvic ring by resort to internal or external fixation or various combinations of these methods is under investigation in our laboratories.

References

1. Brooker, A.F., Edwards, C.C.: External Fixation: The Current State of the Art, Williams and Wilkins Co., Baltimore, p. 3, 1979.

2. Brown, T.D., et al: Personal communication.

3. Carabalona, P., Bonnel, F., et al: Apports des fixateurs externes dans les disjonctions du pubis et de l'articulation sacro-ilque. Montpell.Chir.19, 61-70, 1973.

4. Connes, H.: Hoffman's Double Frame External Anchorage. GEAD, Paris, p. 97, 1973.

5. Edwards, C.C.: Personal communication.

6. Gunterberg, B., Goldie, I., and Slätis, P.: Acta Orthop.Scand. 49, 278-286, 1978.

7. Jenkins, D.H.R., and Young, M.H.: Operative treatment of sacroiliac subluxation and disruption of the symphysis pubis. Injury, 10, 139-141, 1978.

8. Karaharju, E.O., and Slätis, P.: External fixation of double vertical pelvic fractures with a trapezoid compression frame. Injury, 10, 142-145, 1978.

9. Mears, D.C.: Percutaneous pin fixation. In: Materials and Orthopaedic Surgery, Williams and Wilkins, Co., Baltimore, 1979.

10. Mears, D.C.: The management of complex pelvic fractures. In: External Fixation: The Current State of the Art. A.F. Brooker and C.C. Edwards (eds.) Williams and Wilkins, Baltimore, p. 151, 1979.

11. Mears, D.C. and Fu, F.: Modern concepts of external fixation. Clin. Orthop. 151, 65-72, 1980.

12. Mears, D.C. and Fu, F.: External fixation in pelvic fractures. Orthop. Clin. N. Am., 11, 1980.

13. Mears, D.C., Brown, T.D., Fu, F., Stone, P., Rubash, H., and Nelson, D. In press. 1981.

14. Muller, J., Bachmann, B.: Behandlung von instabilen Beckenring-Frakturen mit dem äusseren Spanner nach Wagner. Helv. Chir. Acta 45, 59-61, 1978.

15. Muller, J., Bachmann, B. and Berg H.: Malgaigne fracture of the pelvis: Treatment with percutaneous pin fixation. J. Bone Jt. Surg., 60A, 1978.

16. Muller, K.H., and Muller-Farber, J.: Die Osteosynthese mit dem Fixateur externe am Becken. Arch. Orthop. Traumat. Surg. 92, 273-283, 1978.

17. Patterson, F.P., Morton, K.S.: Neurological complications of fractures and dislocations of the pelvis. J. Trauma, 12, 1013-1023, 1973.

18. Pennal, G.F., and Sutherland, G.O.: Fractures of the pelvis. AAOS, Film Library, 1961.

19. Riska, E.B., et al: External fixation of unstable pelvic fractures. Int. Orthop., 3, 183-188, 1979.

20. Tile, M.: Pelvic fractures: Operative vs Nonoperative treatment. Ortho. Clin. N. Am. 11, 423-463, 1980.

21. Tile, M., and Pennal, G.F.: Fractures of the pelvis. Proc. Seventh Meeting of the Hip Society, pp 313-327, 1979.

22. Trunkey, D.D., et al: Management of pelvic fractures in blunt trauma injury. J. Trauma, 14, 912-923, 1974.

23. Whiston, G.: Internal fixation for fractures and dislocations of the pelvis. J. Bone Jt. Surg., 35A, 701-706, 1953.

24. Wilson, R.F., Mammen, E., and Walt, A.J.: Eight years of experience with massive blood transfusions. J. Trauma, 11, 275-285, 1971.

Pelvic Fracture Stabilization with Hoffmann External Fixation

D. L. Burke and A. Miller

Fractures of the pelvis constitute approximately 3% of all fractures. The majority of these are either of the avulsion type with minimal displacement or single breaks of the pelvic ring. A smaller group, ranging from 10.5 to 30.5% (Slätis and Huittinen, 1972), are of a more serious nature involving major disruptions of the pelvic ring. These correspond to Type III injuries of the Key and Conwell classification. In this group, conservative methods of treatment have been associated with residual deformity, leg length discrepancy, sacroiliac pain and complications requiring prolonged bed rest. Interest in open reduction has been revived by Jenkins (1978) and Mears (1980) in spite of the surgical difficulty, hazards of blood loss, and risk of infection.

Following wide and successful use of external fixation devices in extremity fracture management, interest has been generated in their application to major pelvic injuries (Carabalona et al, 1973; Connes, 1973; Grosse, 1979; Karaharju and Slätis, 1978; Johnston, 1979; Mears, 1980). For the past five years, we have used selectively the Hoffmann External Fixator to manage major pelvic fractures. The method has been successful in facilitating the care of the polytraumatized patients, as well as producing better results than we could obtain by closed methods.

The major objectives were to achieve and/or facilitate: 1) fixation for pain relief; 2) easier nursing care; 3) management of associated injuries; 4) mobility for the patient, and 5) more anatomic results than could be obtained by other methods of closed treatment. Early ambulation was not a major objective.

Materials

Seventeen multiple traumatized patients with unstable pelvic fractures were treated with Hoffmann external fixation between September 1975 and November 1980 at the Montreal General Hospital. There were 13 men and 4 women, ranging from 16 to 65 years of age, with a mean age of 29.8 years. The mechanism of injury involved automobile/pedestrian accidents in 11 patients, motorcycle or bicycle accidents in four patients, one fall from a horse and one suicide attempt by jumping in front of a commuter train. All patients had Type III (Key and Conwell classification) unstable pelvic fractures. Ten "Malgaigne Type" fractures (Type III-B with anterior ring disruption of either ipsi- or contralateral pubic rami or diastasis of the symphysis) and seven severe multiple fractures (Type III-C) constitute the series. The Malgaigne group had hemipelvis ascension of greater than 2.0 cm in six (range 2.0 cm to 6.0 cm) and four had "open-book" displacement with symphysis diastasis of greater than 3 cm. Two injuries were compounded through severe perineal wounds. Symphysis diastasis in the entire series ranged from 2.5 cm to 9.0 cm with an average of 4.5 cm. A compound perineal injury was present in each of the two groups. Associated acetabular fractures occurred in four of the Type III-C injuries and two underwent concomitant open reduction and internal fixation of the acetabular component.

Fifty-nine major associated injuries occurred including 25 lower extremity fractures (3 compound), eight upper extremity fractures or dislocations, four lumbar spine fractures, three urethral tears requiring suprapubic cystostomy, two rectal lacerations requiring defunctioning colostomy, two facial bone fractures, four peripheral neurovascular injuries, five closed chest injuries and six closed head injuries.

The Hoffmann apparatus was applied on the day of injury in seven patients, between 4 and 10 days in six patients, and between 20 and 50 days in four patients. The delays were due mainly to the patients' unfitness for a general anesthetic, delayed transfer and/or failure to maintain reduction by more classical closed techniques.

Method

The patient is positioned supine under general anesthesia. Three threaded half pins are then inserted percutaneously, using a drill brace, into the anteroiliac crest with maximum spacing after first establishing the plane of the inner and outer tables using probe pins. The pilot grips are applied to the pins at skin level and the frame is partially constructed with ball joint units, straight and slider bars, and articulation units. The ball joint grips are applied immediately adjacent to the pilot grips. Reduction is then performed using combinations of manual and skeletal traction forces to correct the triplane deformity. Compressive forces should not be applied before correction of cephalad or posterior displacements of the ilium. Reduction is checked with radiographs following locking of the frame. Skeletal traction, if required for reduction and it feasible, is maintained for up to six weeks.

In this series, only anterior frames of the following configurations were used: 1) single transverse tie bars, 2) quadrilateral (Carabalona, 1973), or 3) trapezoidal (Slätis, 1975). The single transverse bar was used in two "open-book" injuries with symphysis diastasis where simple compressive force was required. The trapezoidal frame was applied in the other two "open-book" injuries, in two with hemipelvis ascension, and two of the multiple fracture group. The quadrilateral frame was used in the other nine cases.

Two cases will be used for illustration.

Case I. A 23-year old male motorcyclist sustained a pelvic injury (Fig. 1) with a fracture of the left superior and inferior pubic rami, a transverse fracture of the right acetabulum, subluxations of the left and right sacroiliac joints and a 9 cm diastasis of the symphysis pubis. Associated injuries included a ruptured membranous urethra, severe perineal laceration involving the rectum, laceration of the right groin with transection of the right femoral artery and a compound fracture of the right femur. Following resusci-

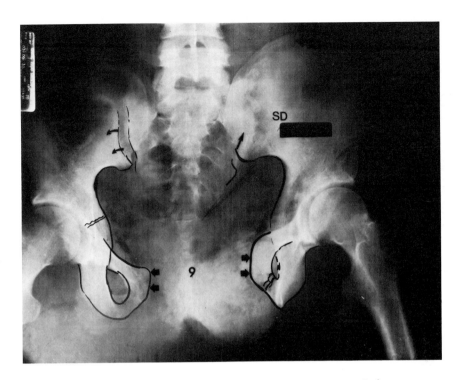

Fig. 1. Case I (SD) - Prereduction radiograph of pelvis.

tation, surgical procedures consisted of debridement, suprapubic cystostomy, defunctioning transverse colostomy, right femoral artery repair, thrombectomy of the right femoral vein, and closed reduction of the pelvic fracture with application of a quadrilateral frame to the pelvis and a femoral external fixator. Anatomic reduction of the pelvis was achieved (Fig. 2). Ten days later, incision and drainage of a groin abscess, repacking of the perineal wound, and cross linking of the pelvic/femoral Hoffmann apparatus were undertaken.

The pelvic fixator was removed at 13 weeks. Ambulation was started at that time. The pelvic fractures were clinically stable. The follow-up radiograph at seven months postinjury is shown in Fig. 3. He returned to work as a laborer 18 months postinjury and is asymptomatic with respect to the pelvic injury.

Case II. A 27-year old male motorcyclist sustained a symphysis diastasis of 4 cm with an "open-book" injury of the left sacroiliac joint (Fig. 4). Associated injuries included a closed head injury, a fracture of the left patella, fracture-dislocation of the left ankle, a laceration of the left groin, and a rupture of the membranous urethra.

296

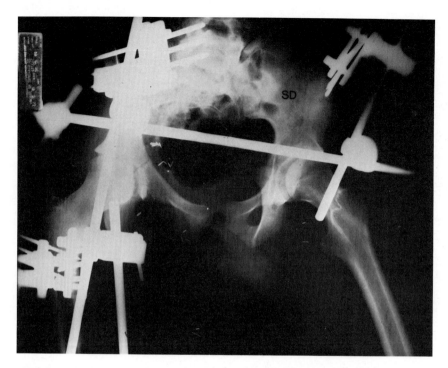

Fig. 2. Case I (SD) – Postreduction radiograph of pelvis.

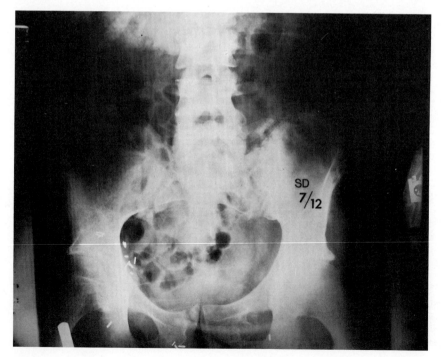

Fig. 3. Case I (SD) - Follow-up radiograph of pelvis.

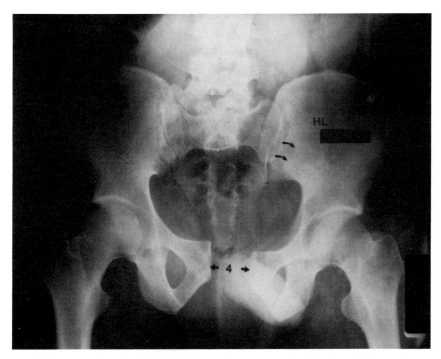

Fig. 4. Case II (HL) - Prereduction radiograph of pelvis.

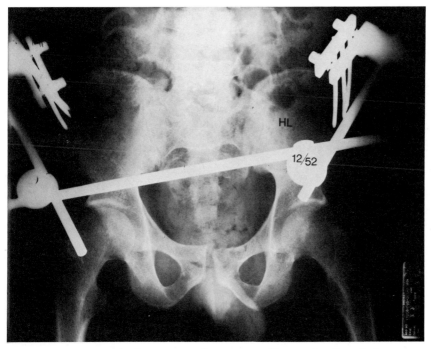

Fig. 5. Case II (HL) - Postreduction radiograph of pelvis.

298

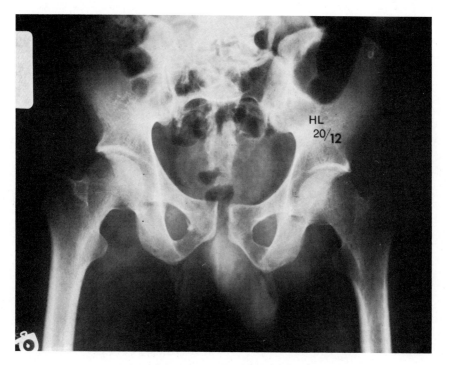

Fig. 6. Case II (HL) - Follow-up radiograph of pelvis.

Initial surgery consisted of closed reduction and Hoffmann external fixation of the pelvis (Fig. 5), open reduction of the left ankle, debridement of the left groin wound and a suprapubic cystostomy.

The apparatus was removed at 12 weeks and ambulation was begun. His final radiograph at 20 months revealed maintenance of anatomic reduction (Fig. 6). The patient has returned to heavy labor and has no complaints related to his pelvic injury.

Results and Discussion

The use of the Hoffmann External Fixator for unstable pelvic fractures in this series of polytraumatized patients has been highly encouraging. All patients tolerated the apparatus well.

At follow-up between six months and $4\frac{1}{2}$ years postinjury, 16 of 17 patients have returned to full activity. Three have mild residual sacroiliac pain on strenuous activity, but two of them continue to work as heavy laborers. Their symptoms do not warrant sacroiliac arthrodesis. One patient developed severe post-traumatic arthritis of his left hip due to an associated comminuted ace-tabular fracture-dislocation which was not amenable to open reduction.

The average duration of fixation was 78.8 days with a range of 55 to 90 days. We feel that a minimum of eight weeks is required even for symphysis diastasis without hemipelvis ascencion; for fractures with hemipelvis ascension or multiple fractures 10 to 12 weeks is recommended. None of the patients in this series was allowed to ambulate before removal of the apparatus. The majority of the patients in this series was incapable of doing so because of restrictions imposed by the associated injuries (extremity and spine fractures and head injuries). Five underwent rereduction within one week of the original reduction. Three required a general anesthetic and two had only parenteral analgesia when further compression was applied to further reduce a symphysis diastasis.

Maximum residual cephalad hemipelvis displacement of 1.5 cm was noted in four patients. Two of these patients had mild sacroiliac pain. The posterior disruptions which could not be anatomically reduced usually had a sacral or iliac bone fragment evident at either the superior or inferior margin of the sacroiliac joint and were seen in the three cases which required early remanipulation. Inability to obtain anatomic-closed reduction of the sacro-iliac component is felt to be due to entrapment of anterior sacroiliac ligaments and bone fragments. Bucholz (1981) has reported on 30 fresh Malgaigne fractures examined and classified at autopsy. He found that infolding of the anterior sacroiliac ligament or interposition of sacral avulsion fracture fragments into the sacroiliac joint prevented anatomic reduction in two out of five of his Group II injuries (posterior sacroiliac ligament complex intact). In his Group III injuries (complete disruption of sacroiliac ligaments with cephalad and posterior displacement and external rotation), anatomic reduction was impossible in 11 out of 11 with external manipulation and traction, but could be approximated if anterior force was applied with a bone hook. After excision of interposed tissue, the fractures could be reduced but were not stable. In contrast, in our series, only four residual cephalad displacements occurred out of a total of 11 with this type of displacement and we therefore consider the overall results excellent. Since the open reduction and exposure of the sacroiliac joint from both posterior and anterior aspects would likely be required to remove the block to complete reductions, open reduction does not seem to be justified when considering the functional end result in this series and the hazards of such extensive surgery.

Average blood replacement in this series was 6.8 units. Two patients underwent successful arterial embolization. The pelvic stabilization resulted in dramatic relief of pain in all patients and facilitated secondary operative procedures. Nursing care was also greatly facilitated due to ease of posturing and allowed better skin care, management of perineal wounds, colostomies and cystostomies. Thrombophlebitis occurred in one patient.

Local infection occurred around one or more pins in 11 patients. *Staphylococcus aureus* was the offending organism in 90% of these superficial infections. All responded to local treatment, but five required systemic antibiotics. In no instances was premature pin removal necessary. Following removal of the Hoffmann apparatus and pins, all pin sites closed with no sequelae of osteomyelitis, ring sequestra, or residual pain.

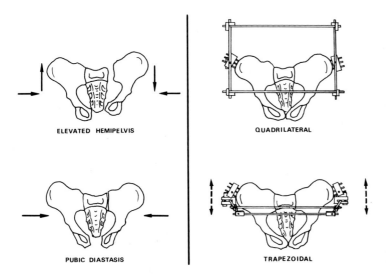

Fig. 7. Schematic diagrams of Malgaigne displacements and frame types.

In conclusion, the use of Hoffmann External Fixators has led to encouraging results in this series of unstable pelvic fractures. Although perfect reductions are impossible to achieve consistently by closed techniques due to local fracture conditions, we have managed to achieve and maintain acceptable reductions using the technique and management program outlined above. The relatively long duration of external fixation and delayed weight bearing may be major factors. Selection of the frame most capable of resisting the displacement which required correction and minimizing the pin length and torsional deformity is another important factor. The schematic diagrams on the left of Fig. 7 illustrate the forces required to reduce the common vertical and rotational displacements of the hemipelvis occurring in the Malgaigne type injuries. In the majority of cases with hemipelvis elevation we have used the quadrilateral frame to take advantage of its greater rigidity in the frontal plane. These applications are illustrated in the corresponding diagrams on the right of Fig. 7. The only major modification that we are considering is the use of additional pins to achieve greater torsional rigidity at the frame to bone link.

References

1. Bucholz, R.W.: The pathological anatomy of Malgaigne fracture-dislocations of the pelvis. J. Bone Jt. Surg. 63-A, 400, 1981.

2. Carabalona, P., Rabichong, P., Bonnel, F., Perruchon, E. and Peguret, F.: Apports du fixateur externe dans les dislocations du pubis et de l'articulation sacro-iliaque. Montpelier Chir. 20, 61, 1973.

3. Connes, H.: Hoffman's Double Frame External Anchorage, GEAD, Paris, 1973.

4. Grosse, A.: Stabilization of pelvic fractures with Hoffmann External Fixation: The French experience. In, External Fixation: The Current State of the Art. Eds: A.F. Brooker and C.C. Edwards, Williams and Wilkins, Baltimore, 1979.

5. Jenkins, D.H.R. and Young, M.H.: The operative treatment of sacro-iliac subluxation and disruption of the symphysis pubis. Injury 10, 139, 1978.

6. Johnston, R.: Stabilization of pelvic fractures with Hoffmann external fixation: The Colorado experience. In, External Fixation: The Current State of the Art. Eds: A.F. Brooker and C.C. Edwards, Williams and Wilkins, Baltimore, 1979.

7. Karaharju, E.O., and Slätis, P.: External fixation of double vertical pelvic fractures with a trapezoid compression frame. Injury 10, 142, 1978.

8. Mears, D.C. and Fu, F.: External fixaxion in pelvic fractures. In, The Orthopaedic Clinics of North America 11-3, 465, 1980.

9. Slätis, P. and Huittinen, V.-M.: Double vertical fractures of the pelvis. A report on 163 patients. Acta Chir. Scand. 138, 799, 1972.

10. Slätis, P., and Karaharju, E.O.: External fixation of the pelvic girdle with a trapezoid compression frame. Injury 7, 53, 1975.

External Fixation of the Upper Extremity with the ASIF Tubular Set and Wagner Apparatus

G. Hierholzer and P.-M. Hax

Introduction

In the upper extremity, external fixation is indicated only in certain
clinically problematic high risk cases. Because of the topographic anatomy
and functional considerations we recommend a clasp or half-pin assembly.
According to our classification, this is Type I external fixation
(Hierholzer, 1978). The Type I assembly can be realized using either the
ASIF-set (Association for the Study of Internal Fixation) or the Wagner
apparatus (Wagner, 1972). The technical principle of the Type I assembly
was described previously (Hierholzer, 1975; 1978; Wagner, 1972).

Clinical Results

Between 1975 and 1980, we performed external fixation of the humerus in
16 patients and in 32 bones of the forearm in 24 patients. Follow-up
examination could be completed for 14 of the humerus and 22 of the forearm
injuries. The average age for the two groups was 30.5 and 32.2 years,
respectively. The indications for external fixation are given in Table I.

Table I. Indications for external fixation (n = 48)

	Humerus (n)	Radius (n)	Ulna (n)
Infected nonunion	11	13	13
Nonunion after previous infection	2	2	1
Open fracture	3	2	1
Σ	16	17	15

The total number of different surgical measures (Table II) and the number
and nature of operative stabilization (Table III) before admission to our
unit in cases of nonunions indicates the severity of the clinical situations.

Table II. Number of preoperations in nonunions

	0	1	2	3	4	5
Humerus (n pat)	-	2	6	3	2	-
Forearm (n pat)	-	6	10	4	1	1

Table III. Nature of pretreatment (stabilization)

	Humerus (n)	Forearm (n)
Nail/rushpin	4	3
Plate	8	24
Cerclage, wire, screw	3	3
External fixator	-	6
Conservative	2	-

Typical examples are presented. The average time for which external fixation was needed is noted in Table IV. Our surgical treatment did not consist only of stabilization of bone, but also in additional surgical measures.
(Table V). The degree of inflammation, contamination and soft tissue damage

Table IV. Average time of stabilization with
           external fixator Type I (months $\bar{x}$)

	Nonunions	Open fractures
Humerus	4.1	4.9
Forearm	3.3	5.0

Table V. Additional operations

	Humerus (n)	Forearm (n)
Primary cancellous bone grafting	9	24
Secondary cancellous bone grafting	7	11
Other secondary surgical interventions	5	10

determines whether bone grafting is indicated primarily or secondarily. In some patients we could not solve the problems of infection and bone defect without additional surgical interventions (Table V).

Control of infection and bone healing could be achieved to date in most patients (Table VI). In four patients, the treatment is not yet finished. An amputation was necessary in one patient. The average time between external fixation and bone union is given in Table VII. Obviously, we have to expect delayed bone healing in these problematic situations. But, if we do not achieve bone consolidation in a reasonable time with external fixation, we change to stabilization by internal fixation, provided the infection has subsided. Table VIII presents the final rate of angular deformity. Judgement of these results has to consider the preexisting severity of the conditions.

Table VI. Bone healing after external fixation Type I.

	Humerus n - 16	Forearm n = 24
Healed	14	21
Amputation	-	1
Not yet healed	2	2

Table VII. Time between external fixation and consolidation

	n pat	months $\bar{x}$
Open fracture - humerus	3	7
Nonunion - humerus	11	6
Open fracture - forearm	1	6
Nonunion - forearm	20	7

Table VIII. Deviation of axis on roentgenograph (A.P./lat. projection)

	Humerus 14 pat	Forearm 21 pat
<10°	6	12
>10° - one plane	7	6
>10° - two planes	1	3

In many cases we have to be content with having achieved our therapeutic objective in the realm of possibility: the control of infection and bone healing. The final functional results are not just those of a bone condition but reflect the associated damage to soft tissue which is usually extensive. External fixation helps us treat the bone to the point where the adjacent muscles and nerves can work to the limit of their capacity.

Summary

External fixation in the upper extremity is a method for the treatment of clinically difficult cases. For stabilization, we recommend the ASIF tubular set or the Wagner apparatus which correspond to assembly Type I of our classification. The results of 48 external fixations are presented with recognition of functional impairment from associated soft tissue damage.

References

1. Hierholzer, G.: Stabilisierung des Knochenbruchs beim Weichteilschaden mit Fixateurs externes. Langenbecks Arch. klin. Chir. 39, 505 (1975).

2. Hierholzer, G., Kleining, R., Hörster, G., Zemenides, P.: External fixation. Arch. Orthop. Traumat. Surg. 92, 175 (1978).

3. Wagner, H.: Technik und Indikation der operativen Verkürzung und Verlängerung von Ober- und Unterschenkel. Orthopadie 1, 59 (1972).

The Treatment of Wrist Fractures with the Small AO External Fixation Device

R. P. Jakob and D. L. Fernandez

Numerous unsatisfactory results have demonstrated the difficulty in the treatment of comminuted fractures of the distal radius. Many of these fractures are unstable even after closed pinning, especially those with metaphyseal and intra-articular comminution. Open reduction has proved difficult, and the exposure required may remove the only surrounding structures holding the bone together. Furthermore, the holding power of the screws is always decreased with the risk of secondary displacement.

Following the principles of Anderson (1944), several authors have during the past years advocated distraction to treat comminuted wrist fractures using an external fixator (Vidal et al, 1978; Grana and Kopta, 1979; Cooney, 1980). They believe that the length of the radius can be maintained only by distraction since the distal radius tends to shorten under the pull of the muscles pivoting the wrist joint around the intact distal ulna. Vidal's term "ligamentotaxis" refers to the principles of distraction in comminuted fractures of various joints like the hip, the knee, the ankle, and the wrist joint, the latter offering the ideal indication. Because of the maintenance of the capsulo-ligamentous apparatus, the pull through the wrist joint is able to maintain the reduction of even multifragmentary fractures. As part of the AO equipment we have developed an external fixator which has proved useful in the management of these difficult fractures over the past four years (Jakob, 1980).

Technique

Under an axillary block, the fracture is reduced under image intensifier control and the wrist is brought into the most stable position. An intra-articular T-fracture may be secured with percutaneous K-wires. If the distraction alone does not result in adequate reduction, the fragments may be levered into position with percutaneous pins. Only exceptionally is it necessary to add a bone graft to hold the reduction. Subsequently, two threaded 2.5 mm pins are inserted proximal to the fracture in the radius, and two further pins are placed in the second metacarpal at an inclination so that they subtend an angle of 40-50° to each other (Fig. 1). A special drill sleeve which is inserted through a 3 mm incision protects the soft

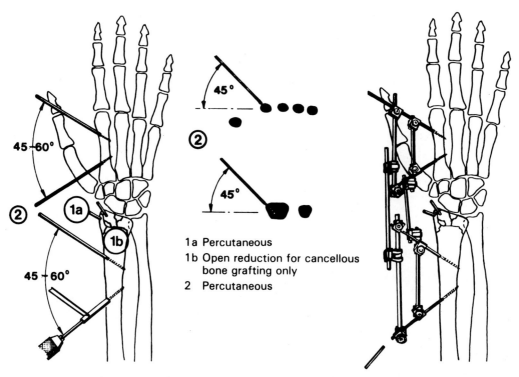

45-60°

② 1a 1b

45-60°

45°

②

45°

1a Percutaneous
1b Open reduction for cancellous
    bone grafting only
2 Percutaneous

Fig. 1. Technique of applying small AO external fixation device.

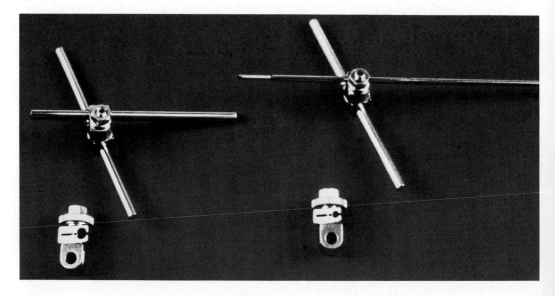

Fig. 2. Two kinds of universal clamps are used to connect the 2.5 mm
pins to the 4 mm rods, and to connect the 4 mm rods.

tissues. The converging direction of the pins increases the holding power in the bone. If reduction cannot be achieved, it may be necessary to insert the distal pins in the distal fracture fragment of the radius using it to lever the articular piece in position (Cooney, 1980). After insertion of the pins in the proper line, they are connected with the 2.5/4 mm clamps to the 4 mm rods of various lengths, creating a parallelogram of forces allowing cast free treatment (Fig. 2). If the fracture is stable in neutral position, a straight frame with long 4 mm rods is used. If it is unstable, a forced angulation at the wrist joint may require a different assembly. Here, the 4/4 mm universal clamps offer the versatility to allow the device to be placed in any desired combination to obtain an optimal position of the hand. In severe injuries of the wrist joint or the hand, the pins may be inserted into any solid stock, thereby obtaining stability. In the after treatment, a volar plaster slab may be used for the first weeks. Roentgenogram control may reveal the need for a secondary reduction which is easily accomplished by increasing the distraction. Normally, marked distraction is not maintained for more than four weeks. It is lessened after that time, but the distractor is usually not removed until six to seven weeks postoperatively. Of great importance is immediate physiotherapy by active and passive mobilization of all finger joints. The tendency toward fixed ulnar deviation is lessened by using an orthoplast splint. Once the apparatus is removed, the recovery of function is facilitated with these positional splints. They are applied dorsally or volarly in alternating fashion.

Material

Since 1977, 40 patients with an average of 38 years have been treated for comminuted fractures of the distal radius. The oldest patient was 66 years of age. In eight patients, the distraction was only applied in cases of secondary displacement after conservative reduction and plaster fixation or percutaneous K-wire fixation.

Results

With the exception of one patient, all fractures healed in the position in which the external fixator was applied. In some patients with marked comminution, and in some fractures which had shown secondary displacement, the quality of reduction was less than perfect. In a 63-year old patient with a proximal metaphyseal fracture consolidation of the fracture did not take place; a plate fixation had, therefore, to be performed two months after the initial trauma.

Four out of 160 inserted pins were associated with infection which, however, did not affect the quality of the end result.

A Sudeck's atrophy was observed in one patient. This complication required intensive physiotherapy and resulted in healing after four months with limitation of finger motion.

The overall clinical results in terms of function, power, pain and deformity

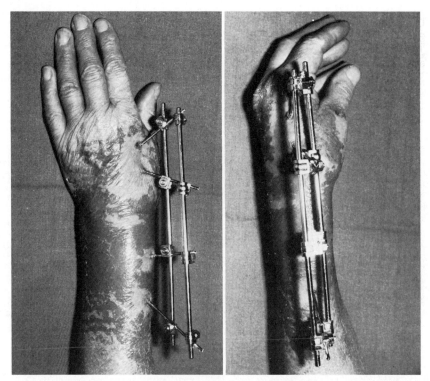

Fig. 3. If the fracture is stable in neutral position, a
straight frame is applied with long 4 mm rods.

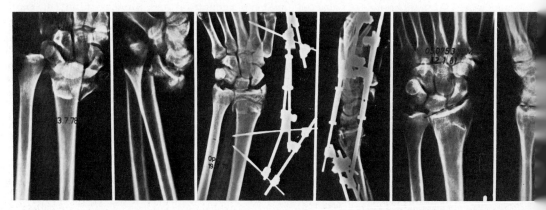

Fig. 4. Multifragmentary fracture which was first treated conservatively and
redisplaced. Secondary reduction after 6 days and external fixation during 6
weeks in slight flexion. Result after 2 1/2 years

Fig. 5. A 27-year old patient, hang-gliding accident, with comminuted distal ▶
radial fracture and severe radial and posterior dislocation. Due to signs of
median nerve entrapment, the anterior compartment and the carpal tunnel had to
be decompressed the day after the fracture was reduced. Radiologic and clinical appearance one year after the injury.

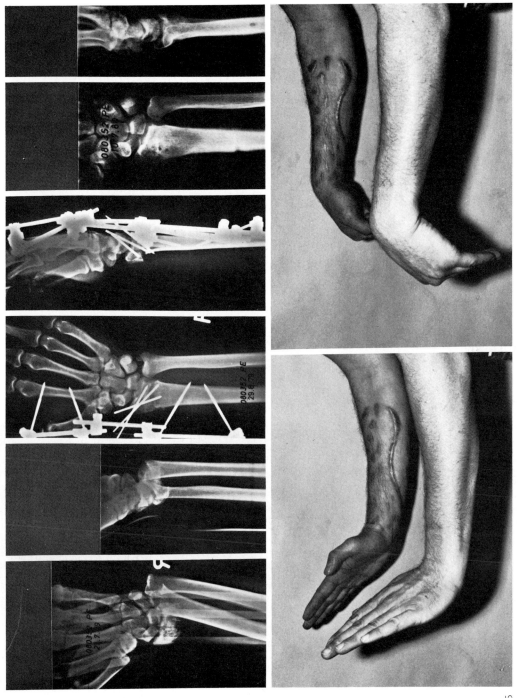

Fig. 5

312

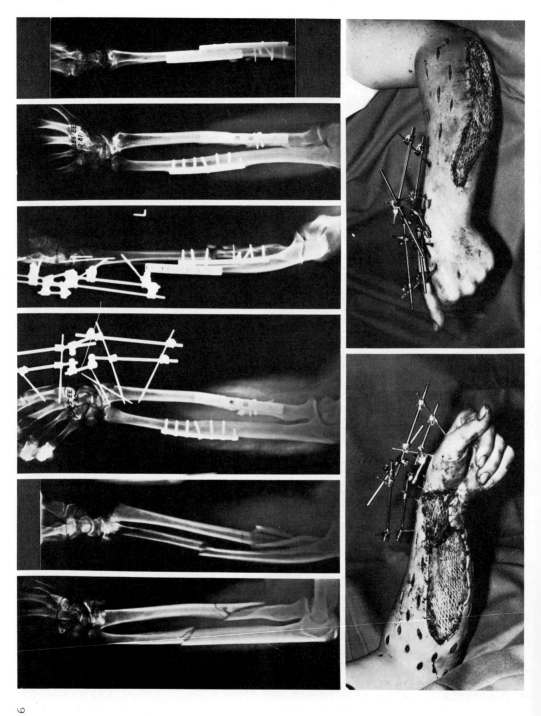

Fig. 6

of the wrist joint were extremely rewarding considering the severity of the
fractures which were selected for this mode of treatment.

Discussion

The fracture types most suitable for external fixation are unstable fractures with metaphyseal comminution lacking a volar or dorsal buttress; the
fracture with secondary displacement in plaster, especially in the young
patient, and the fracture where primary arthrodesis would be the only
alternative.

Due to sufficient stability with the external fixator, a cast-free after-
treatment can be selected without the risk of secondary displacement. The
treatment may be combined with initial percutaneous pinning of the fracture
facilitating reduction or with a cancellous bone graft if necessary. Fixation is possible in any selected position due to the versatility of the
fixator. The use of the hand is facilitated due to free finger and elbow
motion.

External fixation of wrist fractures is extremely helpful in multiple
injury to the upper extremity, especially in dealing with vessel and nerve
lesions, or extensive soft tissue and muscle damage, demanding free approach
to the wound in the postoperative period.

The indication for external fixation is relative in patients over the age
of 65 years with extensive osteoporosis due to delayed consolidation of
the fracture and to the age-inherent risk of Sudeck's atrophy. This tendency is even more prominent if the fixator application is delayed in
cases of a secondary displacement, especially in old patients.

On the whole, our experience with external fixation is favorable in 80% of
the patients, which is in accord with other authors (Vidal et al, 1978;
Grana and Kopta, 1979; Cooney, 1980).

Summary

The distraction of comminuted fractures of the distal radius allows adequate reduction without risk of secondary displacement. It helps avoid
circulatory problems due to immediate hand and finger mobility. Furthermore, it allows free hand function, which is especially useful in bilateral
wrist fractures, and it offers a dependable way to regain pain-free hand
function with good mobility and good power in 80% of the patients. This
technique requires careful follow-up and excellent cooperation from the
patient.

Fig. 6. Crush injury in a 25-year old train worker. Immediate internal fixation of the proximal radius and the midshaft of the ulna. External fixation
of the wrist. Wide anterior fasciotomy and immediate split skin graft in combination with multiple small releasing incisions. Good radiologic and functional result after one year.

References

1. Anderson, R. and O'Neill, G.: Comminuted fractures of the end of the radius. Surg. Gynecol. Obst. 78, 434, 1944.

2. Cooney, W.P.: External mini-fixators: Clinical applications and techniques. In, Johnston, R.M. (Ed.): Advances in External Fixation, Year Book Publishers, Chicago, 1980.

3. Grana, W.A. and Kopta, J.A.: The Roger Anderson device in the treatment of fractures of the distal end of the radius. J. Bone Jt. Surg. 61A, 1234, 1979.

4. Jakob, R.P.: Die Distraktion instabiler distaler Radiustrümmerfrakturen mit einem Fixateur externe - ein neuer Behandlungsweg. Hefte Unfallheilk. 148, 99. Springer Verlag Berling-Heidelberg, 1980.

5. Jakob, R.P.: Ein neuer AO-Fixateur zur Distraktion instabiler distaler Radiustrümmerfrakturen. Internationales Fixateur externe Symposium, März 1980 Duisburg, Herausgeber: G. Hierholzer, Springer Verlag, Berlin (in print)

6. Vidal, J., Buscayret, Ch., and Connes, H.: Treatment of articular fractures by "ligamentotaxis" with external fixation. In, Brooker, A.F. and Edwards, C.C. (Eds.): External Fixation, The Current State of the Art. Williams and Wilkins, Baltimore, 1978.

Mini-Hoffmann External Fixator for Fractures of the Hand

J. J. Bock

Introduction

The Hoffmann mini-external fixator is a simple versatile device that has
been useful in the treatment of many small fractures involving the hand,
foot and maxiofacial injuries. My paper will be confined to its use in
the hand. It has been very valuable for treatment of unstable comminuted
fractures, arthrodeses, conditions associated with extensive bone loss,
comminution and loss of stability, reimplantation and digital lengthening.

Its advantages include the fact that it is a simple versatile device that
provides immediate stability to the fracture site. Compression can be
applied either initially or at a later date. It is valuable for extensive
bone comminution or bone loss. The apparatus can provide distraction to
maintain normal skeletal alignment and position while appropriate bone
grafting procedures can be carried out. Applying the apparatus causes
little tissue trauma. Another hidden advantage is that one can have a
second chance at correction of all deformities that may develop because of
dynamic changes and patient interference either by adjusting the apparatus
and/or by traumatic alteration. One can remove the apparatus and clinically test the stability of healing at will.

Technique

The mini-Hoffmann external fixator is applied after one has carefully prepared the patient's hand for surgery and has appropriately marked the
joints adjacent to the fractured segment. For this, I generally use 23
or 24 gauge needles and insert these into the adjacent joints of the involved phalanx. Following this, using small incisions, I then insert the
mini-Hoffmann pins through a 1.5 mm drill hole. By using the drill guide,
one is able to place parallel pins. I must caution, however, that it is
absolutely necessary to insert these pins in a parallel manner so that the
pin holders can then be applied. Following insertion of two additional
parallel pins and a pin holder at the other extremes of the fractured mem-
ber, one then attaches the pin holder to a simple swivel clamp as well as
a sliding swivel clamp which are applied to a connecting rod of an appropriate length. The fracture is then reduced either clinically or under
direct vision and/or image intensifier control (depending whether the fracture is open or not). After satisfactory correction of alignment, rotation
and angulation are obtained, the frame is tightened. Following this, dis-

traction or compression can be applied to the fracture site with the sliding swivel clamps.

In the case of gunshot wounds with extensive comminution, we have used distraction to maintain the alignment of the skeletal structures of the hand. In some cases of excessive comminuted articular fractures, we have used a combination of internal and external fixation in an effort to better align the fracture fragments. In general, the stability obtained has permitted early motion of the joints provided that immobilization was not necessary due to adjacent soft tissue injuries.

Management

Attempts have been made to protect the digit and the mini-fixator with the use of a soft dressing to avoid injury to the patient where the apparatus could get caught in clothing, bed covers, etc. (The mini-Hoffmann apparatus has multiple projections that could get caught in various things during the activities of daily living.) The soft tissue wrap has been found helpful to prevent injury to the apparatus, the digit and the patient. All patients are told to keep the pin sites dry and clean. Only one patient out of 20 has had any significant pin tract infection that required removal of the apparatus. This occurred with a patient who had a preexisting infection that recurred after application of the Hoffmann apparatus. It did eventually require early removal of the apparatus.

Postoperatively, I have also been able to adjust the apparatus where, because of dynamic changes and patient injury, the alignment of the skeletal structures was unsatisfactory. Under such circumstances it is possible, using digital block anesthesia, to loosen the frame, to realign the fracture fragments, and then to reapply and tighten the frame. This technique also permits us to apply compression as stability is obtained in severely comminuted fractures where initially it would not be possible to apply compression because of severe comminution and instability at the fracture sites.

Vascularized versus Conventional Bone Grafts in the Treatment of Bone Loss of Extremities

J. Melka and J. Vidal

Severe injuries to the extremities causing bone and skin loss present difficult problems in reconstructive surgery.

The external fixator of Hoffmann, which we have been using for over ten years, has permitted us to solve satisfactorily the problems of osseous union in these severe injuries (Connes, 1975).

The external fixator, however, is not a treatment by itself. It is the basic structure which enables us to perform, step by step, all the necessary surgical procedures.

Conventional methods of bone loss reconstruction require surgery directed to skin and bone. The question is how much have microsurgical anastomoses of bone transplants improved the situation and at what price? We believe that our technique can reduce the number of surgical procedures as well as the incidence of delayed union.

Conventional Techniques

Forty-seven cases of bone loss treated by conventional methods were reviewed. Bone loss was subdivided as follows: partial bone loss - 21 patients (bone loss affecting at least two cortices but osseous union maintained at the level of one cortex); total bone loss - 26 patients (all three cortices are affected and no bony contact exists; these cases resemble a resection of the diaphysis).

Bone loss in the femur occurred in 12 patients, in the leg in 27 patients, and at the upper extremity in 8 patients. Conventional procedures were used to attempt skin and bone healing.

1. Skin coverage

The problem exists only at the level of the leg where the tibia is poorly protected, particularly at its anteromedial aspect. Obviously, the first step is prevention of infection.

In previous publications, we have described our approach to control infections (Connes, 1975; Vidal, 1976). The first step is excision of all infected and necrotic tissues. The second step is continuous irrigation with a detergent solution, followed by a solution to promote granulation and, thus, skin healing. Skin coverage occurs either spontaneously or is achieved by thin skin grafts. This technique, however, leads to poor skin coverage which does not permit later surgical procedures directed to the bone. Only cutaneoplasties, using a thick covering, can resist trauma and repeated surgical procedures necessary to obtain bone healing.

We generally use the cross leg method. The skin flap taken from the other leg must cover the entire skin defect. Some basic principles must be applied, such as the preservation of the saphenous vein. Here again, the external fixator of Hoffmann is an important aid to maintain the correct position of the crossed legs. It prevents an accidental avulsion of the flap and reduces the discomfort associated with that position.

We have never used local muscle and musculocutaneous flaps from the same leg. In fact, these flaps are usually taken from the posterior aspect of the leg, a zone which we like to preserve for possible later bony reconstruction (bone grafts between tibia and fibula).

2. Conventional bone grafting

We do not intend to describe here in detail the surgical technique of the various procedures. Generally, three different techniques have been used:

i.   A bone graft replacing diaphyseal bone loss, either through interposition or apposition. Good skin coverage is essential and, particularly in the leg, a cross leg skin coverage is often indicated.

ii.   Interposition of a bone graft between tibia and fibula.

iii. The Papineau technique, now considered a standard treatment, in which a surgical excision precedes open grafting with spongy bone. An interval of 15 to 21 days between the two stages should elapse to permit development of granulation tissue (Papineau, 1973).

3.   Results of conventional methods

Results of reconstructive procedures will be listed according to the anatomic sites since different sites give rise to different technical problems.

Femur. Of the 12 patients suffering from a femoral bone defect, three were treated by the Papineau technique whereas in nine patients we used a diaphyseal corticospongious bone graft either interposed or apposed.

The Papineau technique led to a bony consolidation in all patients, on the average within eight months. In one patient, however, the fistula persisted.

With respect to bone grafts, healing was obtained in seven out of nine patients, usually after eight months. Unfortunately, numerous complications arose:

Total or partical resorption of the bone graft
necessitating a new graft . . . . 3 times

Refracture . . . . 3 times

Recurrent infections . . . . 3 times

Finally, in three patients, bony consolidation was achieved but at the cost of severe shortening (5, 7 and 11 cm), the surgeon therefore not achieving his goal of reconstructing the bony defect.

Leg. In a group of 25 patients, 15 were treated with the Papineau technique, nine with a tibiofibular graft, and one with a major interposition bone graft spanning a defect of 17 cm of both bones.

In seven of 15 patients, the Papineau technique led to consolidation. In the other eight patients, resorption of the bone graft was observed in the presence of a satisfactory skin cicatrization. It is worth noting that in all patients with a total bone loss over 7 cm, the Papineau technique did not succeed (5 out of 8). In these patients, the bone loss occurred at the lower part of the leg where no muscle attachment exists (2 cases: middle third; 6: lower third). In all nonunions, a new procedure became necessary. In six patients, a bone graft between tibia and fibula permitted full weight bearing seven months after surgery. In the two remaining patients, a full bone transfer with microvascular anastomosis was performed.

Conversely, the success rate differed in bone grafting six partial and one total loss at the level of the proximal part of the leg (2: proximal third; 2: middle third; 1 distal third). Here, muscle insertion promotes healing. Consolidation was achieved eight months after the second stage of the Papineau technique.

Finally, in five of 11 patients a shortening of more than 3 cm was observed. This was most probably due to insufficient distraction by the external fixator or to premature weight bearing.

The bone graft between tibia and fibula was performed six times (distal third: 2; middle third: 4). In four patients bone loss was total. Bone healing occurred on an average of eight months.

In three patients, this procedure was associated with an interpositional bone graft of the tibia. Here, the bone loss was always total, more than 4 cm at the middle third, and associated with an important skin loss at the anteromedial and anterolateral aspect.

Patients close to traumatic amputation are treated by the extreme method. Skin coverage is achieved after granulation by a cross leg flap. Bone loss is treated early during the first stage by a tibiofibular graft. This posterior bridge is later supplemented by an interpositional bone graft approaching the tibia through a thick, strong skin flap. Three patients with this technique healed in 11 months. It is interesting to note that we used the tibiofibular graft in most patients with a bone loss exceeding 3 cm.

Tibiofibular grafting as a first procedure, or following a failure with the Papineau technique, led to a bony consolidation in 10 patients. Three patients with major bone loss were successfully treated with an inter-positional bone graft. In five of 13 patients (38%), the tibiofibular grafting had to be repeated, markedly prolonging the time of consolidation.

In summary, the indication for the Papineau technique seems questionable in patients with a major (more than 3 cm) or total bone loss (diaphysectomy). The tibiofibular graft, if correctly applied, assures bone healing in the shortest time with less risk of recurrent bone infection.

Free Microvascular Bone Transplants

The increasing use of microvascular techniques during the last 10 years has opened a promising avenue in the treatment of major bone losses of the extremities.

It is now possible to transfer an osteoperiosteal segment to a receptor site with arterial and venous anastomoses.

Precise anatomic studies have determined several donor sites, in particular at the fibula, the iliac crest, and the ribs. It is also possible to leave attached to the bone graft a skin flap revascularized by the same vascular pedicle.

The advantage of this technique is a more rapid consolidation requiring less procedures. It does require, however, an experienced surgical team.

1. Anatomic considerations of free microvascular transplants.

The anterior inguinoiliac flap. This unit is composed of inguinoiliac skin and the anterior portion of the iliac crest. Vascularization of both components was thought to be derived from the superficial circumflex iliac artery, a branch of the femoral artery, 2 cm distal from the femoral arcade. The vessel has a rather small diameter (1.5 cm; Daniel, 1973).

As Taylor has recently demonstrated (1979), however, the flap is completely revascularized by the deep iliac circumflex artery, a branch of the external iliac artery originating just proximal to the femoral arcade. The diameter of this vessel is more than 2 mm; it is accompanied by veins of equally large diameters. Its role in the vascularization of the anterior part of the iliac crest and the overlying skin has been disputed for a long time. The definitive results of Taylor's studies have apparently settled this controversy. We, as well as other teams, have successfully adopted this approach, retaining the deep iliac circumflex artery for the vascularization of the bone-skin flap.

The vascularized fibular transplant. The blood supply to the fibula is
derived essentially from branches of the arteria fibularis. The fibula
is supplied by a nutrient artery which penetrates at the middle third,
and by musculoperiosteal vessels, usually three, all situated posteriorly.
Whether the supply comes predominantly from the endosteal or the periosteal vessels is still a matter of controversy. Since no definite conclusion can be reached at the present time, it is advisable to preserve
both supply routes during the removal of the fibular graft (Melka, 1979).
While removing the middle third of the fibular, care should be taken to
preserve the periosteum and the posterior collateral arteries as well as
1 to 2 mm of muscle insertion.

2. Results

Ten patients with bone loss over 8 cm were treated by this method. In
four patients with skin and bone loss of the leg, we used the anterior
inguinoiliac flap technique. This method led to consolidation in only
two patients, 4 and $3\frac{1}{2}$ months respectively after the procedure, calculated from the time of removal of the external fixator and the application
of a walking cast permitting full weight bearing. We must point out that
one patient removed his cast without our knowledge and consent, and refractured his iliac graft during a fall on a staircase. Following closed
reduction and application of a long leg cast, consolidation of the fracture occurred in two months.

The two failures of the vascularized flap were caused by an early thrombosis. One failure in a young healthy patient occurred six hours after
surgery secondary to a hematoma causing vessel occlusion. The other
failure occurred in a 68-year old patient who had evidence of arteriosclerosis at the receptor site. The anastomosis was not functioning.

The free transfer of the fibula was used in six patients, twice at the
femur, three times at the leg, and once in the forearm.

Bone healing was achieved in five of six patients on an average within
5 months. In the sixth patient, an infection at the contact site flared
up. Radiologically, resorption cavities were noted and we had to return
to the conventional treatment method.

Discussion

We have observed that conventional bone grafts result in some complications. The most important of these are resorption of the graft, recur-
rence of infection, and refracture.

Obviously, without blood supply the conventional bone graft will undergo
necrosis. The dead bone will gradually be replaced by living bone. This
replacement is preceded by vascular invasion and resorption. The osteoid,
formed at varying rates, separates the blood vessels from the necrotic
bone, thus causing incomplete or partial replacement only. The large
amount of necrotic bone remaining at the site explains the mechanical weak-

ness of the graft (stress fracture) and its susceptibility to infection (Enneking, Morris, 1972).

It appears that the success of any bone grafting depends on the revascularization of the graft. Early revascularization by means of vascular microanastomoses seems to solve this problem.

The value of microsurgical procedures, however, must be assessed after careful evaluation of their advantages and disadvantages, and in comparison with conventional methods.

Disadvantages of vascularized bone grafting

Length of operating time is the greatest disadvantage. Six to 8 hours are required for an anterior inguinoiliac skin bone flap and 4 to 6 hours for a fibular transplant.

We have also observed that, in certain cases, the age of the patient may be a risk factor. Arteriosclerosis, for example, can lead to early thrombosis at the site of anastomosis. The vascular state of the receptor site must also be taken into consideration. In fact, the original trauma sometimes disrupts blood flow in one or more arteries. Therefore, an arteriogram of the site of bone loss will assist in deciding whether conservative or conventional treatment should be carried out. It will also help to determine the number of remaining arteries and to select the receptor artery. During surgery, it is not unusual to find vessels embedded in dense fibrous tissue. In these cases, one should not hesitate to proceed with a surgical dissection of these tissues of several centimeters. In freeing the artery from constricting fibrosis, the blood flow is improved. More difficulties are sometimes encountered when dissecting the receptor veins. The dissection should be done with extreme care since the vessel walls are fragile, especially when surrounded by dense fibrosis.

Furthermore, a surgical team highly trained in microsurgical procedures must always be available during the first postoperative days in case reoperation should become necessary.

Finally, there is the evident risk of failure necessitating a return to conventional methods. Failures can be expected soon after surgery in cases of thrombosis. We have observed thrombosis as a consequence of hematoma formation within the pedicle. These complications seem to occur almost exclusively in free inguinoiliac grafts where vascular drainage occurs mostly through spongy bone and not through venous channels. Realizing the origin of these hematomas, we now drain the raw surfaces of the graft and make 4 to 5 peripheral loose stitches. This prevents an accumulation of blood and consequently hematoma formation.

The internal fixation of grafts is another important factor causing problems. In patients with complete and extensive bone loss, it is difficult to maintain bone interposition with an external fixator. With fibular transplants one must be sure that the graft is placed in line with the diaphysis. The use of a screw at each end will help to stabilize the position. Should compression be impossible and instability result, the use of a large guide pin will help to orientate the compressive forces of the external fixator.

Advantages of vascularized bone grafting

There are numerous advantages: The complete treatment of bone loss takes place during one sitting. Rigid postoperative observation of the patency of the anastomosis is imperative. Besides dressings, no other specialized care is needed. Prolonged immobilization in an uncomfortable position (cross leg) is not required.

The quality of vascular perfusion of the graft is superior to that of conventional grafts. The risk of massive resorption and delayed union is decreased, thus shortening the time of total incapacity.

In the presence of a well vascularized graft, the danger of a flare-up of infection is minimized. On the other hand, we have observed fractures of revascularized iliac grafts. The iliac crest, being much more fragile than the fibula, seems to take longer to attain a solid incorporation.

Although progressive hypertrophy of the fibular graft after implantation in the diaphyseal axis of the tibia has been reported frequently, we did not observe this generally. As a preventive measure, we recommend adding spongy bone chips, since it is well known that spongy bone incorporates faster than compact bone, especially when in contact with a vascularized graft (Phemister, 1914).

At the leg it is possible to complete the fibular graft by filling the tibiofibular space with bone.

The donor sites, either at the pelvis or leg, heal satisfactorily. The scars do not interfere with conventional bone graft removal at the pelvis, femur or tibia. Thus, in case of failure, removal of a conventional bone graft is still possible.

References

1. Connes, H.: Le fixateur externe en double cadre: méthode, application et résultats à propos de 160 observations. Edition GEAD, Paris, 1975.
2. Daniel, R.K., and Taylor, G.I.: Distant transfer of an island flap by microvascular anastomosis: a clinical technic. Plast. Reconstr. Surg. 52, 11, 1973.
3. Enneking, W.F., and Morris, J.L.: Human autologous cervical bone transplants. Clin. Orthop. 87, 28, 1972.
4. Melka, J.:Traitement des pertes de substance osseuse des membres. Méthodes conventionnelles et transferts libres en microchirurgie. Thèse de Doctorat en Médecine. Université de Montpellier (Montpellier, France), 1979.

5. Papineau, L.J.: L'excision greffe avec fermeture retardée délibérée dans l'ostéomyélite chronique. Nouv. Presse Méd. 41, 2753, 1973.

6. Phemister, D.B.: The fate of transplanted bone and regeneration of its various constituents. Surg. Gynec. Obst. 19, 303, 1914.

7. Taylor, G.I., Townsend, P., and Corlett, R.: Superiority of the deep circumflex iliac vessels as the supply of free groin flaps; experimental work. Plast. Reconstr. Surg. 64, 595, 1979.

8. Taylor, G.I., Townsend, P., and Corlett, R.: Superiority of the deep circumflex iliac vessels as the supply of free groin flaps; clinical work. Plast. Reconstr. Surg. 64, 745, 1979.

9. Vidal, J., Buscayret, Ch., Connes, H., Paran, M., and Allieu, Y.: Traitement des fractures ouvertes de jambe par le fixateur externe en double cadre. Rev. Chir. Orthop. 62, 433, 1976.

Indication and Technique of Knee Joint Arthrodesis

S. Weller and K. Weise

Introduction

Arthrodeses of the knee joint performed in 109 patients from 1969 to 1980
at the Workmen's Compensation Board Hospital, Tübingen, West Germany,
demonstrate that results achieved with this technique compare favorably
with results of alloarthroplastic knee joint replacements. Arthrodesis
was first described and performed by Albert approximately 100 years ago.
Originally, this procedure was mainly confined to tuberculous, poliomye-
litic or tabetic joints. As increasing experience was gained in the control of these conditions, this procedure was gradually extended for the
treatment of rheumatic and post-traumatic joint disorders. Today, surgical
ankylosis of the knee joint is indicated in patients with serious limb
impairment associated with painful and restricted motion, recurrent inflammatory conditions or irreversible ligament instabilities.

Indications

The largest group of patients necessitating arthrodesis of the knee suffered
from post-traumatic or postinfectious damage to the articulating surfaces,
especially open knee joint injuries and/or intra-articular fractures. Infected or loosened endoprotheses also necessitated arthrodesis. Massive
resection of bone, necessary for the insertion of joint components, present
technical problems when arthrodesis has to be performed. Furthermore, large
pseudarthrosic gaps as well as en bloc resections for benign or semimalignant tumors in the vicinity of the joint may constitute an indication for
arthrodesis. To summarize, arthrodesis is indicated in the following conditions:

1) post-traumatic gonarthroses

2) rheumatic gonarthroses

3) degenerative gonarthroses

4) inflammatory destruction of the joint (open injury, iatrogenic damage,
    arthritis)

5) neuropathic joint diseases

6) benign or semimalignant tumors

7) pseudarthroses in the vicinity of the joint.

The decision whether to perform arthrodesis rests between surgeon and patient, especially when no other reasonable surgical options exist to restore joint mobility. In older patients, total joint replacement may be a preferred procedure provided it does not involve too great a risk.

Arthrodesis is the method of choice in younger patients with joint damage because of the high stress exerted on total prostheses and the durability of the protheses in that age group. In our opinion, total joint replacement is particularly contraindicated in the presence of infection or a history of infection.

Before performing a knee arthrodesis the condition of the adjacent joints of the same leg and, above all, of the opposite hip and knee joint must be taken into consideration. Another important factor is the condition of the lumbosacral spine. It is an accepted fact that a fused knee may in the long term have a negative impact on these structures, either inducing or aggravating an arthrosis.

Advantages of knee arthrodesis:

- stability
- load-bearing capacity
- freedom from pain

Disadvantages of arthrodesis:

- shortening of the leg
- loss of mobility
- strain on neighboring joints

This situation must be discussed with the patient in depth preoperatively to enable him to become aware of the condition to be anticipated. This will prevent disappointments and lack of cooperation during follow-up treatment.

Concomitant physiotherapy and occupational therapy are essential for achieving a good functional result. In our opinion, the following regimen should be ordered:

- Physiotherapeutic exercises aimed at strenghtening the muscles in both legs.

- Intensive gait training aimed at gradually eliminating walking aids; gymnastics.

- Adaptation of the arthrodesed joint to the function of the supporting limb.

- Orthopedic adjustment of shoes with subtotal length equalization.

Special consideration should be given to length. A slight shortening of the arthrodesed leg improves the gait since it permits a normal movement of the leg from the hip joint. Leg length discrepancies which are too large inevitably damage the vertebral column due to pelvic tilt. The patient's gait may be severely distorted by foot drop at the ankle joint of the same leg or flexion deformity of the opposite knee joint if the length discrepancy is not compensated. After surgical arthrodesis, the patient should be followed closely since, otherwise, the positive results of the operation could be lost.

Technique

Surgical techniques used in the past, such as stabilization of arthrodesis by means of crossed Kirschner wires according to Lexer and Lange, two-wire traction clips according to Greifensteiner and Wustmann, and nailing according to Küntscher, with percutaneous destruction of the articular cartilage, are only of historical importance today. Moreover, the various modifications of joint surface resections for optimal interlocking combined with long-term plaster cast immobilization are rarely performed today. Double-plate osteosynthesis with AO-implants is also considered an exceptional indication in our hospital (Fig. 1). External fixation with the AO tubular system yielded the best results and has become the standard procedure in our institution. This assembly can be adapted to the individual situation. In our opinion, external fixation, which was first described by Key and subsequently improved by Charnley and Müller, entails optimum stability and thus relatively rapid bone healing (Fig. 1).

Supplementary methods are anterior longitudinal resection or, preferably, the sectional incision according to Textor. Initially, the ligamentum patellae is severed, the patella enucleated and, later if necessary, used again as autologous cancellous bone graft or as a gap-filling, cortico-spongious peg (Fig. 2a). Thereafter, tight joint structures must be sufficiently released to permit a mobilization of the knee to an angle of 90°.

Resection of the articular surfaces is then performed with an oscillating saw or, preferably, with a chisel, while the knee joint is bent at an angle of 90° (Fig. 2b). Resection of the joint surfaces has to be carried out in such

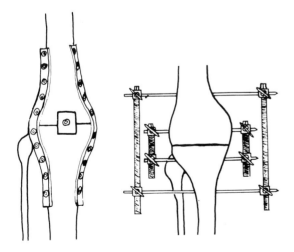

Fig. 1. Possibilities of knee joint arthrodesis. Left: double-plate arthrodesis, internal fixation (exceptional indication!). Right: compression arthrodesis according to Charnley with 2 external tensors and 4 Steinmann pins.

328

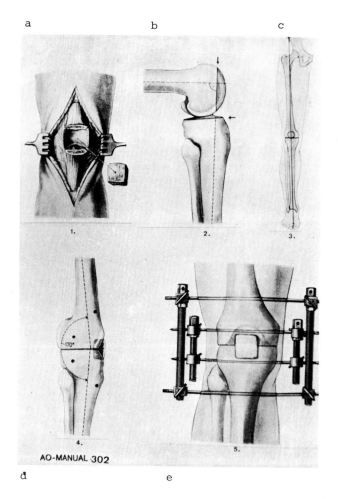

a   b   c

1.   2.   3.

4.   5.

AO-MANUAL 302

d   e

Fig. 2. a) Removal of the patella for the purpose of subsequent corticospongious peg fixation. b) Resection surfaces of the femoral condyles and tibial plateau. c) Correct axis in A.P. projection. d) Correct axis in lateral projection. Note flexion of the knee at 10° and the position of the Steinmann pins. e) Complete assembly and peg fixation.

a way that the arthrodesed knee is in a flexed position of 10°, a valgus position of approximately 5°, and an external rotation of 10-15° (Fig. 2c, 2d). A direct line between anterosuperior iliac spine, middle of the knee joint and interdigital fold between the first and second toe may serve as a guideline for adjusting rotation.

Following close adaptation of the cancellous surfaces, two parallel Steinmann pins 4.5 mm thick are driven into the femoral condyles and the head of the tibia adjacent to the osteotomy in a frontal plane. Before starting this procedure, the respective holes are predrilled after small skin incisions, the pins themselves being inserted with sharp hammer blows to avoid thermal damage. Subsequently, two other Steinmann pins must be inserted more anteriorly and more distantly from the osteotomy site, leaving approximately 6 to 8 cm between pin holes and osteotomy. Similar to the more posteriorly inserted pins, they have to be connected with an external tubular system. Afterwards, axial compression can be exerted to the surfaces of resection by means of a specially-designed threaded compressive device. To attain an even better degree of stability, we recently resorted to a three-dimensional assembly combined with two Schanz screws (Fig. 3).

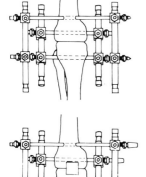

Fig. 3. Diagramatic representation of assembly with external clamps in three-dimensional arrangement and the additional Schanz screws used in a sagittal plane.

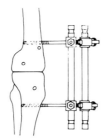

Wound closure is carried out after suture of the ligamentum patellae; two Redon drains are left in place. Thorough hemostasis is imperative. Depending on the condition, the patella is either discarded or inserted as a cancellous bone graft or a bridging peg. Finally, in the operating theatre, a broadly fenestrated long leg plaster cast is applied and the patient is confined to bed. Special attention should be paid to the vessels located in the popliteal fossa when joint surfaces are resected, especially in the presence of flexion deformities needing correction. An overstretch of the vessel/nerve bundle may occur in the latter case because the arthrodesis is performed in a more extended position. This can be avoided by wider resection.

Provided undisturbed healing progresses, bone union is complete after approximately seven to nine weeks, permitting removal of the external fixator and subsequent immobilization in a walking cast for two to three weeks. The above-described physiotherapy combined with occupational therapy will then be carried out as an obligatory follow-up treatment.

Results

The results of 109 knee joint arthrodeses, performed in our hospital between 1969 and 1980, reveal that in approximately four-fifths of these patients the indication for this procedure was severe post-traumatic joint changes, some with associated infections. The remainder consisted principally of patients with rheumatic gonarthroses and another group with infected loosened total knee implants.

With the exception of two patients, arthrodesis was performed by external fixation according to Charnley-Müller. In all cases, a stress-resistant bony fusion could be obtained (Fig. 4a, 4b; 5a, 5b, 5c). Osseous healing was achieved also in the two special cases where a double-plate arthrodesis

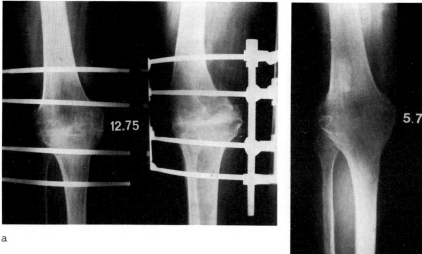
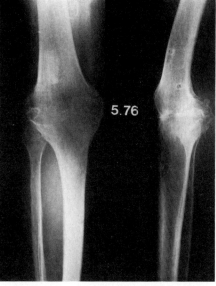

a

b

Fig. 4. a) Arthrodesis by means of external clamps in a 64-year old patient suffering from empyema of the knee joint. b) Complete bone union in a favorable position after 7 months.

was performed. Good functional results were obtained in most patients with respect to the position of arthrodesis, its load-bearing capacity, and walking ability. These results were especially favorable in younger patients. The results were less impressive in older patients after removal of a total knee prosthesis;differences in leg length and a decreased capacity to adapt to the new condition account for these less favorable results.

Discussion

Growing sophistication of total joint replacement necessitates more definitive indications for knee arthrodesis. According to our experience, either of the two methods are of value. Surgical ankylosis, however, is undisputedly the preferred method for younger patients with post-traumatic or rheumatic knee joint arthrosis and limited motion. As a general rule, for patients over 60 years of age partial or total prosthetic joint replacement is performed. It maintains their mobility and eliminates problems associated with ankylosed knee joints. Any history of infection constitutes an absolute indication for arthrodesis even in older patients.

Good functional results can be obtained in spite of the known disadvantages of knee arthrodesis, provided most exacting techniques are carried out, concomitant physiotherapy is provided, and adequate equalization of leg length is achieved.

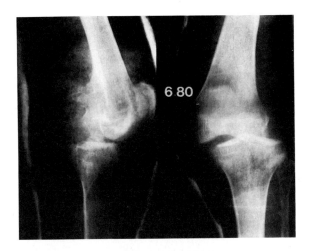

Fig. 5

a) 42-year old patient with an unstable knee joint following complete traumatic dislocation.

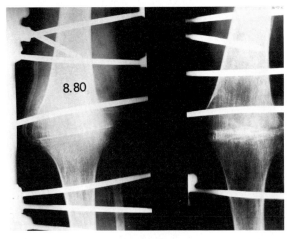

b) Arthrodesis by means of external clamps and Schanz screws in threedimensional arrangement.

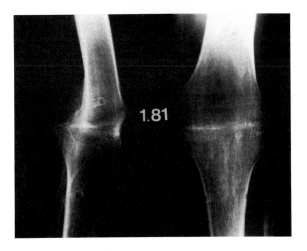

c) Picture of the degree of restoration in a functionally favorable position after 5 months.

Summary

Arthrodesis of the knee is mainly indicated in post-traumatic changes and changes resulting from infections. Less frequent indications are ligament instabilities, loosened total joint implants, tumors, and pseudarthroses in the vicinity of the joint.

Arthrodesis by means of external clamps according to Charnley in a valgus position of 5° and a flexion of 10° is our preferred method. Double-plate arthrodesis is considered an exceptional technique. Subsequent physio-therapy and occupational therapy are important for gait training and ad-justment to shortening of the affected extremity.

Favorable results of restoration of function of the lower extremity were achieved with these methods in a series of 109 knee joint arthrodeses between 1969 and 1980 at the Workmen's Compensation Board Hospital, Tübingen, West Germany.

References

1. Bessenbach, M.: Unsere Erfahrungen mit der Arthrodese, destruierter Kniegelenke infolge chronischer Polyarthritis. Beitr. Orthop. Traum. 17, 763, 1970.

2. Brattström, H., and Brattström, M.: Kniegelenksarthrodese bei Patienten mit rheumatoider Arthrosis. Orthopäde 2, 92, 1973.

3. Brückner, L.: Spätergebnisse der Kniearthrodese. Beitr. Orthop. u. Traumatol. 26, 1979, H6

4. Charnley, J.C.: Positive pressure in arthrodesis of the knee joint. J. Bone Jt. Surg. 30B, 478,1948 .

5. Greiffensteiner, H.: Kompressionsarthrodese des Kniegelenkes. Z. Orthop. 83, 406, 1953.

6. Holz, U., and Weller, S.: Möglichkeiten der äusseren Fixatur Chirurg. 46, 97, 1975.

7. Holz, U.: Indikation and Technik der Kniegelenksarthrodese. Vortrag 5, Reissensburger Workshop zur klinischen Unfallchirurgie, 26-28, Feb. 1976.

8. Key, J.A.: Positive pressure in arthrodesis for tuberculosis of the knee joint. 8th. med. J. 25 909, 1932.

9. Pfister, U.: Die Arthrodese des Kniegelenkes. Vortrag Unfallmed. Arbeitstagung Baden-Baden 18/19. Oct. 1975.

10. Schreiber, A., et al: Sonderdruck aus "Hefte z. Unfallheilkunde" H. 126, 2. Deutsch-Österreichische - Schweizerische Unfalltagung in Berlin 1975. Die Kniearthrodese heute.

External Fixation of High Tibial Osteotomies and Proximal Metaphyseal Fractures of the Tibia

D. L. Fernandez and R. P. Jakob

Introduction

Metaphyseal osteotomies and joint fusions consolidate after five to seven
weeks when a large contact surface is submitted to important axial compression forces, provided that the local cancellous bone is well vascularized. For this reason, external fixation devices are used in metaphyseal areas as compression frames and are a reliable definitive method of
osteosynthesis. The advantages of external fixation for compression
arthrodeses of the shoulder, knee and ankle were first reported by Charnley
in 1948 and 1951. In 1952, M.E. Mueller (1977) applied the same principles,
not only for joint fusions but also to stabilize metaphyseal osteotomies.
Intertrochanteric osteotomies in dysplastic hips and coxa vara were fixed
with two Shanz screws, connected with two threaded rods and set under axial
compression. This first AO external fixation device was subsequently used
for stabilizing high tibial osteotomies, third degree open fractures, and
infected nonunions of the tibial shaft. Until 1975, high tibial osteotomies
were stabilized with a simple compression frame connected to one Steinmann
pin in each bone segment at either side of the osteotomy (Fig. 1a). With
the introduction of the AO Tubular System in 1976, stability was increased
by applying two Steinmann pins in the shaft and one in the metaphysis
(Fig. 1b). In most cases, however, where a simple frame was used, an
additional postoperative plaster splint or a cylinder cast after removal
of the implants was necessary. This residual instability was probably due
to insufficient neutralization of rotatory moments by the simple frame.

With the development of new double clamps in 1978 (to be used with the "old"
threaded rods), it was possible to introduce two Steinmann pins in each bone
segment, resulting in a considerable increase of stability which permitted
full weight bearing of the operated extremity without need for additional
plaster immobilization. The external fixation device consists of two
threaded rods (or spindles), two longitudinal threaded double clamps for
the diaphyseal segment, and two free-gliding transverse double clamps for
the metaphyseal area (Fig. 2a).

The introduction of an anterior and a posterior Steinmann pin in the sagittal plane of the tibial metaphysis permits a greater and more even distribution of the axial compression forces on the whole osteotomy surface, thus
increasing impaction of the cancellous bone and eliminating micromovements
at the osteotomy site. The introduction of the third and fourth Steinmann
pins through the clamps is considerably simplified by using a special aiming device (Fig. 2b and 2c).

334

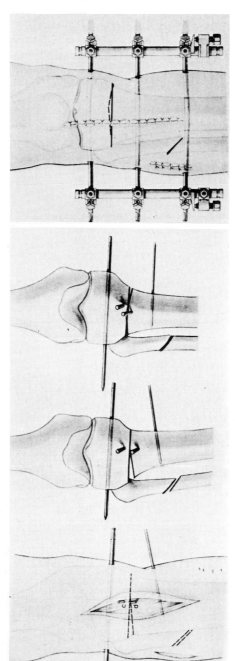

Fig. 1. a) Simple compression frame in bone model for external fixation of high tibial osteotomies used until 1975. b) Technical steps of application of the AO Tubular system with one pin above and two below the osteotomy to increase stability.

External Fixation of High Tibial Osteotomies

The ideal indication for a high tibial osteotomy is the early, primary, predominantly monocompartimental osteoarthritis of the knee, mostly due to varus-valgus malalignment of the lower extremity. The majority of the cases are painful varus knees showing progressive degenerative changes in the medial compartment, not infrequently following a medial meniscectomy performed 10 to 15 years before. Considerable limitation of the range of motion of the knee joint (less than 80-90° of active flexion) contraindicates high tibial osteotomies. The site of corrective osteotomies about the knee is decided after careful analysis of long preoperative roentgenograms taken with the patient standing. Surgical correction should be undertaken at the site of the main deformity: supracondylar, high-tibial,

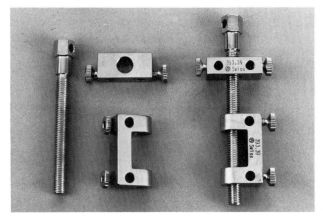

a

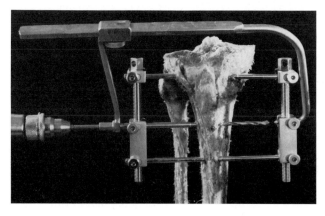

b

Fig. 2. a) New external fixation device for high tibial osteotomies and ankle and knee fusions, showing threaded rods, transverse gliding double clamps, and longitudinal threaded double clamps. Fixation screws for Steinman pins can be tightened by hand. Also shown: a hexagonal AO screwdriver. b) A special aiming device permits accurate drilling for the introduction of the third and fourth Steinmann pins through the double clamps.

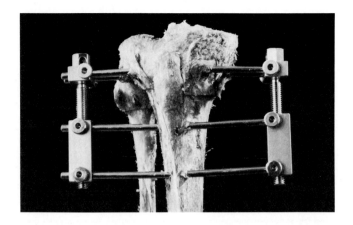

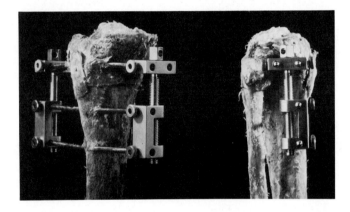

Fig. 2 (continued)
c) Anterior, oblique, and lateral views of the external fixator in place. Notice high fibular osteotomy and partial osteotomy of the tibial tubercule which acts as a vascularized bridging bone graft. Fixation screws on the medial clamps are excentric so that the sharp pointed tips of the Steinmann pins remain within the clamps avoiding unnecessary skin lesions of the opposite leg.

or both (in cases of complex deformities), based on the relation of the knee axis to the mechanical axis and the physiologic angles of the distal femur and proximal tibia in relation to the anatomic longitudinal axis of these bones.

It is important to consider also the degree of unilateral collapse of the joint space in the standing roentgenograms, which is directly proportional to the cartilage defect. Therefore, during preoperative planning, the amount of collapse should be added to the correction angle of the osteotomy. Analysis of the failures of high tibial osteotomies at the University of Berne has shown that they were mostly due to insufficient overcorrection of this unilateral collapse of the joint space. In cases with complex deformities, especially rotatory malalignment, the exact amount of malrotation is best determined with a preoperative CAT study.

Technique

The leg is prepared and draped in such a manner that a visual control of the long axis of the lower extremity is guaranteed. Usually, a long Steridrape,

as used for total knee replacements, is applied. The limb is exsanguinated
and a tourniquet applied. A 10 cm anterolateral longitudinal straight incision is made, beginning just proximal to the joint space and is centered
at a midpoint between the bony prominences of the tibial tuberosity and the
head of the fibula. Through this incision it is possible to expose both
the lateral and anterior aspects of the proximal tibia and the head and neck
of the fibula. The anterolateral insertion of the anterior tibial muscle is
detached, exposing the lateral aspect of the tibia, and then the anterosuperior insertion of the peroneus longus muscle is incised and the head and
neck of the fibula are exposed subperiosteally by separating the proximal
attachment of the peroneus longus muscle laterally and distally. The common
peroneal nerve does not need to be identified, since it lies posterior to the
peroneus longus muscle. The fibula is osteotomized at the head-neck level,
and a small lateral wedge is resected if a valgus osteotomy is planned.

The great advantage of the high fibula osteotomy 10 to 12 cm below the joint
space, compared with the one formerly used, is that it allows greater mobility of the distal fragment. It is useful in cases where complex corrections are to be performed, ie, forward replacement of the shaft to ventralize
the tibial tuberosity in patients with associated patellofemoral osteoarthritis, or to correct important rotatory malalignments. If a low fibular osteotomy is used, free motion of the tibial shaft is somewhat limited by the
strong proximal attachments of the interosseous membrane to the proximal
third of the fibula.

Fig. 3 shows the different steps of the operation based on the preoperative
planning of a high tibial valgus osteotomy:

1. Oblique osteotomy of the fibula, 10 cm below the joint line for simple
    corrections in the frontal plane, or high fibular osteotomy for complex
    osteotomies as explained above, which also has the advantage that it is
    done through the same skin incision.

2. A 2 mm drill hole is made 5 cm distal to the planned osteotomy site,
    through the anterior cortex and perpendicular to the long axis of the
    tibia in the frontal plane. A 2 mm Kirschner wire (a) is introduced
    in this hole.

3. A 4.5 mm Steinmann pin is introduced 1 or 2 cm distal to the joint space
    and anterior in the sagittal plane, after drilling the hole with a 3.5 mm
    drill bit. Its position in relation with K-wire (a) represents the angle
    of correction. In the coronal plane, this Steinmann pin is slightly
    oblique from anterior to posterior, to provide enough room in the proxi-
    mal tibia for the posterior Steinmann pin which will lie just in front
    of the head of the fibula.

4. The proximal part of the tibial tuberosity is osteotomized and elevated
    together with the patellar tendon using a flat osteotome.

5. Partial transverse osteotomy of the tibial metaphysis about 2.5 cm below
    the articular surface, using flat osteotomes and oscillating saw.

6. Two Kirschner wires (c and d) are drilled from the front to the back
    above and below the osteotomy line, and parallel to each other to con-
    trol rotation.

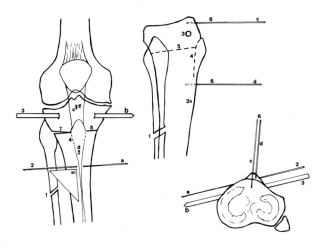

Fig. 3.

a) Preoperative planning and tactical steps of the bone procedure. The steps are numbered and correspond to those explained in the text.

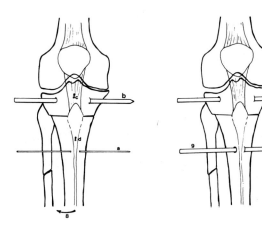

b) Realignment of the leg after completion of osteotomy and introduction of 2nd Steinmann pin distally.

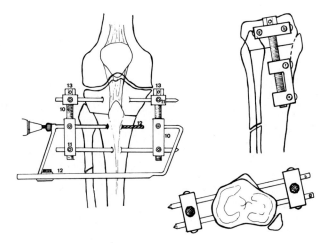

c) External fixator adjusted over Steinmann pins. Diagram shows use of aiming device and position of external fixator in the sagittal and coronal planes.

7. The osteotomy is completed with the knee held in flexion to relax the posterior tibial neurovascular bundle. A small lateral wedge is then removed if we are dealing with hard cancellous bone.

8. The leg is reduced to obtain the desired corrections. At this point, Steinmann pin (b) and the K-wire (a) should be parallel to each other. The K-wire (a) is removed and the 2 mm hole overdrilled to 3.5 mm.

9. The second 4.5 mm Steinmann pin (e) is introduced from lateral to medial.

10. The external fixation device is placed by sliding the transverse gliding double clamps onto the proximal Steinmann pin, and the longitudinal threaded double clamps on the distal Steinmann pin.

11. The alignmnent of the leg is checked and the fixation screws for the Steinmann pins slightly tightened.

12. Once the correction corresponds to the preoperative planning, the holes for the introduction of the third and fourth Steinmann pins are pre- pared with the 3.5 mm drill bit. For this purpose a special aiming device (Fig. 2b), which permits drilling the holes exactly parallel to the first two Steinmann pins, is placed with the 3.5 drill guide within the free holes of the double clamps. Then, Steinmann pins (f) and (g) are introduced through the clamps.

13. By tightening the threaded rods on both sides, the osteotomy is set under axial compression.

The tourniquet is released, careful hemostasis is performed, and the wound is closed. Special attention must be given to skin tension around the Steinmann pins. Small relaxing incisions are made to prevent secondary necrosis, thus avoiding the risk of pin-tract infections. Postoperatively, a conventional sterile dressing is applied and the patient is instructed on careful daily disinfection of the wounds. Full weight bearing and early joint motion is allowed as soon as the postoperative edema has subsided. Secondary corrections in the frontal plane can be undertaken in the post- operative period through unilateral tightening of one threaded rod. The device is removed 5-6 weeks after surgery, once bone union has been confirmed clinically and radiographically.

Clinical Profile

In 1979, a clinical control of the first 12 high tibial osteotomies which were stabilized with this system was carried out. Eleven were primary early osteoarthritides of the knee with significant axial malalignment, and one patient had a post-traumatic valgus deformity. The following corrections were performed: 8 valgus osteotomies, 3 varus osteotomies and 1 derotation osteotomy. In three patients, correction in the frontal plane was combined with extension in the sagittal plane to correct extension lags not exceeding 15°. In one patient with associated femoropatellar osteo- arthritis and lateral subluxation of the patella, the tibial tuberosity was medialized and displaced anteriorly. The average consolidation time of this series was 6.5 weeks. Type and degree of corrections performed and postoperative function achieved are presented in Table I. Ten patients (83%) could fully bear weight within the first two weeks after surgery.

Table I.

Patient	Year of birth	Operation	Correction	Consoli-dation	Postop. active function Flexion/Extension
1. N.A.	1924	July 78	Valg. 10°	6 W	130-5-0°
2. B.T.	1901	Jan. 79	Var. 10° Ext. 10°	7 W	120-0-0°
3. B.M.	1927	Feb. 79	Valg. 12° AR 25°	5 1/1 W	110-10-0°
4. A.O.	1906	March 79	Valg. 15°	8 W	115-5-0°
5. C.E.	1906	June 79	Var. 15°	6 W	110-0-0°
6. S.T.	1959	June 79	Var. 10°	7 W	110-0-0°
7. S.H.	1907	June 79	Valg. 15° Ext. 10°	8 W	100-0-0°
8. K.H.	1924	June 79	AR 30°	9 W	130-0-0°
9. B.F.	1917	Aug. 79	Valg. 15° AR 30°	delayed union	80-10-0°
10. R.A.	1923	Sept. 79	Valg. 10° Elmslie	7 W	120-0-0°
11. P.P.	1933	Sept. 79	Valg. 10° Ext. 5°	6 W	120-30-0°
12. H.A.	1920	Sept. 79	Valg. 10°	5 W	105-0-0°

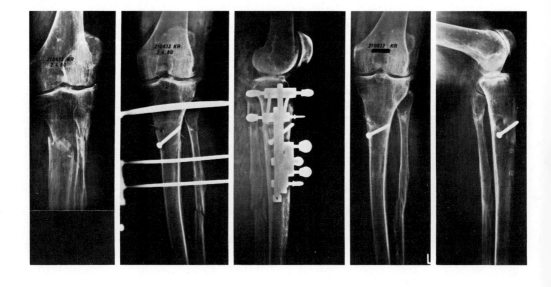

Two pin tract infections were observed: in 1 case a distal Steinmann pin got infected. This localized infection healed with local treatment three weeks after removal of the implants, after the osteotomy had healed. The second patient had a pin tract infection of one of the proximal pins, from which *Staphylococcus aureus* was cultured. This patient had a valgus osteotomy of 12° combined with a derotation of 25° due to internal tibial torsion. Derotation led to important skin tension and secondary necrosis favoring local contamination. Undisturbed bone healing was observed in 11 cases. The second infected case showed delayed union due to loosening of the proximal pins at the time of the follow-up study in September 1979.

Other indications

The same system has now been introduced and used routinely for compression arthrodesis of the ankle and knee joints. The indication has been extended for the stabilization of proximal metaphyseal fractures of the tibia where the plane of the fracture is transverse or slightly oblique, therefore suitable for primary axial compression (Fig. 4).

Summary

Current clinical experience with the new AO external compression device with double clamps in high tibial osteotomies and certain proximal fractures of the tibia has revealed that with a double Steinmann pin fixation placed in different planes, a considerable increase in stability is achieved. The patients have practically no postoperative pain, and early rehabilitation of the arthritic knee and full weight bearing after wound healing is guaranteed (Fig. 5). Additional postoperative plaster splints or external supports after removal of the external fixation device are no longer necessary.

References

1. Charnley, J.: Compression arthrodesis of the ankle and shoulder. J.Bone Jt. Surg. 33B, 180, 1951

2. Fernandez, D.L. and Mueller, M.E.: Neue AO-Fixateur Externe Osteosynthese bei der Tibiakopfosteotomie: Technik und Ergebnisse. Read at the International Symposium on External Fixation, Duisburg, Germany, March 1980.

3. Mueller, M.E., Allgoewer, M., Schneider, R., Willenegger, H.: Manual der Osteosynthese, Zweite Auflage, Springer Verlag, 1977. Berlin-Heidelberg-New York.

◄ Fig. 4. Short oblique metaphyseal compound fracture of the tibia and segmental fracture of the fibula in a 68-year old patient. Fixation by means of one lag screw, after anatomic reduction and application of compression frame with double clamps. Roentgenographic appearance of healed fracture at 12 weeks.

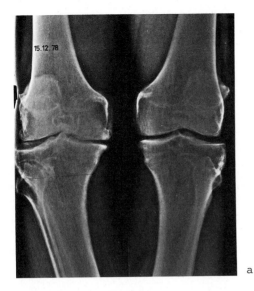

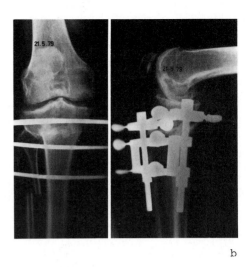

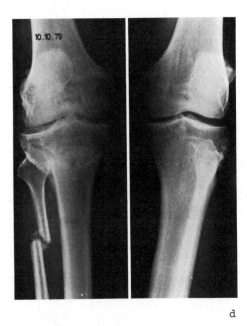

Fig. 5. a) Degenerative changes mostly localized in the medial compartment and varus malalignment of the right knee following medial meniscectomy. b) Postoperative roentgenograms after high tibial valgus osteotomy fixed with new external fixation device. c) Photograph of same patient fully weight bearing 12 days after surgery, with external fixation device in place. d) Roentgenograms after 4.5 months, showing correct axial realignment and healed osteotomy.

Arthrodesis of the Ankle Joint

K. Weise and S. Weller

Introduction

A high percentage of patients with ankle injuries experience secondary
arthrosis, discomfort while weight bearing, and difficulty in walking despite most exacting surgical reconstruction procedures. These conditions,
considerably reducing the patient's mobility and ability to work, are
partly due to the severity of the injury, but occasionally also due to
unsatisfactory surgical procedures which fail to restore an anatomic position of the fragments. Besides post-traumatic osteoarthritis, infections
of the ankle joint, congenital foot deformities, and unfavorably positioned,
essentially ankylosed joints associated with paralysis constitute indications for arthrodesis.

The opinion expressed by Vulpius over 50 years ago that arthrodesis is a
case of an *operatio pauperum* can no longer be shared today. Neither the
lifelong provision of an orthesis nor the talocrural alloarthroplasty,
which has not yet given satisfactory results, can, in our opinion, be considered a useful alternative. We believe that a properly placed, arthrodesed ankle joint with an orthopedically designed and fitted shoe offer
the best conditions for the patient as far as weight bearing of the affected
extremity is concerned.

A great variety of surgical procedures has been described, such as Lange's
interlocking method, the removal of cartilage and peg implantation according to Merle-d'Aubigné, Mittlemeier's osteotomy plate, rotational ankylosis
according to Roeren, and Greifensteiner's two-wire traction clip. From the
point of view of bony consolidation, however, correct position of the foot
and early stability to enable exercise, compression arthrodesis by means of
external clamps according to Charnley stands out distinctly among these
methods.

Internal compression arthrodeses appear to us too dangerous, frequently
damaging soft tissues, especially in the presence of poor blood supply.
Besides, indications for bone peg and interlocking operations, and surgery
involving the removal of cartilage followed by protracted plaster cast
immobilization, appear questionable to us in view of the difficulties in
obtaining union and maintaining a proper foot position.

Indications

As to the timing of ankle fusion after an accident involving talocrural
articulation, we propose the following classification:

1) Primary arthrodesis

2) Early arthrodesis (up to one-half year after the accident)

3) Late arthrodesis

Primary arthrodeses are carried out in our hospital only in exceptional cases where reconstructive surgery is impossible as a result of fractures of the pilon tibiale and severely comminuted fractures of the talus. In patients with fracture dislocations of the ankle joint, this procedure is only indicated when the injury is associated with extensive damage to the joint surfaces. The main advantage of primary arthrodesis is the prevention of disuse changes of neighboring joints. Also, complications usually do not occur, such as dystrophy followed by osteoporosis or disturbances resulting from lack of blood supply to bones.

Early arthrodesis should be performed when primary osteosynthesis fails and there is no suitable alternative for correction. Early arthrodesis seems to be the best method, especially in the event of infection of the joint following a compound injury, or in the event of postoperative infection; it enables the patient relatively early weight bearing on the affected extremity.

By far the greatest number of patients with severe changes in the talocrural articulation are treated with *late arthrodesis*, which is carried out when a patient suffers increasing discomfort and insists on the treatment himself. Secondary damage to neighboring joints, foot bones, and soft tissue constitute a distinct disadvantage of late arthrodesis. By then, the tarsal joint is frequently affected by a more or less marked arthrosis and the tarsal area often shows degenerative changes. Swelling and impaired blood circulation are other unfavorable factors of late arthrodesis, deteriorating subjective and objective results. Bony fusion and maximum weight bearing may thus be delayed, particularly since poor positioning will often necessitate a correction at the same time. Occasionally, arthrodesis of the ankle joint has to be extended to the subtalar joint; moreover, corrective osteotomy in the tarsal region has sometimes to be carried out. Despite these difficulties, arthrodesis permits full weight bearing of the affected extremity with little or no pain, thereby improving the patient's ability to work. Concomitant intensive physical and occupational therapy contributes significantly to success and thus merits special attention.

Technique

Under tourniquet, a skin incision is made over the distal end of the fibula, and the fibula is osteotomized subperiosteally and obliquely two fingerbreadths proximal to the joint line. The distal end of the fibula is removed and kept for subsequent peg fixation. The osteotomy of the medial malleolus is performed through a small, separate incision. Removal of cartilage from the distal end of the tibia and the joint surfaces of the talus is carried out with an oscillating saw or, still better, to prevent heat necrosis with a broad chisel, in such a way that flat spongeous surfaces are created to allow afterwards placing of the foot in a right-angled position (Fig. 1a).

Existing varus and valgus deformities as well as a possible equinus position must be considered during resection. We do not believe that a certain degree

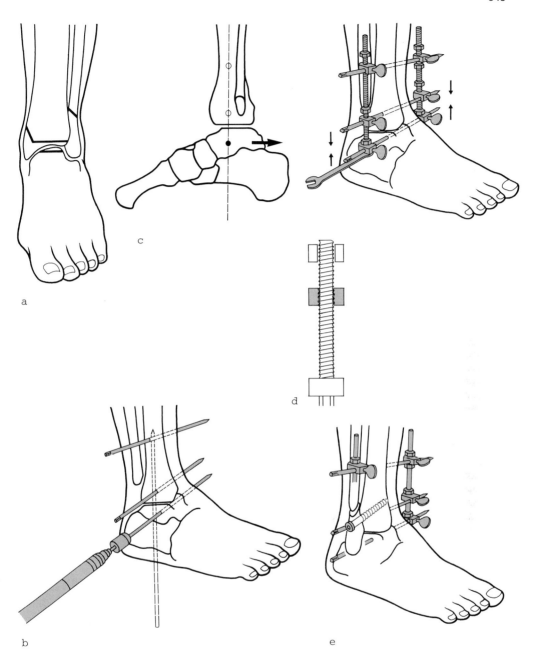

Fig. 1. a) Resection lines. b) Temporary fixation of the arthrodesis position with a Steinmann pin from the heel into the distal end of the tibia. Localization of the 3 Steinmann pins applied parallel through the distal end of the tibia and the talus. c) Backward displacement of the foot. d) Compression in the area of the resectioned surface by means of external clamps. e) Bridging with the distal end of the fibula freed of cartilage used as a bone peg; fixation by means of a screw.

of equinus, once considered desirable in women, is any longer called for because of the plantar range of movement of the talonavicular joint. After dorsal displacement of the foot, the corrected position can be temporarily maintained by means of a Steinmann pin driven through the heel. Following preliminary drilling with a 3.5 mm bit, three 4.5 mm Steinmann pins are inserted through small, separate incisions into the skin, two in the tibia and one into the talus. Care should be taken to place the Steinmann pins parallel to one another and perpendicular to the shaft axis, in the tibia at a distance of approximately 10 and 3 cm from the osteotomy surface, and in the talus at a sufficient distance from the ankle joint so that the pins do not cut through the soft, osteoporotic bone during application of tension (Fig. 1b and 1c).

After assembly has been completed with external clamps, sufficient pressure is applied to the osteotomy surfaces. The arthrodesis is completed by lateral apposition and screw fixation of the corticocancellous end of the fibula, freed of any articular cartilage (Fig. 1d and 1e). In the presence of infection, additional internal fixation is not carried out.

Following release of the tourniquet and careful hemostasis, the incisions are closed after insertion of two separate Redon drains. After a postoperative roentgenogram, immobilization is effected by a circular, fenestrated plaster cast applied to the lower leg. The patient is confined to bed, the leg being held in the elevated position on splints.

Following the operation, we prescribe physiotherapy with gradual mobilization and walking exercises, progression depending on the individual patient (Fig. 2). With good compression and good adaptation of the osteotomy surfaces, consolidation will take place within 6-12 weeks. During the last phase of plaster cast immobilization, a walking heel may be applied, the clamps having already been removed by this time. If advanced union can be observed on roentgenograms, the patient can be temporarily discharged. Plaster cast removal, supply of proper footware and physiotherapy, however, necessitate rehospitalization. In cases of pronounced dystrophy, corrective orthopedic footware is fitted as quickly as possible, assuring that the foot is properly placed and the sole permitted to roll from heel to toe. On the other hand, the mobility of the tarsal, metatarsal and forefoot areas must be given consideration. When the footware is ready, intensive walking exercises are begun.

Results

A clinical study involving 135 arthrodeses of the ankle (Schmelzeisen, 1975) from October 1969 to April 1975 at the Workmen's Compensation Board Accident Hospital, in Tübingen, West Germany, clearly demonstrates the superiority of results achieved by employing the modified Charnley method over results of subsequently published series (Fig. 3a, 3b; 4a, 4b, 4c; 5a, 5b, 5c). The following arthrodeses were performed:

Primary arthrodesis	4
Early arthrodesis	23
Late arthrodesis	94
Rearthrodesis (6 from our clinic, 8 from elsewhere)	14
Total	135

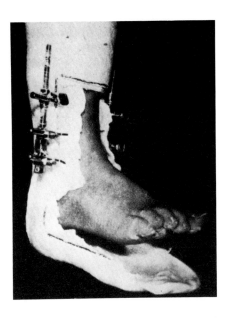

Fig. 2. Therapeutic exercises in a padded plaster cast applied to the lower leg of patients confined to bed.

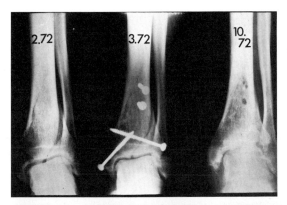

Fig. 3.

a) 43-year old patient with a fracture of the pilon tibiale of the left leg. Inadequate repositioning and fixation by means of screw osteosynthesis. Severe arthrosis associated with osteolysis as a result of infection.

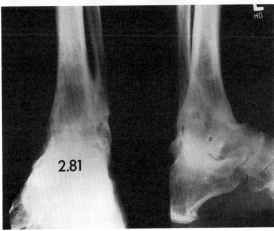

b) Arthrodesis in the presence of infection with external clamps using a modified Charnley technique. Result of healing process after 9 months.

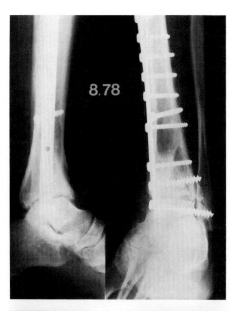

Fig. 4.

a) 43-year old patient with a pilon fracture of the tibia. Treatment by primary arthrodesis of the talocrural articulation using a plate in an unfavorable position. No bone healing occurred.

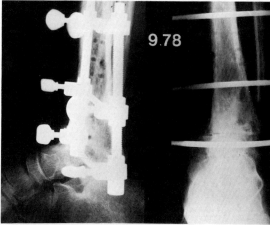

b) Rearthrodesis with external clamp and resection of the joint surfaces.

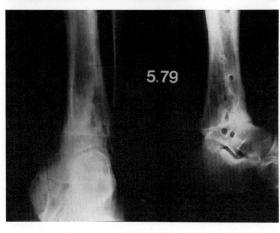

c) Radiograph showing excellent position and union after 8 months.

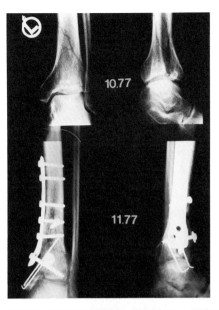

Fig. 5.

a) Fracture of the pilon tibial of the
left leg in a 51-year old patient. Inadequate treatment by means of osteosynthesis with screws; development of
a severe post-traumatic secondary arthrosis associated with malposition.

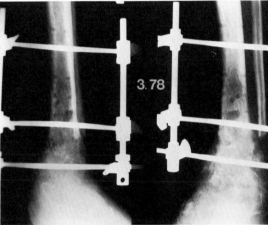

b) Arthrodesis by means of external clamps.

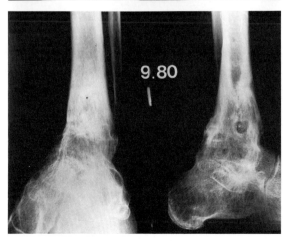

c) Healing process resulting
in complete union in a good
position.

Arthrodesis of the ankle joint was performed in 120 patients. In eight
patients the subtalar joint was simultaneously fused. In seven patients,
pseudarthrosis of the tibia was treated at the same time. Our results can
be tabulated as follows:

Primary union	127
No bony union	8
Solid after rearthrodesis	6
No rearthrodesis	2
Total	135

These results compare favorably with a similar series reported in the literature.

Complications during the postoperative period were as follows:

No ankylosis	8
Wound infection	4
Fistula around the screw	6
Drainage around Steinmann pins	12
Hematoma	3
Necrosis of the margin of the wound	2
Malrotation	2
Decubitus	2

It should be mentioned that in the presence of an infection, internal fixation of the bone-peg by means of a screw is rarely performed today. If
the soft tissues are of a poor quality, we consider the internal fixation
methods contraindicated. Some of the complications may also have resulted
from previous infections.

Discussion

If the results of 94% primary arthrodesis using external clamps are compared
with those of other techniques of arthrodesis, it is apparent that compression arthrodesis by means of external clamps, a modification of the Charnley
and AO techniques, offers definite advantages. This is especially apparent
when considering the time factor and success rate of union, even in the presence of soft tissue damage and displacement.

Meticulous surgical techniques, careful treatment of soft tissue damage and
intensive occupational and physiotherapy will generally provide all the
essential elements to achieve not only healing but also weight bearing under
strenuous conditions.

Summary

Post-traumatic secondary arthrodesis following injuries to the ankle joint accompanied by restricted mobility and pain on exercise is the main indication for surgical ankylosis.

We prefer a modification of the Charnley technique, a fixation by means of external clamps. An exact resectioning of the joint surface of the distal end of the tibia and the talus is of prime importance. A distinction is made between primary, early and late arthrodeses depending on the timing of surgery. Concomitant therapy involving physiotherapy and supply of orthopedic footware is of great importance for the functional outcome.

Between October 1969 and April 1975 we performed 135 arthrodeses of the ankle joint at the Workmen's Compensation Board Hospital, Tübingen, West Germany. Primary union was achieved in 127 patients. Six patients in whom the arthrodesis had failed achieved bony union after a second procedure.

References

1. Boltze, W.-H., Fernandez, D.L., Schatzker, J.: The External Fixator (Tubular System). Official Publication of the Swiss Association for the Study of Internal Fixation.

2. Bürkle, de la Camp, H.: Zur Resektion und Arthrodese des oberen Sprunggelenkes. Z.Chir. 86, 912, 1961.

3. Charnley, J.: Compression arthrodesis of the ankle and shoulder. J.Bone Jt.Surg. 33B, No. 2, 180, 1951.

4. Dahmen, G., and Meyer, H.: Über die verschiedenen Methoden zur Arthrodese des oberen Sprunggelenkes. Arch. orthop. Unfall-Chir. 58, 265, 1965.

5. Holz, U., and Weller, S.: Möglichkeiten der äußeren Fixation. Chir. 46, 97, 1975.

6. Kossyk, W., and Kern, R.: Klinische Ergebnisse bei Arthrodesen des Sprunggelenkes. Arch. orthop. Unfall-Chir. 80, 177, 1974.

7. Meinhardt, U.: Indikation, Technik und Ergebnisse der posttraumatischen Arthrodese des oberen Sprunggelenkes. Act.Traumatol. 3, 177, 1973.

8. Mittelmeier, H., Hort, W., and Diehl, K: Interne Kompressionarthrodese des oberen Sprunggelenkes (einschließlich vergleichender Stabilitätsuntersuchungen). Arch. orthop. Unfall-Chir. 81, 57, 1974

9. Rimoldi, M.: Spätergebnisse bei oberen Sprunggelenksarthrodesen nach Charnley. Act.Traumatol. 7, 315, 1977.

10. Schmelzeisen, H.: Arthrodesen nach schweren Gelenkverletzungen im Bereich des Fußes . Vortrag Unfallmed. Arbeitstagung, Baden-Baden, 18/19, October 1975.

11. Speiser, P.: Die Kompressionsarthrodese des oberen Sprunggelenkes. Arch. orthop. Unfall-Chir. 51, 187, 1959.

12. Thom, H.: Spätergebnisse nach 81 Arthrodesen des oberen Sprunggelenkes. Z. Orthop. 111, 446, 1973.

External Skeletal Fixation of the Lower Thoracic and the Lumbar Spine

F. Magerl

Introduction

By far the most common level of spinal injury is the thoracolumbar junction.
In our experience (Magerl, 1980), 22% of the thoracic and 8% of the lumbar
injuries had significant neurologic involvement. About 9% of all thoracic
and lumbar fractures required surgical intervention with different methods.

The goals of surgical treatment are: efficient decompression of neural tissue; healing of the spine without deformity and instability; early ambulation and functional aftercare; facility of nursing care. The operative
method should permit the surgeon to meet these goals; otherwise it would
offer little benefit over conservative measures.

Widely known methods of surgical stabilization include Harrington instrumentation (Dickson et al, 1978; Flesch et al, 1977; Jacobs et al, 1980);
plate fixations (Roy-Camille et al, 1979; 1980); and various composits of
implants and bone cement. Using these methods for the treatment of thoracolumbar and lumbar fractures, early mobilization without rigid external
support generally is not possible. Moreover, a major disadvantage is the
need to include five vertebrae in the segment to be stabilized to achieve
adequate results.

We have investigated an external fixation procedure for stabilization of
the spine based on several reasons which will be discussed in detail. In
addition to the versatility of the external fixation system, one of the
main reasons was the advantage of achieving nearly the same initial but
apparently a more durable stability while requiring immobilization of
fewer intact segments than with the other methods. For instance, in treating an unstable fracture of L3 we need only immobilization from L2 to L4,
as opposed to the routine L1 to L5 immobilization with other methods. This
makes an important difference regarding function.

Experience with plate fixation has shown that screws can securely be introduced and anchored into the pedicles and the vertebral body. It seemed to
be advantageous and the insertion of Schanz screws in an external fixation
device is not more difficult than other methods.

Method Description

The external fixation device

The original ASIF external fixator with threaded bars was used in the first
12 cases. A new device, specifically designed for the spine with improved

adjustability, was developed in collaboration with F. Schläpfer* and used
in subsequent cases. Basically, the fixator consists of four Schanz screws
and a connecting mechanism. This mechanism, shown in Fig. 1, is fully adjustable and easy to handle. The special Schanz screws have a posterior
diameter of 6 mm and an anterior of 5 mm. They are sharp-pointed and self-
tapping.

Operative technique

A complete description of the operative technique is beyond the scope of
this paper but has recently been published (Magerl, 1981). Only a brief
review of the essential points is given here.

Over the course of this study some improvements and refinements of the
technique have been made. The current standard procedures are outlined
in Fig. 2-8.

Closed reduction is performed in the anesthetized patient unless this
maneuvre would risk neurologic damage. The final correction is obtained
by the open method, and Schanz screws as well as the external fixator can
be used to aid the reduction. In this case the fixator is preliminarily
assembled in the open wound.

The Schanz screws can be inserted through the open wound or by a closed
method. An image intensifier is always required for correct positioning
of the screws as they must enter the vertebral body through the pedicle
and should not penetrate its anterior wall. In the closed technique the
position of the pedicle is identified with the patient in the prone position and the image intensifier in the vertical position. The table is then
tilted until the pedicle appears as a sharply defined oval ring. At the
center of the ring the self-tapping Schanz screw is vertically inserted into
the bone.

----

*Laboratorium für experimentelle Chirurgie, Davos, Switzerland

Fig. 1. The assembled external fixator. a) The Schanz screws, inserted into
the vertebrae, are fixed with connectors to the transverse bars. Three rods
with counter rotating threads connect the bars in the longitudinal direction.
Adjustability in all planes of motion is provided by ball and socket joints
between the rods and bars. For secure locking of the final position between
bars and rods, triangular plates with three setscrews are threaded into the
ends of the rods and the screws tightened. b) Close-up showing the ball and
socket joint before placement of the triangular plate. The rod with the balls
attached is introduced through the larger portion of the holes in the plates
and secured into the smaller socket portion by means of setscrews.

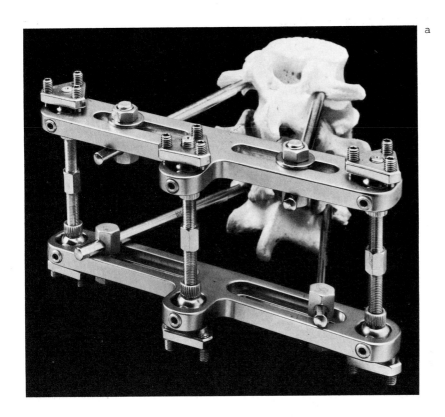

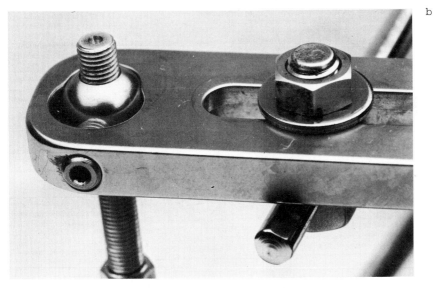

Fig. 1. (Legend see previous page)

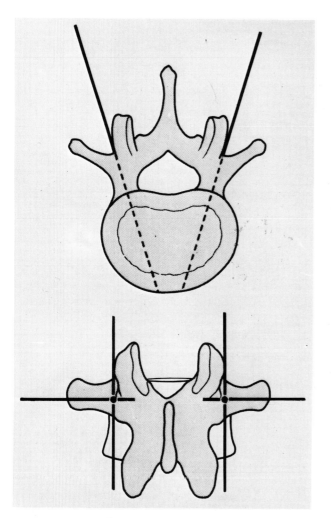

Fig. 2. Point of entry and direction of the Schanz screws.

a) The point of entry is the central axis of the pedicular tube indicated by the intersection of the two lines. The vertical line touches the lateral border of the superior articular process, the horizontal line bisects the base of the trans- verse process.

b) The direction of the Schanz screws is 10°-20° convergent toward the sa- gittal plane (see text).

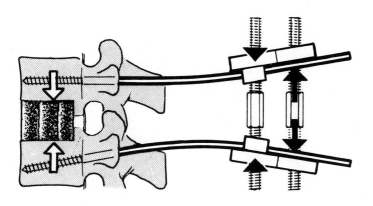

Fig. 3. The fixator used in compression for stabilization of an anterior inter- body fusion. For adequate anchorage the inferior screws are directed into the inferior part of the vertebral body. In this case, the Schanz screws are inserted by the closed technique (see text).

Nearly all patients who are suitable for operative stabilization of the spine
have definite damage to the intervertebral disc or facet joints and require
a posterior or, rarely, an anterior fusion. In most cases, therefore, the
Schanz screws can be applied by the open method. Recently, to shorten operative time, the Schanz screws have been inserted by the closed method after
wound closure.

The safety and effectiveness of the procedure is dependent on the accurate
placement of the Schanz screws. Fig. 2 shows the point of entry and the
direction of the screws. They pass through the pedicle, approximately
parallel to the end plate and with an inclination toward the sagittal plane
to about 10° at the lower thoracic levels, increasing up to 15-20° at L5.
In the lower lumbar levels the larger size of the pedicles (Saillant, 1978)
gives more margin of safety for placement of the screws.

According to the mechanical demands, the fixator can be applied in compression (Fig. 3), distraction (Fig. 4, 6, 7, 8) or in a neutral position
(Fig. 8). Continuous compression or distraction is provided by elastic deformation of the Schanz screws. For this important preloading of the
screws a constant counterforce is necessary. This counterforce is provided
by the screw fixation of the facet joints and/or by the wire loop around
the spinal processes when the fixator is preloaded in distraction (Fig. 6).
In an anterior interbody fusion (Fig. 3) this force acts at the corticocancellous grafts.

When the fixator is prestressed in distraction, the principal fulcrum is at
the threaded rods close to the skin. The fusion provides a supplementary
fulcrum (Fig. 6) for the Schanz screws which is beneficial for stability
when the axial compression load exceeds the pretension of the Schanz screws.

For screw fixation of facet joints at the thoracolumbar junction and the
lumbar spine, a translaminar screw fixation as shown in Fig. 5 is recommended (Magerl, 1980). It is important to emphasize that the screws are
not inserted as lag screws. King's technique (Crenshaw, 1971) is used
where the facet joints are oriented toward the frontal plane (L5-S1).

In the treatment of osteomyelitis (Fig. 8), the suction irrigation system is
used for three days followed by suction alone for about five days. The
patient can be mobilized after irrigation is discontinued. For stage 2,
the same surgical approach is used as for the anterior debridement in
stage 1. Delay of stage 2 of more than three weeks is avoided to prevent
difficulties of exposure secondary to adhesions. At the present time, for
stage 2, the fixator is applied in the neutral mode if the anterior graft
is pressure resistant and if an interspinous H-graft has been inserted.

Postoperative care

To enable the patient to lie supine, we use a foam mattress with a hole to
accommodate the fixator. A compressive dressing prevents window edema
which could occur during supine sleep. Patients are mobilized as comfort
permits, usually after four days. A short molded plastic brace with a
rigid box houses the fixator and protects it from damage. Pin tract care
instructions are given before discharge. Outpatients are followed biweekly.

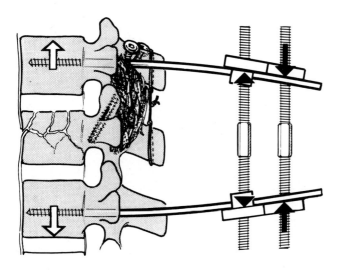

Fig. 4. Stabilization of a wedge fracture with damage to the upper disc. After reduction of the fracture, posterior fusion with screw fixation (see text and Fig. 5), occasionally supplemented by a tension band wire loop, is performed only at the level where the fracture of the end plate has damaged the intervertebral disc. The fixator is prestressed in distraction. This mechanical system continues to allow some motion at the un-fused level due to the elasticity of the Schanz screws.

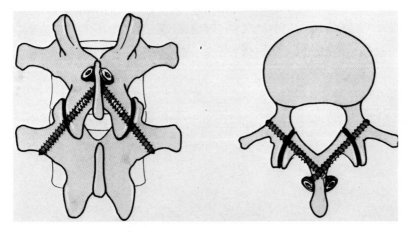

Fig. 5. The translaminar screw fixation of facet joints at the thoracolumbar junction and the lumbar spine where the facet joints are oriented toward the sagittal plane (see text).

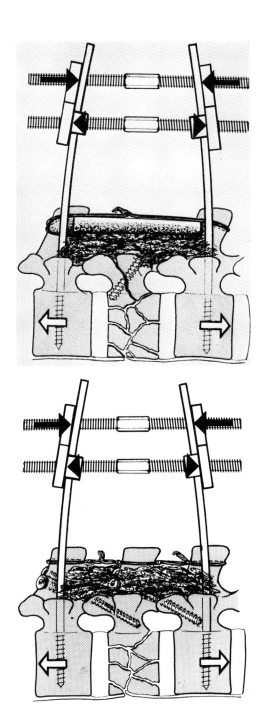

a

b

Fig. 6. Stabilization of a fracture with damage to both adjacent discs or facet joints.
a) When the bony integrity of the posterior elements is maintained, or a suitable fracture configuration exists, dorsal fusion with screw fixation of the facet joints is carried out over the
two levels of involvement and is supplemented by a tension band wire loop. The fixator is prestressed in distraction. Rigid fixation of the facet joints provides a solid bony fulcrum for
the Schanz screws (see text).   b) When screw fixation of the facet joints is impossible due to
the fracture configuration of the posterior elements, a corticocancellous H-graft secured with
a wire loop provides the fulcrum. Again, the dorsal fusion is carried out over the two levels of
involvement. Structurally significant fractures of posterior elements are fixed with lag screws
to increase stability and to prevent potentially dangerous dislocation of fragments. In both
instances, a and b, an important function of the wire loop is to provide the counteracting force
for the pretension or, in other words, to prevent overdistraction when the pretension is applied
to the Schanz screws.

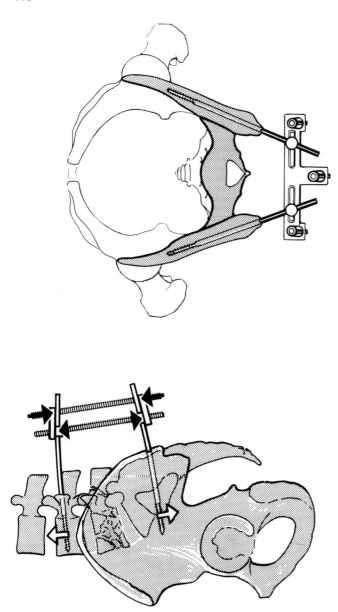

Fig. 7. Stabilization of a fracture of L5 requires placement of the lower screws under direct vision into the sufficiently exposed posterior iliac wing. Iliac grafts
for the fusion (not shown) are obtained from the area anterosuperior to the placement
of the Schanz screws.

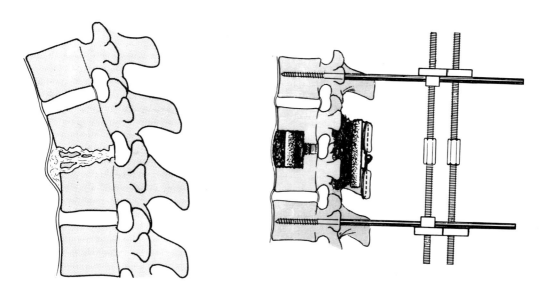

a

c

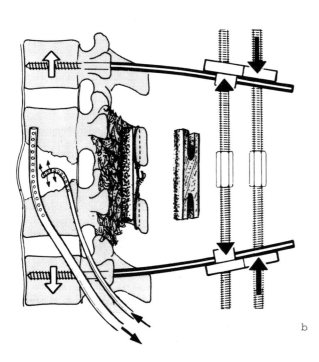

b

Fig. 8. Treatment of
osteomyelitis of the
spine at the lowest
thoracic and the lumbar
levels using external
fixation. a) Abscess,
sequestra and kyphotic
deformity. b) First
stage: Posterior graft-
ing, application of the
fixator in distraction,
followed during the same
anesthesia by anterior
debridement and instal-
lation of a suction-ir-
rigation system. c)
Stage 2, 2-3 weeks lat-
er: Interbody fusion
after clinical subsi-
dence of the infection.
The distraction has been
released, the fixator
is in neutral position
(see text).

Normally, the fixator is removed as an outpatient procedure, without anesthesia, as soon as the fracture and/or fusion is healed, confirmed by roentgenograph. If further protection seems to be indicated, patients wear a lumbar corset or brace. At the present time, a plaster body jacket is used only on the rare occasion when the fixator is removed earlier than scheduled.

Materials and Methods

Since 1977, external skeletal fixation has been used in 39 patients (32 fractures, 5 osteomyelites, 2 dorsal fusions) for stabilization of the spine from T10 to L5.

Thirty of these patients (24 men, 6 women), treated before the end of 1980, are included in this study. Their age ranged from 16 to 68 years (average 33 years).

Indications and operative treatment

Acute fractures. Twenty-six patients with acute trauma had the following injuries:

- 44 fractured vertebral bodies (30 major, 14 minor fractures); 18 fractured posterior elements; six facet dislocations

- positive neurologic findings, ranging from some sensory loss to incomplete conus or cauda equina syndrome were present in 18 patients

- eight patients had significant associated injuries.

The main indications for operative treatment were: anterior wedging in nine patients (20°-35°, average 29°); instability in 10 patients; instability and severe neurologic compromise in seven patients.

Operative treatment consisted of: external fixation without fusion in four early cases; external fixation and posterior fusion in 21 patients; external fixation and anterior fusion in one patient. In three patients the closed method was used. Concurrent laminectomy was necessary in three patients.

Osteomyelitis of the spine. Two patients had hematogenous osteomyelitis caused by *Staphylococcus aureus* (L2-3, L4). They had mild neurologic findings and were in a poor medical condition after failure of conservative treatment.

Operative treatment consisted in the first patient of anterior debridement followed three weeks later by posterior fusion and external fixation. The second patient was treated by the two-stage procedure previously described.

Dorsal fusion. Two patients needed stabilization of a dorsal fusion: one at L3-4 after previous laminectomy and anterior fusion from L4 to S1; the other from L1 to L3 because of progressive neurologic deficit due to post-traumatic adhesions necessitating extensive laminectomy and neurolysis.

Operative treatment consisted of a posterior fusion with H-graft and external fixation.

Number of intervertebral spaces bridged with the fixator. One space was bridged in two patients, two spaces were bridged in 24 patients, three spaces in one patient and four spaces in three patients.

Postoperative course

Time of ambulation: 29 of the 30 patients began ambulation between day 2 and day 14; one patient after six weeks.

Hospital stay: The average hospital stay for 24 patients was 23 days (13-37 days). Two patients with fractures were hospitalized for seven weeks; the four patients with osteomyelitis and dorsal fusion were discharged after two to 15 weeks.

Duration of external fixation: The external fixator was removed after 12-24 weeks, in the last 10 patients on an average of 16 weeks.

Treatment after removal of the fixator: No further support was necessary in 13 patients. Seven patients wore a lumbar corset and two a brace for an average of six weeks each. A plaster body jacket was used for four to eight weeks in four patients early in this series, one due to loss of reduction and one due to early removal on the patient's request.

Results

All 30 patients were followed closely until the fracture or fusion had solidly healed. No fracture or fusion failed to unite.

Twenty-nine of 30 patients were personally evaluated, both clinically and radiographically, over an average follow-up period of 25 months (6-45 months). In no case did a further loss of reduction occur during the period from bony union until final follow-up. All 18 neurologic deficits showed improvement; 16 patients had essentially complete neurologic recovery. We also evaluated pain and function. Of the 25 patients with fractures, 11 had an excellent result. Nine patients had minor symptoms without disability and a good result. Three patients had symptoms sufficient to cause change of occupation and a fair result. In two patients the result was poor. In nine patients with anterior wedging, an average final correction of 16° was obtained. If we exclude the three patients with early loss of reduction, listed as complications, the average final correction was 19°.

In both patients with osteomyelitis the result was excellent. Of the two patients with dorsal fusion, one had a fair and one a poor result.

Complications: Fourteen complications have occurred in 10 of our 30 patients:
- partial loss of reduction at the vertebral body in three patients. The final kyphosis did not exceed 20°. Two of these patients required interbody fusion because of pain. A plaster body jacket was used for eight weeks for the third patient.

- superficial wound infection, hematoma at the donor site, seroma in one patient each. Treatment consisted in evacuation and aspiration. The course was uneventful.

- pin tract irritation in eight patients resolved without treatment.

No death and no serious complications related to the treatment of the spinal injury have occurred so far.

Discussion

Experience over the past four years with 39 patients has proven that external skeletal fixation offers some unique characteristics beneficial in operative stabilization of the spine.

When using plates or Harrington distraction rods the mobile connection between plates and screws, or hooks and bone, makes fixation across five levels mandatory for adequate stability. Since all connections in the external fixation system are absolutely rigid, immobilization may be restricted to one level above and below the fracture site. The stability of the external fixation is enhanced by preloading the Schanz screws in distraction or compression.

The structural elasticity of the fixator seems to be an advantage rather than a disadvantage because it absorbs energy, thus protecting screw anchorage from overload and also preventing stress raisers.

Versatility of the system allows application in distraction, compression or in a neutral mode depending upon the mechanical requirements of the individual case. If multiple levels are to be stabilized, the system will adapt to allow bridging of as many levels as necessary. The ability of secure fixation into the ilium is a great advantage in the otherwise difficult immobilization of L5.

In external fixation no large implant obscures the site for bone graft. Fusion may be restricted to the involved segments.

The insertion of Schanz screws into the vertebral body is no more difficult than placing plate screws and also can be done by a closed method. The screws can be removed as an outpatient procedure without anesthesia.

The scope of external fixation of the spine is limited proximally by the excursion of the scapula and attached posterior musculature. We therefore have not attempted insertion of Schanz screws above T9.

Early mobilization is generally possible. In principal, external support is unnecessary while the fixator is in place; however, a special brace must be used for protection of the protruding device.

In three early cases with wedge fractures there was partial loss of reduction before bone healing. The first case was due to a technical error in application of the fixator. In the other two patients the fixator was removed too early (12-14 weeks). We have learned that in wedge fractures it is necessary to wait until the defect in the vertebral body, present after reduction, has refilled with bone and until the anterior cortex is healed. In one patient this has taken as long as 24 weeks.

We have encountered no deep infection and pin tract irritation has not been a problem.

Indications for external skeletal fixation are the same as for other operative stabilizations, but the patient must be able to cooperate. We still do not apply external fixations in spinal lesions with complete paraplegia.

The results obtained with external fixation in cases of severe spinal injuries or osteomyelitis have been most encouraging. The additional advantages of a short period of immobilization, brief hospitalization, and the possibility of a fully functional aftercare, even in patients with osteomyelitis, may be regarded as a distinct improvement in treatment.

Summary

Since 1977, external skeletal fixation has been used in 39 patients for stabilization of the lower thoracic and the lumbar spine. A special device has been developed for this purpose. Indications for operative treatment were kyphotic deformity and unstable fractures (32 patients), osteomyelitis of the spine (5 patients) and dorsal fusions (2 patients). The method is briefly described. The results in the first 29 patients with sufficient follow-up are presented. No serious complications were encountered. Of the 25 patients with fractures, including 18 with neurologic involvement, 20 had an excellent or good result. The method is felt to be especially beneficial in the treatment of osteomyelitis of the spine.

References

1. Crenshaw, A.H.: Internal fixation in spinal fusion. In, Campbell's Operative Orthopaedics, 5th Ed., vol. 2, p. 1171. C.V. Mosby Co., Saint Louis, 1971.

2. Dickson, J.H., Harrington, P.R., Erwin, W.D.: Results of reduction and stabilization of the severely fractured thoracic and lumbar spine. J. Bone Jt. Surg. 60A, 799, 1978.

3. Flesch, J.R., Leider, L.L., Erickson, D.L., Chou, S.N., Bradford, D.S.: Harrington instrumentation and spine fusion for unstable fractures and fracture-dislocations of the thoracic and lumbar spine. J. Bone Jt. Surg. 59A, 143, 1977.

4. Magerl, F.: Verletzungen der Brust- und Lendenwirbelsäule. Lanbenbecks Arch. Chir. 352 (Kongressbericht), 427, 1980.

5. Magerl, F.: Clinical application on the thoracolumbar junction and the lumbar spine. In, External Skeletal Fixation. Ed, D.C. Mears. Williams & Wilkins, Baltimore, 1981 (in press)

6. Roy-Camille, R., Saillant, G., Berteaux, D., Marie-Anne S.: Early management of spinal injuries. In, Recent Advances in Orthopaedics, Vol. 3, p 57. Churchill Livingstone, Edinburgh - London - New York, 1979.

7. Roy-Camille, R., Saillant, G., Marie-Anne, S., Mamoudy, P.: Behandlung
    von Wirbelfrakturen und -luxationen am thorakolumbalen Uebergang.
    Orthopäde 9, 63, 1980.

8. Saillant, G.: Etude anatomique des pédicles vértebraux, applications
    chirurgicales. Revue de Chirurgie, Orthopédie et Traumatologie 62,
    151, 1976.

Stabilization of the Lower Thoracic and Lumbar Spine: Comparative in Vitro Investigation of an External Skeletal and Various Internal Fixation Devices

F. Schläpfer, O. Wörsdörfer, F. Magerl, and S. M. Perren

Introduction

In spinal surgery, an external skeletal fixation technique has been in use
for four years, primarily for instabilities in the thoracolumbar and lumbar
spine caused by fractures and infections. According to clinical experience
it is an advantageous alternative to various internal fixation systems
(Magerl, 1979; 1981). Adequate stability has been achieved and no failure
of skeletal anchorage encountered. The area of fixation is limited to the
vertebrae adjacent to the spinal lesion. It is applicable in the presence
of infections.

It is of interest to investigate its mechanical behavior to see how far the
external fixation device is an advantageous alternative to internal systems.

In this investigation we compared _in vitro_ the rigidity and strength of fixation in the lumbar spine provided by the Harrington rod systems and by
plates. The spine, instrumented with the various systems, was deformed in
flexion.

Materials and Methods

We compared the newest design of the external fixation devices called the
ESF-device (External Spinal Fixation device)(Fig. 1), the conventional
Harrington distraction rod system (shortened HDR-system)(Fig. 6), a modi-
fied HDR-system (Fig. 5a) and a modified Tinturier plate system (Fig. 5b).

The ESF-device (Magerl, 1978; 1981; Schläpfer, 1980) (Fig. 1) consists of
an external frame and four Schanz screws which connect the frame with the
spine. They affect, for the most part, the rigidity of fixation: In the
investigations their free length (distance from the external frame to the
spine) was 100 mm. Over the posterior 90 mm their diameter was 6 mm. The
anterior part of the screws had a diameter of 5 mm.

The conventional HDR-system (Benner et al, 1977; Flesch, et al, 1977;
Hannon, 1976; Yosipovitch, et al, 1977) (Fig. 6) consists of two partly
notched rods and four hooks connecting the rods with the lumbar spine.

The length of the rods was 168 mm, the outside diameter 6.2 mm and the diameter within the notches 4.6 mm.

The modified HDR-system (Jacobs, et al, 1980a; 1980b) (Fig. 5a) also consists of two rods and four hooks. In contrast to the conventional system, the connection between the hooks and the rods is locked in rotation. The length of the rods of the tested system was 185 mm and the diameter 8 mm.

The investigated plate-system consisted of two modified 9-hole Tinturier plates (Fig. 5b). The plates were 115 mm long, 11 mm wide and 6 mm thick. Cortical bone screws, 4.5 mm, attached the plates to the spine.

The investigations were carried out on thawed cadaver spine specimens. They consisted of seven vertebrae (T11-L5), with intact discs and ligaments. On both sides of the specimens the outermost vertebrae were embedded in a cold-hardening plastic material (Beracryl).

Two different fracture situations in the lumbar spine were produced:

Model 1 represented a combined anteroposterior injury: A wedge-shaped part of the vertebral body of L2 was removed with integrity of the posterior wall and the anterior longitudinal ligament. The capsules of the facet joints of the motion segment L1/L2, the inter- and the supraspinous ligament and the ligamentum flavum were dissected.

Model 2 represented the same injury with additionally disrupted anterior longitudinal ligament: In addition to model 1, this ligament was dissected.

Six lumbar spines each per injury model were stabilized with the ESF-device and the various internal fixation systems as follows:

The ESF-device immobilized three vertebrae (L1/L2/L3) (Fig. 1). The Schanz screws were inserted through the pedicles of L1 and L3. The ESF-device was tested with and without screw fixation of the L1/L2 facet joints.

Before installation of the internal fixation systems, the rods of the modified HDR-system and the plates were fitted to the spinal lordosis (Fig. 5). The rods of the conventional HDR-system could not be shaped for the following reason. When the adapted system was mounted, an abrupt rotation of the rods around their longitudinal axis could be observed when loading the instrumented lumbar spine in flexion. The rods rotated in such a way that their curvature was opposed to the spinal lordosis. The hooks disengaged. In case of the modified HDR-system the same problem did not exist, because the connection between the hooks and the rods does not permit rotation.

The hooks of the two rod systems were anchored in the laminae of the second vertebrae above and below L2 (Fig. 5a, 6). The systems preloaded model 1 in distraction. Because of the dissected anterior longitudinal ligament, model 2 could not be preloaded.

The plates immobilized five vertebrae (two above and two below L2). They were used in the same manner as the Roy-Camille plate system (Roy-Camille, et al, 1976). Cranial and caudal of the unstable area cortical bone screws were alternatively inserted into the pedicles and the facet joints of vertebrae (Fig. 5b).

The lumbar spine specimens were tested in flexion on a Rumul test machine (Mikrotron 654K). The caudal embedded end of the spines was rigidly fixed on the bottom of the frame of the test machine. A bar was mounted on their cranial end. Parallel to the longitudinal axis of the spine two opposite forces of the same value were acting. Their points of application on the bar had the same distance from the center of the spine. This disposition of the forces resulted in a pure bending load on the spine specimens. The forces were produced by a rope mechanism connecting the bar with the test machine (Fig. 2). A load cell measured the sum of the two forces acting on the bar.

For determination of the angular motion in the defect of L2 the two angles of L1 and the caudal part of L2 were measured with inductive goniometers (Fig. 2). The two angles were registered in dependence on the bending moment by an X-Y-recorder (Sefram T2Y). The difference of the angles was calculated by a calculator (Wang 600) and recorded as a function of the bending moment by a plotter (Wang 612). The slope of the plots is characteristic for the stability achieved by the fixation systems. The measurements are evaluated as to stability or failure of the anchorage of the systems.

Results

Stability (Fig. 3)

Both fracture models stabilized with the ESF-device showed, with additional screw fixation of the cranial facet joints (Fig. 4b), one-third better stability than achieved without screw fixation (Fig. 4a). In model 1 the stability achieved with the conventional HDR-system was up to 1 Nm, similar to that of the intact nonstabilized lumbar spine specimens. With increasing load it increased for the short period up to the failure of its skeletal anchorage to a value similar to the modified HDR-system. The latter provided stability up to 10 Nm, identical to that of the plate system. With higher load it rapidly decreased. Both models instrumented with the plate system showed twice the stability as achieved with the ESF-device with screw fixation of the cranial facet joints.

Failure of the skeletal anchorage (Fig. 3)

Both diagrams indicate no failure of the skeletal anchorage of the ESF-device with and without screw fixation of the facet joints (tested up to 40 Nm). In model 1, the moment of failure of the conventional HDR-system was 5.9 ± 0.5 Nm (SE) with an angular deformity in the defect of $3.3 \pm 0.4°$ (SE). At this load the upper hooks disengaged. The same observation was made in model 1 with the modified HDR-system at a moment of failure of 19.5 ± 2.5 Nm (SE) with $3.6 \pm 0.3°$ (SE) deformity. In model 2 the conventional and the modified HDR-systems failed to work. The upper hooks disengaged. The statistical evaluation of the moments of failure of the plate system in model 1 and 2 showed no significant difference. For that reason the results of both models were combined: 29.5 ± 2.5 Nm (SE) with 3.2 ± 0.2° (SE) deformity. The screws came out.

Discussion

In vivo, by flexing the intact spine, in relation to the intervertebral discs the weight of the trunk produces a constant axial force and an anterior bending moment. The latter increases with increase of the angular deformation of the spine. Roughly summarized, the flexion is thereby controlled actively by the dorsal muscles and passively by the geometry of the facet joints and limited by the posterior ligaments. The muscles and ligaments produce an axial force and posterior bending moment also acting in the intervertebral discs. The latter is balancing the bending moment resulting from the weight of the trunk. The axial forces produced by the weight of the trunk and the muscles are supported by the spinal column. In case of an anteroposterior spinal lesion the spine is no more able to bear axial load. An artificial support is produced by stabilizing the unstable spine with external or internal fixation systems. Provided it is anterior to the dorsal muscles, the muscles are able to balance the anterior bending moment as before. In case of a support posterior to them, the bending load on the instrumented spine is increased. The muscles still try to balance the bending moment. In this way they produce in relation to the support an anterior bending moment in addition to that of the body weight.

As to the internal systems, eg, rods or plates, they produce an internal support anterior to the dorsal muscles. The supporting element of the ESF-device is its external frame. It is posterior of the dorsal muscles. Depending on the type of spinal lesion an additional support can exist in the stabilized area. In view of the flexibility of the Schanz screws and the distance from the spine to the external frame, an internal support is desirable. If there is none, it can be produced by screw fixation of the facet joints of the unstable motion segments, or, if not possible (eg, in case of laminectomy), by a dorsal H-shaped cortical bone graft or, better, by a ventral spondylodesis with corticocancellous grafts. In the case of spinal instabilities, as simulated in our *in vitro* investigations, the internal support is given by the remaining part of the defective vertebra. It is stiffened with screw fixation of the cranial facet joints.

In our *in vitro* investigations we assumed that an internal support existed in the spine specimens stabilized with the various systems. In such a way the *in vitro*-applied anterior bending moment corresponded to the difference of the bending moments produced *in vivo* by the body weight and the dorsal muscles. This difference results *in vivo* in spinal flexion, corresponding to the *in vitro* effect. Contrary to the bending moments, the axial forces also produced by the muscles and the body weight were not considered in this study. They would be borne for the most part by the internal support within the stabilized area. We assume that the support was so rigid that the axial forces would not significantly contribute to the deformation affecting the results of the *in vitro* investigations. The two rod systems are an exception. In this study, the neglected axial forces would increase the moment of failure of their skeletal anchorage. Nevertheless, the *in vitro* investigations give a qualitative picture about the mechanical behavior of all systems *in vivo* as described below.

ESF-device

The ESF-device was used immobilizing three vertebrae only, one each above and below the defect (Fig. 1). The flexibility of the Schanz screws of the ESF-device allowed an axial dislocation and an AP-rotation of the vertebrae adjacent to the defect towards each other. As a result of the integrity of the posterior wall and the caudal end plate of L2, the axial dislocation produced a posterior rotation of the remaining part of L2 (Fig. 4a, b). As long as the cranial facet joints were not fixed with screws, the nucleus of the disc caudal of L2 was the center of rotation (Fig. 4a). Because of the mobility at the intact facet joints L2/L3 the rotation was hardly obstructed by their capsules. When the cranial facet joints were fixed, the axis of rotation was formed by them (Fig. 4b). The facet joints and the disc immediately cranial of the defect were limiting the rotation. For that reason a significant increase of the stability could be observed. A further improvement may be achieved with the screw fixation of the cranial and caudal joints inside the stabilized area. This situation was not tested. We assume that in this case the stability obtained is similar to or better than that achieved by the plate system. But according to clinical observation it seems that it is not necessary to block the caudal facet joints, provided the caudal motion segment immobilized by the ESF-device is still intact.

Internal spinal fixation systems

In the case of internal systems the stability in flexion could only be achieved together with the spine. Five vertebrae were immobilized (two intact vertebrae each cranial and caudal of the defect). With the exception of the conventional HDR-system, which will be discussed below, the internal systems were fitted to the spinal lordosis. In such a way the anterior bending moment was transformed in a pair of opposite AP-forces supported by the systems. The anterior one was acting on the hooks, respectively on the outermost cortical bone screws, and the posterior one on the rods, respectively the plates, at the level of the vertebrae adjacent to the defective one (Fig. 5a, b).

In the case of the modified HDR-system, the remaining possible motion of the vertebrae adjacent to the defect can be separated into an axial dislocation and an AP-rotation towards each other. The main motion was axial dislocation along the rods. In the nonpreloaded model 2, the intact posterior wall of L2 obstructed the axial dislocation. It thus effected a lifting of the cranial vertebral laminae in the hooks resulting in the prompt failure of the system. The dislocation of the hooks was further increased by the anterior force acting on the hooks. As a result of the intact anterior longitudinal ligament, model 1 could be preloaded by the rod system. In this way the discs connecting the defective vertebra with the adjacent ones were vertically extended. As long as this situation continued, the intact posterior wall of L2 did not obstruct the axial dislocation. As soon as the axial dislocation was larger than the extension of the discs, it also resulted in lifting of the vertebral laminae placed in the hooks. Together with the anterior force acting on the hooks and the position of the laminae, the hooks becoming increasingly bent with increasing load, the hooks finally pulled out.

As to the plate system, the remaining motion was above all AP-rotation. The axis of rotation was formed by the corresponding pair of heads of the screws inserted through the plates into the pedicles and the vertebral body (Fig. 5b). The rotation was mainly the result of the uneven surface of the spine under the plates. It was hardly obstructed by the remaining part of L2. The failure of the system was caused, for the most part, by the anterior force. The outermost screws had come out.

In the case of the conventional HDR-system the remaining possible motion of the vertebrae adjacent to the defect can be separated in an axial dislocation and an AP-rotation towards each other and a posterior dislocation towards the rods. The latter could not be prevented because the rods were not fitted to the spinal lordosis (Fig. 6a). In model 2, which could not be preloaded, the intact posterior wall caused lifting of the cranial vertebral laminae in the hooks, resulting in their dislocation with a small anterior bending moment. By preloading model 1 the lumbar spine was deformed in such a way that the defective vertebra touched the rods at L2 (Fig. 6b). The ligaments connecting it with the adjacent ones were tightened and the adjacent discs vertically extended. The adjacent vertebrae were not yet touching the rods. Nevertheless, because of the tightened ligaments and the extended discs, a reduced stability was achieved (Fig. 3). With increasing load the adjacent vertebrae moved toward the rods. After touching them, the same mechanical situation was produced as in the case of the adapted modified HDR-system (Fig. 5a, 6c). For that reason the stability increased to a similar value as achieved by the modified system (Fig. 3). The lumbar spine, however, already showed a kyphotic deformation (Fig. 6c). The system therefore failed to work on the lumbar spine with a significant smaller anterior bending moment than the modified one, although the same mechanical situation existed.

Conclusions

The significance of the *in vitro* investigations is in the description of the mechanical behavior of the various fixation systems mounted on the lumbar spine when the latter is deformed in flexion.

The ESF-device immobilizing only two motion segments (the defective one and the intact one caudal to it) is able to provide a certain stability in flexion by itself. Its ability to work is independent of the condition of the anterior longitudinal ligament. Due to the flexibility of its Schanz screws, the stability obtained is also influenced by the mechanical interaction between the spine and the device. It can be improved by screw fixation of the

facet joints of the unstable motion segments. Because of their flexibility
the Schanz screws are able to adsorb energy. For that reason the skeletal
anchorage of the Schanz screws is protected against load peaks. Based on
the *in vitro* investigations and clinical observations, failure of the skeletal anchorage of the Schanz screws need not be anticipated. The ESF-device
is used without additional external support permitting a permanent training
of the muscles and the mobility of the back. A brace is used only for the
protection of the device.

Contrary to the ESF-device, the internal systems have to immobilize a minimal number of five vertebrae to be able to produce stability. Therefore,
they have to be fitted to the spinal lordosis. Furthermore, to function
satisfactorily in the lumbar spine the conventional and the modified HDR-
systems have to preload the spine in distraction. Consequently, a ruptured
anterior longitudinal ligament is a contraindication for both systems.
Furthermore, the conventional rod system cannot be fitted to the spinal
lordosis without the rods springing out of their spinal bed. For that reason it is not able to resist a significant flexion deformation in the lumbar spine.   In the case of the plate system, best stability was achieved
regardless of the condition of the anterior longitudinal ligament. But to
provide stability, screws must also be inserted into the facet joints of
the intact motion segments, thus damaging them (Fig. 5b).

Based on *in vitro* investigations and clinical observations (Yosipovitch
et al, 1977), failure of the skeletal anchorage of the internal fixation
systems in the lumbar spine can occur in certain situations. For that
reason using internal fixation systems in addition to external supports
(eg, brace, cast) is recommended (Benner et al, 1977; Flesch et al, 1977;
Yosipovitch et al, 1977) to prevent flexion.

Summary

External fixation of instabilities of the lumbar spine permits limiting the
fixation to the vertebrae adjacent to the spinal lesion. A study of the
mechanical quality of external fixation compared with internal methods has
been undertaken using human cadaver spines. Flexing the spine with an anterior bending moment, angular motion in the fracture area occurred least
with a modified Tinturier plate system followed by the external fixation
device, a modified rod system and the conventional Harrington distraction
rod system. In direct contrast to internal fixation systems, no failure of
the skeletal anchorage of the external skeletal fixation device was observed.

References

1. Benner, B., Moiel, B., Dickson, J., Harrington, P.: Instrumentation of
    the spine for fracture dislocations in children. Child Brain 3, 249,
    1977.

2. Flesch, J.R., Leider, L.L., Erickson, D.L., Chou, S.N., Bradford, D.S.:
    Harrington instrumentation and spine fusion for unstable fractures and
    fracture dislocations of the thoracic and lumbar spine. J Bone Jt Surg
    59A, 143, 1977.

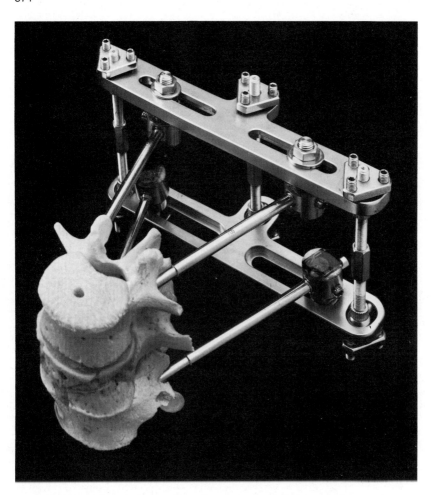

Fig. 1. External skeletal fixation device used for stabilization of lower spine instabilities. Four Schanz screws are inserted through the pedicles into the vertebral body of the vertebrae adjacent to the unstable segment. The cranial and caudal pair of screws are connected with a plate each. The plates are attached by three threaded rods. The junction plate-rod is a ball and socket joint rigidly fixed by six safety-discs.

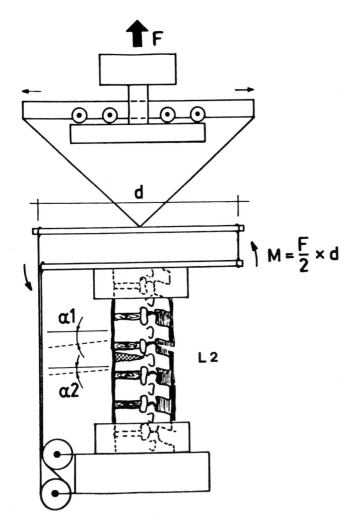

$$M = \frac{F}{2} \times d$$

Fig. 2. Test apparatus for deforming spine specimens in flexion with a pure bending moment. The special arrangement of the cables transforms the force (F) to a bending momemt (M) applied on the spine specimens. The two uppermost cables connect the upper horizontal bar with a sled. The sled prevents shear load when the spine is flexed. Two injury models were proposed. In both a wedge-shaped part of the vertebral body L2 and the posterior ligaments at this level were removed. The posterior wall and the caudal end plate of L2 were intact. In model 2 the anterior longitudinal ligament was additionally divided (not shown in the figure). The two flexion angles of L1 (α1) and of the caudal part of L2 (α2) were measured. Their difference describes the interfragmentary angular deformation.

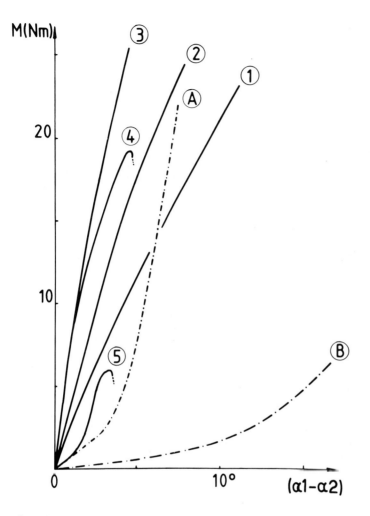

Fig. 3. Results of the investigations made on fracture
model 1. The flexion moment (M) is plotted as a function
of the difference of the two measured flexion angles
$(\alpha 1-\alpha 2)$ (Fig. 2). The plots describe the mechanical behavior in flexion of the intact spine (A), the spine
with an anteroposterior defect (B) and the spine instrumented by the following fixation systems: external fixation device without (1) and with (2) screw fixation of
the facet joints, a modified Tinturier plate system (3),
a modified (4) and the conventional Harrington distraction rod system (5). In fracture model 2 (not shown in
the figure) (1), (2) and (3) showed the same mechanical
behavior as in model 1. (4) and (5) failed to work at
beginning of the test. Their cranial hooks disengaged.

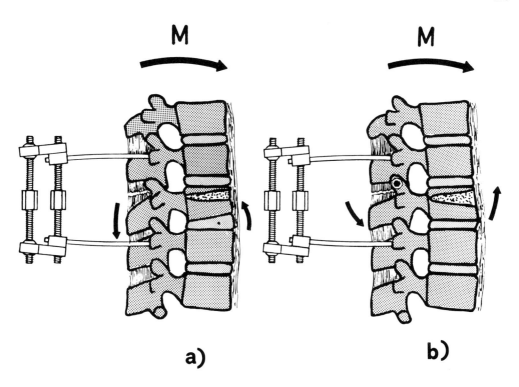

Fig. 4. Mechanical interaction between the external skeletal fixation device and the spine. a) Stabilization without screw fixation of the injured
facet joints. An internal support is given by the remaining part of L2. Its
points of contact with the adjacent vertebrae are the intact posterior wall
on the cranial and the disc on the caudal side. Because they are not on the
same perpendicular, axial dislocation of the adjacent vertebrae towards each
other results in a posterior rotation of L2. Center of rotation is the nucleus of the caudal disc. b) Stabilization with screw fixation of the injured
facet joints. Points of contact of L2 are the blocked facet joints on the
cranial and the disc on the caudal side, resulting in a similar mechanical
situation as previously described. The axis of rotation is formed by the
stabilized facet joints. The caudal adjacent disc and the ligaments limit
the rotation.

378

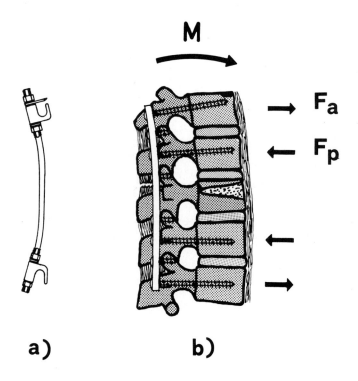

a)   b)

Fig. 5. Modified Harrington distraction rod system:
The hooks are anchored in the laminae of the second
vertebra above and below L2. The connection between
the rods and the hooks is stable in rotation. The
system can thus be fitted to the lumbar lordosis
without risk of rods springing out of their spinal
bed when the system is loaded in flexion. b) Modified Tinturier plate system: It immobilizes five
vertebrae. Cranial and caudal to the defect, screws
are alternatively inserted into the pedicles and the
facet joints. It is adapted to the lumbar lordosis.
Due to their adaptation to the spinal curvature both
systems transform the flexion moment in a pair of AP-
forces assisted by the spine. The anterior force (F_a)
is acting on the hooks and the posterior (F_p) on the
rods respectively; the plates at the level of the
vertebrae adjacent to L2. Only in this way can they
support a flexion moment.

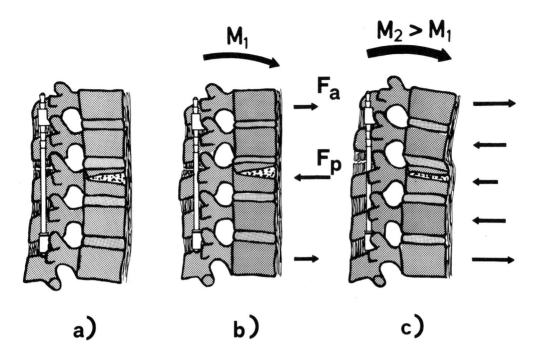

Fig. 6. Conventional Harrington distraction rod system. It is efficient
when axial forces are acting on it. To support anterior bending moments,
the rods have to touch the vertebrae within the stabilized area. In the
lumbar spine it cannot be fitted to spinal lordosis without rods springing
out of their spinal bed when the instrumented spine is loaded in flexion.
Preloading the instrumented spine in distraction, the central vertebra
touches the rods, enabling the system to resist a certain bending moment.
a) Nonadapted rod system mounted in the lumbar spine. The spine is not yet
preloaded. The rods are not in contact with the spine. b) Preload of the
lumbar spine with the rod system results in a kyphotic deformation. L2 is
pressed against the rods, thus the flexion moment is transformed in an anterior force (F_a) acting on the hooks and a posterior one (F_p) acting on
the rods at the level of L2. The vertebrae adjacent to L2 are not yet touching the rods. The flexion moment moves them to the rods. c) Provided the
bending moment is big enough, the adjacent vertebrae touch the rods. A
similar mechanical situation has occurred as in the case of the adapted
modified rod system (Fig. 5a). In addition to the posterior force in Fig. 6b
a posterior one each is acting at the level of the adjacent vertebrae. Due
to the initial mobility of the adjacent vertebrae, a big kyphotic deformation of the lumbar spine has been produced.

3. Hannon, K.M.: Harrington instrumentation in fractures and dislocations of the thoracic and lumbar spine. Southern Med J 69, 1269, 1976.

4. Jacobs, R.R., Schläpfer, F., Mathys, Jr., R., Perren, S.M.: A new spinal instrumentation system for dorsal-lumbar spinal fractures. J Biomech 13, 801, 1980a.

5. Jacobs, R.R., Schläpfer, F., Mathys, Jr., R., Nachemson, A., Perren, S.M.: A new instrumentation system for fracture-dislocations of the dorsal-lumbar spine. Proc 15th Annual Meeting of the Scoliosis Research Society, Chicago. 1980b (in press).

6. Magerl, F.: Die Behandlung von Wirbelsäulenverletzungen. 19. Tagung der Oesterreichischen Chirurgengesellschaft Kongressbericht. Hrsg.: Waynand, E., Brücke, P., Bd II, 859. Ed.: H. Egermann, Vienna 1979.

7. Magerl, F.: Clinical application on the thoracolumbar junction and the lumbar spine. In, External Skeletal Fixation. Ed.: D.C. Mears. Williams and Wilkins, Baltimore 1981 (in press).

8. Roy-Calmille, R., Saillant, G., Berteaux, C., Salgado, V.: Osteosynthesis of thoraco-lumbar spine fractures with metal plates screwed through the vertebral pedicles. Reconstr Surg Traumat 15, 2, 1976.

9. Schläpfer, F., Wörsdörfer, O., Magerl, F., Perren, S.M.: Development of an external skeletal fixation device for the lumbar spine and in vivo load measurements. Proc. 7th Annual Meeting of the Internat Soc for the Study of the Lumbar Spine, 1980 (in press).

10. Yosipovitch, Z., Robin, G.C., Makin, M.: Open reduction of unstable thoraco-lumbar spinal injuries and fixation with Harrington rods. J Bone Jt Surg 59A, 1003, 1977.

The Use of External Fixators in the Polytraumatized Patient

B. F. Claudi and V. Mooney

Application of external fixators in the management of severe fractures has
become an important part in the management of polytraumatized patients.
Parallel to the development and presentation of new external fixators during recent years we have been confronted with numerous publications on
where and how these fixators might be used. Over the past years, it has
been increasingly accepted that the corrent application of external fixators requires a sound understanding of the mechanical characteristics of
these devices; furthermore, it became obvious, mainly following a number
of disappointing clinical results, that masterful skills in surgical techniques are absolutely essential. As demonstrated best by workshops on
external fixators held during the last three years in North America, this
issue has become very complicated for the majority of common orthopedic
surgeons, and even confusing with regard to the basic mechanical data
available about biomechanical results. How can highly specialized knowledge of a small aspect match the needs for a sound integrated knowledge
of the various problems in the management of a polytraumatized patient?
Some of us have found an answer to that question in that we try to escape
involvement in the emotionally exhausting treatment of multiple - injured
patients. The others who must share the responsibilities for the treatment
of these patients are frequently confused, particularly when reading recent
publications on indications for external fixators stressing the fact that
there is nowadays almost no skeletal part which cannot be successfully
managed by external devices. This, we believe, implies a risky management
of musculoskeletal injuries in polytraumatized patients, since opportuni-
ties for definitive and appropriate fracture fixation often will be missed.

Thus, this course should help to outline how useful external fixators really
are in the management of polytraumatized patients.

Indications, as they are widely accepted, for the use of external fixators
in polytraumatized patients are:

- pelvic fractures
- fractures associated with burns
- gunshot fractures
- other open fractures (2° and 3°)
- comminuted wrist fractures
- ipsilateral long bone fractures of upper or lower extremity.

Certain common advantages of external fixators have increased the use of these devices. In our opinion, these fixators are applied to the best advantage for:

- appropriate reduction and stabilization of the fracture site;
- maintenance of extremity length;
- protection of soft tissues by providing rigid skeletal fixation;
- ease of general nursing care, particularly transfer in and out of bed;
- ability to perform secondary procedures in fracture treatment.

Without doubt, the disadvantages as related to the type of fixator and technique of its application are obvious. Since a few of the negative aspects have been published and described before, we like to stress some of the shortcomings as far as they remain a problem in long-term fracture treatment.

Obviously, certain advantages of external fixators cannot be generalized for all fractures. We can qualify this statement by an example of the use of external fixators in an open tibia fracture compared with an open femur fracture. The use of an external fixator in a Grade III open tibia fracture has been shown to be the method of choice even when used for prolonged periods. In contrast, we might consider the treatment of a Grade III open femur fracture. With a few exceptions, these fractures can be managed by means of internal fixation provided enough vascularized soft tissue cover is available. Unquestionably, soft tissues benefit from adequate fracture stabilization. Here, by choosing a primary internal fixation device we try to avoid certain shortcomings of prolonged external fixation in femur fractures, such as shortening and angulation of the bone and interference with muscle function. The quadriceps muscle is particularly prone to irritation by pin insertion through muscle fibers, often preventing early intensive postoperative care.

A true disadvantage of external fixators, when used for the wrong indication and kept on for too long, is well known to most of us - the nonunion of the tibia being a perfect example. Another problem in the external fixation treatment of polytraumatized patients is the dilemma of whether the fixator should be applied as a temporary or permanent device.

Practical considerations, gained from experience in polytraumatized patients over the last ten years, have given us some basic guidelines for the management of certain conditions.

We regard an external fixator as a permanent device in a polytraumatized patient as long as it is not expected to be replaced by an internal fixation device. We do not, however, exclude replacement by a different external fixation device, such as a plaster cast, braces, or other orthotic devices.

As a definitive device, we consider the external fixator applied in patients with:

- anterior instability of pelvic fractures (open book type lesions),
- fractures calling for primary arthrodesis,
- comminuted wrist fractures,
- open fractures (in exceptional cases),
- acetabular fractures associated with pelvic fractures (in exceptional cases).

Instability of the anterior pelvis by a disrupture of the symphysis pubis, with or without an incomplete ligamentous lesion of the sacroiliac joint, can be easily managed by an anterior frame. Other methods, such as plating, might be even more convenient for the patient and still be of comparable efficiency.

Primary arthrodesis, rarely accepted as the primary method of choice in a severely damaged joint, might be indicated as an emergency procedure only, with special attention to other serious problems usually seen in polytraumatized patients.

External fixation for comminuted wrist fractures has been proven very effective and, due to the principles of ligamentotaxis, is often superior to other techniques.

Open fractures should be kept in external fixators only as long as indicated, depending on the soft tissue condition. Undoubtedly, many open fractures can benefit from a changeover from external to internal fixation. Mastering this challenge, however, demands sound judgement and experience. If properly executed, it usually shortens the time of fracture healing. We have to admit, however, that some open fractures can be treated only with an external fixator until bone union has occurred.

A similar position can be taken with regard to the management of acetabular fractures associated with pelvic fractures. As long as the acetabular displacement remains minimal after reduction or the patient's general condition does not permit a major surgical procedure to restore the hip joint, one should stay with the external fixator. On the other hand, there is no contraindication to a delayed reconstructive procedure with internal fixation, even after several weeks, if not contraindicated by gross displacement of joint components causing early and permanent disability.

As a temporary device we prefer the external fixator for:
- open fractures and fracture dislocations;
- pelvic fractures with posterior instability;
- isolated or associated acetabular fractures;
- ipsilateral femur/tibia fractures (floating knee type injury);
- ipsilateral humerus/forearm fractures (floating elbow type injury).

With regard to open fractures, the external fixator is an excellent means to initiate treatment. Successful treatment of these fractures includes, however, continuous adaptation to the actual needs of a healing course, which sometimes demands additional procedures such as increasing compression on the fracture site, bridging of defects by bone grafting, and others. Thus, the question should always be asked: What can be done to facilitate the healing process, at the same time minimizing the risks of future disabilities? Until proven otherwise, there is currently no contraindication to changing from an external to an internal device, provided that this procedure is technically meticulously carried out to improve fracture healing.

The posterior instability of pelvic fractures remains a serious problem as to the best way to achieve stability and proper reduction. Most of the pelvic frames currently recommended have left this problem unsolved or, if solved, with an extremely inconvenient fixator assembly for the patient. The urgency of early fixation of unstable pelvic fractures is best achieved by external fixators, thereby decreasing the tremendous blood loss and obtaining the best possible reduction. In cases of persisting posterior instability, an initially applied external fixator should be replaced or supplemented by internal fixation of the sacroiliac joint area. Since the surgical approach to this area seems to be one of the easier procedures in orthopedic surgery, one should not hesitate to aim for a stable posterior fixation, using screws and washers or plates.

Single or associated acetabular fractures are treated best by anatomic reduction and stable fixation, thus allowing early functional treatment of this important joint. The earlier the fixation can be carried out, the easier the procedure will be technically.

Ipsilateral femur and tibia fractures, causing a floating knee, or fractures with major bone defects are temporarily treated best with an external fixator until the definitive procedure can be carried out, as soon as the patient's general or local conditions permit. This temporary treatment may sometimes include the bridging of joints by means of an external fixator to provide initially the best possible stability. If a femur has to be put temporarily in an external fixator, we strongly recommend the use of the half-pin technique, connecting the preloaded pins by means of two laterally placed bars, thus avoiding interference with the quadriceps muscle. For the same purpose one may use, if available, a Wagner apparatus.

Ipsilateral humerus and forearm fractures due to gunshot injuries are best treated with an external fixator until the soft tissues permit a permanent procedure, usually consisting of bone grafting combined with plate fixation.

From our experience during the past years we have come to the following conclusions:

- An external fixator is a useful device in the management of polytraumatized patients, but it is not a panacea.

- The application of an external fixator demands outstanding skills in operative fracture treatment.

- When applying an external fixator, it must be remembered that it might be the one and only chance to stabilize a fracture, thus determining the course of fracture healing and its final result in a polytraumatized patient.

- Sound knowledge of application and outstanding technical ability in internal and external fixation procedures are essential for the successful use of these devices.

- Ignorance of the basic principles of internal fixation does not justify excessive propagation of external fixators for polytraumatized patients.

- Whenever possible, an external fixator should be regarded as a temporary device in the course of fracture treatment of a polytraumatized patient.

References

1. Boltze, W.H., Fernandez, D.L., and Schatzker, J.: The External Fixator
    (Tubular System). AO-Bulletin, November 1976, Bern.

2. Brooker, A.F., Jr.: The use of external fixation in the treatment of
    burn patients with fractures. In, External Fixation: The Current State
    of the Art. Williams & Wilkins, Baltimore/London, 1979. pp. 225-237.

3. Claudi, B., Rittmann, W.W., and Ruedi, Th.: Anwendung des Fixateur
    externe bei der Primaerversorgung offener Frakturen. Helv. Chir. Acta
    43,, 469, 1976.

4. Edwards, Charles C.: Management of the polytrauma patient in a major
    U.S. center. In , External Fixation: The Current State of the Art,
    Williams & Wilkins, Baltimore/London, 1979. pp 181-201.

5. Hoffmann, R.: L'ostéotaxis: Ostéosynthèse transcutanée par fiches et
    rotules. Gead, Paris, 1951.

6. Hierholzer, G.: Stabilisierung des Knochenbruchs beim Weichteilschaden
    mit Fixateurs externe. Langenbecks Arch. Chir. 339, 505, 1975.

7. Mears, D.C., and Fu , F.H.: Modern concepts of external skeletal fixation
    of the pelvis. Clin. Orthop. 151, 65, 1980.

8. Pfister, U.: Fixateur externe bei Arthrodesen. Akt. traumatologie
    6, 91, 1976.

9. Slätis, P., and Karharju, E.O.: External fixation of the pelvic girdle
    with a trapezoid frame. Injury 7, 53, 1975.

10. Tile, M., and Pennal, G.F.: Pelvic disruption: Principles of management.
    Clin. Orthop. 151, 56, 1980.

11. Trentz, O.: Notversorgung von frischen Verletzungen mit dem Fixateur
    externe. Akt. traumatologie 6, 76, 1976.

External Fixation and Pedicled Muscle Flaps in Complex Open Tibia Fractures

R. E. Jones, G. Cierny, III, and S. Byrd

The patient with a complex open fracture of the tibia presents a difficult problem. The high energy traumatic forces cause displacement and comminution of the bone and soft tissue damage with associated skin loss, all of which complicate treatment. Wound healing in these complex injuries implies healing of the soft and hard tissues. The concept of the open fracture wound, which involves the bone, the periosteum, the muscle, the fascia, and the skin, emphasizes the interrelated healing process of the soft and the hard tissues (Jones and Cierny, 1980). Management of such complex open tibia fractures by external skeletal fixation stabilizes the fracture and allows ready access for soft tissue wound observation. Karlstrom and Olerud (1975) documented less wound healing disturbances when Type II or Type III open tibia fractures were treated with external rather than internal fixation. They hypothesized that the creation and maintenance of a favorable mesenchymal milieu accomplished by transportation of pedicle muscle flaps would enhance soft and hard tissue healing in Type III tibia open fracture wounds.

Our report describes experience gained at the Orthopedic and Plastic Surgical Division of the University of Texas Health Science Center with a prospective management protocol for the treatment of Type III tibia open fracture wounds by external fixation and myoplasty or myocutaneous coverage.

Materials and Methods

From July 1, 1978 to June 30, 1979, 18 patients with 20 Type III open tibial fracture wounds were hospitalized either at Parkland Memorial Hospital or the Veterans Administration Medical Center in Dallas Texas, and were entered into the prospective management protocol.

The Type III open fracture wounds were defined as resulting from high energy forces causing a significantly displaced fracture pattern with severe comminution, segmental fracture, or bone defect with extensive skin loss and muscle damage. A subgroup, Type IIIA, included limbs with open fracture wounds and with a significant vascular deficit such as a concomitant vascular injury requiring repair, high velocity gunshot or shotgun wound, or history of crush or degloving injury.

The initial management of the patient in the emergency room was wound assessment, culture, and sterile dressing to prevent further contamination. The limb was held by cast splintage to align the hard and soft tissues and to provide decompression of any marginally vascularized areas. Parenteral cephalosporin antibiotics were administered before a roentgenogram was taken and tetanus prophylaxis was given if indicated. In the operating room, approximately five hours after admission to the emergency room, radical debridement and thorough jet lavage irrigation were performed. Transfixing pins were placed above and below the fracture site and reduction of the fracture was accomplished with the external fixation device. Supplemental coronal plane stabilization by additional fixation in the sagittal plane was performed in patients with severe instability or segmental bone loss. Soft tissue damage was then assessed and any further nonviable tissue removed. Wet, compressive dressings were placed on the open fracture wound and the limb was elevated.

The patients were returned to the operating room three to five days after the injury for further assessment of the open fracture wound by the orthopedic and plastic surgical services. Depending on the severity of the injury, surgical debridement was repeated at three to five day intervals until the wound was judged to be clean and viable. At this point, either myoplasty or myocutaneous flap coverage was performed. Meshed split thickness skin graft of exposed muscle was also accomplished. Following discharge, the patients were regularly checked in the outpatient clinic until fracture union was obtained, which was defined as that point when no clinical motion at the fracture site could be detected, when painless, unprotected weight bearing was possible, and when radiographic evidence of union was present.

Results

The patients' ages ranged from 18 to 58 years, with a mean age of 29 years. Thus, most patients were young adults. The cause of injury was pedestrian auto accidents in six limbs, motor vehicle accidents in six limbs, motorcycle accidents in five limbs, high energy missiles in two limbs, and a fall from 20 feet in one limb. Associated multiple systems injuries were present in 15 of the 18 patients, further complicating their management. Popliteal artery injury requiring repair was documented by arteriography in two limbs with ipsilateral supracondylar fractures. Injury to the peroneal nerve was present in three limbs.

Three limbs had segmental fractures and one limb had a bony defect of 6 cm. The area of the fractures was predominantly at about the middle-third of the tibia with the wound site being in the proximal third in two limbs, the proximal-middle junction in four limbs, the middle-third in eight limbs, and the middle-distal junction in six limbs. Sixteen limbs had open fracture wounds classified as Type III and four limbs were classified Type IIIA.

The average time from injury to flap coverage was nine days, ranging from two to 27 days. Soft tissue coverage was accomplished with a soleus muscle flap in eight limbs, a medial gastrocnemius myocutaneous flap in eight limbs, a lateral gastrocnemius myocutaneous flap in three limbs, and a crossleg medial gastrocnemius myocutaneous flap in one limb.

Three of the four limbs with Type IIIA wounds had significant complications. One amputation below the knee was performed 14 days after the injury and ten days after a soleus muscle transfer, for muscle necrosis and infection. The patient had been wounded at close range with a 12-gauge shotgun missile. In the 19 remaining limbs, one infection persisted in a patient with a popliteal artery laceration, resulting in delayed union.

The average time to union was $18\frac{1}{2}$ weeks, ranging from 12-35 weeks. The external skeletal fixation device was the primary mode of treatment for an average of six weeks. Patients were placed in a walking cast after removal of the external fixation device and were followed up until union occurred.

Four limbs required secondary operations to stimulate the bone healing process. Posterolateral bone grafts were performed in three limbs and a fibula protibia operation in one limb with segmental defect.

The alignment of the tibia at the time of union was assessed clinically and radiographically. Clinical malalignment did not occur in this series. Radiographic alignment was normal in ten limbs; in three limbs there was posterior deviation at the fracture site of 5°, and anterior deviation of the fracture site of 5° in one limb. Three tibias showed medial deviation at the fracture site of 10° while one limb had 10° of lateral deviation at the fracture site.

Discussion

The proponents of open fracture care (Gregory, 1975) emphasize that management of the soft tissue wound is of primary concern. If the requirements for soft tissue wound healing are met, stabilization of the fracture should be beneficial to post-traumatic osteogenesis. Rhinelander (1974) has shown that bone and the surrounding soft tissue share numerous vascular micro-anastomoses. The proliferation of vessels supplying the muscles and periosteum is responsible for the elaboration of the fracture callus in limbs with displaced fractures, especially in the presence of interruption of endosteal blood supply. Holden (1972) clearly showed a lag phase in the healing of complex open fractures and that initiation of callus depended on restoration of soft tissue vascularity. The healing process in bone was initiated by neovascular ingrowth from the gradually revascularized muscle and periosteum. During the lag phase required for restoration of blood supply to the soft tissue, there was no endosteal circulation seen in Holden's experimental model.

This prospective study was undertaken based on the hypothesis that if a viable soft tissue envelope could be placed around the compound fractured tibia largely devoid of soft tissue, healing could be initiated without prolonging the revascularization phase. We attempted to create a favorable mesenchymal milieu to hasten open fracture wound healing by maintaining a live wound with muscle flaps.

Numerous reports have described the use of pedicle muscle flaps in the management of acute and chronic soft tissue defects of the leg (Ger, 1970; 1971; Jones, 1980; McCraw, 1978; Vasconez, et al, 1974), giving details of the surgical techniques employed. Ours is the first report, however, of a prospective study designed to assess the treatment of complicated open tibia fractures with pedicled muscle flaps.

Myoplasty or myocutaneous flap coverage was performed according to the level of the open fracture wound. First line coverage was provided by the gastrocnemius muscle in the proximal half of the leg. Because the myocutaneous gastrocnemius flap is no more complicated to perform than a local gastrocnemius myoplasty, it is preferred in most situations. Either the medial or the lateral head of the gastrocnemius can be pedicled with the directly overlying skin; the skin distal to each head can be expected to survive on its musculocutaneous unit to a distance approximately equal to the width of each head. Twelve of the 20 flaps in this series were gastrocnemius myocutaneous units. The remainder were soleus muscle flaps which were primarily used in defects of the middle or middle-distal junction of the leg.

Traditional treatment of complex open fractures has been debridement and healing by secondary granulation tissue or skin grafting. While such traditional methods may provide satisfactory early results, the skin is frequently directly adherent to bone in the pretibial area and susceptible to recurrent trauma and breakdown. Hicks (1975) presented a ten-year follow-up of 54 tibia fractures with skin breakdown over the anterior-medial surface treated by debridement and skin grafting or secondary granulation healing over bone. While the early results showed 90% successful wound healing, the ten-year results showed that only 60% of the limbs had remained healed. The skin directly over the bone was delicate, friable, unstable, and trivial trauma caused breakdown of the adherent scar. Failure of proper management in these conditions, such as coverage of exposed, dead cortical bone and tendinous or neurovascular structures, result in poor blood supply to adjacent tissues and a severely compromised outcome.

None of the wounds in this series developed breakdown in the pretibial area. In fact, the soft tissue cover was stable with no adherence of skin to bone. The transposed muscle did atrophy, usually about one-third of the mass, as the wound matured. No wound problems were encountered in the walking cast after external fixation was removed.

The classification system used in this prospective series was designed to emphasize the concept of open fracture wound healing. The classification took into account the soft tissue wound and the radiologic appearance of the fracture fragments, a key to the amount of energy dissipated. Type III open fracture wounds were defined as high energy forces causing a significantly displaced fracture pattern with severe comminution, segmental fracture, or bone defect with extensive skin loss and muscle damage. A subclassification of Type IIIA included those open fracture wounds that had concomitant vascular injury requiring repair, high energy gunshot or shotgun wound or a history of a crush or degloving injury. There were four such wounds in this series. This subclassification was made because the ischemia resulting from vascular injury, blast injury or crushing, causes severe breakdown of all the tissues of the limb. Essentially, a Type I fracture pattern with minimal soft tissue damage secondary to the trauma could be converted to a Type IIIA fracture in cases of associated vascular injury or extensive devitalization of soft tissue.

In this prospective series, both limbs with disturbance of open wound healing had associated popliteal artery transections requiring repair. The ischemic interval before restoration of distal perfusion was seven and nine hours, respectively. In one limb a crush injury had destroyed the entire posterior compartment. A crossleg medial gastrocnemius myocutaneous flap was used to provide coverage. Because of the severe circumferential crush, however, and the associated popliteal artery interruption, complete envelopment of the bone was not possible and union was delayed. In the other limb, distal perfusion after arterial repair was inadequate. Consequently, both the initial soleus muscle flap and a subsequent latissimus dorsi free flap failed in providing soft tissue coverage of the wound defect. The fracture of this patient did not progress to union and a chronic infection persisted.

The limb which underwent amputation below the knee was injured by a high energy, close range, 12-gauge shotgun blast and was classified as a Type IIIA. Soleus muscle transfer was performed four days after the injury but a repeat debridement was not done. The transposed muscle was also damaged by the blast, and an error was made in not repeating debridement of this limb. The blast injury caused necrosis of the crural muscles and the patient developed a gangrenous limb. An amputation below the knee was performed ten days after attempted flap coverage and 14 days after injury.

In this series, union of the fractures occurred between 12 and 35 weeks. The external fixation device was maintained for an average of six weeks. When stress testing showed some stability at the fracture site, the external fixation device was removed. The patients were then placed in a well molded patella tendon-bearing walking cast and followed up until union. The $18\frac{1}{2}$ weeks average union time in this series was much shorter than the 31 weeks reported by Widenfalk (1979) for a series of Type II and Type III open tibia fractures treated by external fixation without myoplastic coverage.

Both limbs with failures of union also had a popliteal artery injury with ipsilateral open supracondylar fractures. The initial postulate seems to be justified, that osseous healing response of Type III open fractures depends on a well vascularized soft tissue envelope. A posterolateral bone graft was performed after six months in one of the limbs. Clinical and roentgenographic evidence of progression of union was seen over the next three months. The patient, however, fell from a height and refractured the limb three months after bone grafting. Reoperation was performed and fixation achieved by means of a Lottes nail, supplemented by a posterolateral bone graft which led to union. The other patient with a nonunion did not come for his appointments for four months. He has since refused bone grafting and is being maintained in a lightweight plastic ankle-foot orthosis.

There was only one chronic infection in the 19 limbs. This infection occurred in the patient with popliteal artery transection and poor vascular
flow to the entire limb. The ischemic interval was nine hours and both a
soleus myoplasty and a latissimus dorsi free flap failed. It is believed
that the chronic infection was due to our inability to establish circumferential vascularity to the limb.

The incidence of persistent infection in this Type III open fracture is
about the same as that reported by Karlstrom and Olerud (1975). They included only 14 Type III fractures in their report on external fixation
management. Comparison of the current series with other studies is somewhat
difficult because a clear delineation of Type III open tibia fractures has
not been established. Edwards (1965) found a close correlation between
soft tissue injury and infection, particularly skin necrosis, in open tibia
fractures. Tonnesen (1975) also showed the relationship between loss of
skin cover and failure of union. He was the first to suggest stable external fixation supplemented by myoplasty for the management of Type II and
Type III open tibial fractures. With this approach, overcaution in debridement or concern about coverage of exposed bone is unnecessary. The surgeon
can perform radical debridements, secure in the knowledge that coverage can
be obtained with soft tissue flap procedures. Therefore, the highlights
of this protocol management were radical wound debridement combined with
systemic cephalosporin antibiotics, copious jet lavage, and external fixation for easy wound care.

No significant functional deficits were identified in these patients. Toe
walking was possible. Limitation of ankle motion is a common sequela of
tibia fracture and interpretation of the functional deficits of patients
after myoplasty must be tempered in view of the overall deficits usually
seen in Type III open fractures.

The two failures of union and the single incident of infection occurred in
patients with arterial injury to the limb proximal to the fracture. In
spite of surgical repair of the arterial damage, there was no perfusion of
the muscular tissue during an average of eight hours. The purpose of the
pedicled muscle flap to provide a favorable mesenchymal milieu for open
fracture wound healing was therefore thwarted by lack of vascular perfusion.
Otherwise, the good results confirm the initial hypothesis: complete debridement of the open fracture wound accompanied by early provision of a vascularized myocutaneous envelope about the osseous tissue maintains a live,
closed wound. When combined with stable external skeletal fixation, soft
tissue coverage can be expected to vastly improve the treatment of complex
open tibia fractures.

References

1. Edwards, P.: Fracture of the shaft of the tibia. Acta Orthop. Scand.,
    Suppl. 76, 1965.

2. Ger, R.: The management of open fracture of the tibia with skin loss.
    J. Trauma, 10, 112-121, 1970.

3. Ger, R.: The technique of muscle transposition in the operative treat-
    ment of traumatic and ulcerated lesions of the leg. J. Trauma, 11,
    502-510, 1971.

4. Gregory, C.F.: Open fractures. In Fractures. Eds: Rockwood, D. and Green, D., J.B. Lippincott, Philadelphia, 1975.

5. Hicks, J.H.: Long term follow-up of a series of infected fractures of the tibia. Injury, 7, 2-7, 1975.

6. Holden, C.E.: The role of the blood supply to soft tissue in the healing of diaphyseal fractures. J. Bone Jt. Surg. 54A, 993-1000, 1972.

7. Jones, R.E. and Cierny, G.C.: Management of complex open tibial fractures with external skeletal fixation and early myoplasty or myocutaneous coverage. Canad. J. Surg. 23, 242-244, 1980.

8. Jones, R.E.: External fixation: soft tissue coverage. In, AAOS Instructional Course Lectures, C.V. Mosby, St. Louis, 1980 (in press).

9. Karlstrom, G. and Olerud, S.: Percutaneous pin fixation of open tibial fractures. J. Bone Jt. Surg. 57A, 915-924, 1975.

10. McCraw, J.B.: The versatile gastrocnemius myocutaneous flap. Plast. Reconstr.Surg. 62, 15-23, 1978.

11. Rhinelander, F.W.: Tibial blood supply in relation to fracture healing. Clin. Orthop Rel. Res. 105, 34-81, 1974.

12. Tonnesen, P.A., et al: 150 open fractures of the tibial shaft: The relation between necrosis of the skin and delayed union. Acta. Orthop. Scand. 46, 823-835, 1975.

13. Vasconez, L.Q., Bostwick, J., and McCraw, J.: Coverage of exposed bone by muscle transposition and skin grafting. Plast. Reconstr. Surg. 53, 526-530, 1974.

14. Widenfalk, B., Penten, B., and Karlstrom, G.: Open fractures of the shaft of the tibia: Analysis of wound and fracture treatment. Injury, 11, 136-143, 1979.

Indications for the Hoffmann Fixator in Severely Injured Patients

Ch. C. Edwards and B. D. Browner

Patients with severe injuries to the musculoskeletal system are often vic-
tims of high energy trauma. Whereas some fall from heights and others
suffer industrial injuries, the great majority suffer motor vehicle accidents. Many are either struck by or thrown from motocycles or automobiles.
These patients usually have major soft tissue injury, comminuted fracture
patterns, fractures in more than one bone, often with associated head, chest
or abdominal injuries.

Because of the complex nature of high energy fractures and the frequency of
associated injuries, these patients require a fracture fixation system that
is sufficiently versatile to treat a wide variety of fracture patterns and
which permits unlimited mobilization. Patient mobilization is important for
at least two reasons: Firstly, it is necessary for the prevention and
treatment of respiratory complications. Due to direct chest contusion,
abdominal or head injuries, or the physiologic derangements following massive trauma, respiratory distress syndrome is a frequent complication. Unrestricted patient turning in bed and sitting is needed to maximize the
ventilation-to-perfusion ratio and promote adequate drainage of all pulmonary
segments. Secondly, mobilization facilitates the general management of the
patient. Due to the prevalence of soft tissue and associated injuries, these
patients must be returned to the operating room frequently for wound debridement and coverage procedures and for treatment of nonorthopedic injuries.
They may also have to be moved from their beds for axial tomography, arteriography and other diagnostic studies.

Both primary internal fixation and primary external fixation may be versatile enough to manage complex fractures and permit unrestricted patient
mobilization. When combined with open wound management, both methods are
probably superior to former traction or plaster casting techniques in the
multiply-injured patient. The routine use of primary internal fixation,
however, for the treatment of open fractures complicated by major soft
tissue wounds raises a number of concerns:

1. Is it possible for most surgeons to identify all contaminated or necrotic
   bone and adjacent tissues before metal implantation?

2. Doesn't the required dissection, stripping, and retraction for internal
   fixation further disrupt the already marginal vascularity of the edema-
   tous injured tissues?

3. Do laboratory studies showing suppressed host antibacterial activity in
    the presence of metal (Brown et al, 1976; Schurman et al, 1974) have
    clinical relevance to the treatment of open fractures?

Based on these concerns, we feel that primary external fixation might be a
more physiologic first step in the treatment of fractures complicated by
major open wounds.

We have found the Hoffmann external fixation system sufficiently versatile
to stabilize complex fractures in most bones while permitting maximum patient mobilization and providing good access to soft tissue observation and
for subsequent reconstruction. Our team of orthopedic surgeons at the University of Maryland Hospital and Trauma Center has now treated over 500 major
open injuries with this system. From this experience, we can identify seven
general indications for the use of Hoffmann external fixation in the severely
injured patient.

I   Major Pelvic Disruptions

Pelvic disruptions with bleeding

Bleeding associated with unstable pelvic fractures is a major and sometimes
life-threatening problem. Because of the extensive collateral circulation
in the pelvis, surgical intervention alone is often unsuccessful and wrought
with complications (Kane, 1975). Arterial embolization (Ring et al, 1974)
and G-suits or Mast trousers (Flint et al, 1979) can be used with some success in selected cases. We have found that rapid stabilization of the pelvic ring using the Hoffmann external fixator can also decrease bleeding. We
have hypothesized that stabilization of the pelvis with an external frame
might reduce bleeding in three ways:

1. *Reapproximation of soft tissues.* In the severely disrupted pelvis, the
    two sides of the bony pelvis are generally spread apart. When these
    bones are brought together to restore the pelvic ring, disrupted tissues
    and vessels are also brought closer together to facilitate clotting.

2. *Establishment of rigid walls for tamponot.* External fixation fixes the
    pelvic ring bones. To some degree, this limits the potential space for
    clotting blood and hence, may promote tamponot.

3. *Reduction of motion.* Even a simple anterior Hoffmann frame will reduce
    gross motion in a severely disrupted pelvis (Koraharju and Slätis, 1978;
    Riska et al, 1979). This should minimize clot disruption and further
    bleeding as the patient moves or is moved about.

The following case illustrates the value of pelvic fixation in controlling
hemorrhage. A patient was admitted in shock with multiple injuries, including severe pelvic disruption with 7 cm lateral displacement of the right
hemipelvis. She required nine units of blood to maintain a palpable pressure
during the first half hour in the admitting bay of our trauma center. Follow-

ing manual reduction of the pelvis, a pelvic Hoffmann frame was applied as quickly as possible in the adjacent operating room. Following pelvic stabilization, the patient's blood pressure was easy to maintain and rose to 100/60 following blood transfusion of seven additional units over the next hour. Since significant bleeding is often due to arterial disruption (Ring et al, 1974), external fixation alone will not always yield such dramatic results as in this case. Nevertheless, it does provide a low risk first step in the treatment of pelvic bleeding and can be supplemented with the other methods outlined above when bleeding fails to subside.

Does primary external fixation of the pelvis preclude needed intrapelvic or abdominal surgery? On the contrary; stabilization of the bony pelvis in a relatively anatomic position reduces bleeding during surgery as well and makes soft tissue relationships more predictable according to our general surgeons. The frame can be tilted caudally to facilitate anterior abdominal exposure. Following surgery, the frame can be returned to its proper cephalad orientation.

Pelvic disruption with ring instability

Treatment of pelvic ring disruption with pelvic slings blocks all patient mobility and is completely unsatisfactory for the polytraumatized patient. Most authors associate primary internal fixation for major pelvic ring disruptions with a high rate of surgical complications (Kane, 1975). Placement of external fixation half pins in both ilia provides a handle for the surgeon to effect a closed reduction using supplemental extremity traction on a fracture table when necessary. The pin groups can be attached to the appropriate Hoffmann frame to maintain reasonable fixation for most pelvic fractures. The frames are constructed with standard Hoffmann components: ball joint pin clamps without rods, adjustable rods, free rods and couplings. The Slätis style "A" frame is satisfactory for open-book or Bucholz Type II (Bucholz, 1978) pelvic ring fractures. Additional pin groups (Mears and Fu, 1980) or supplemental short-term leg traction may be necessary for displaced Malgaine or Bucholz Type III fractures. The resultant pelvic fixation permits excellent early patient mobilization and greatly decreases pain.

Open pelvic disruption

Open pelvic fractures and pelvic fractures with bladder ruptures have a mortality between 30 and 45% reported in the literature (Kane, 1975). Death usually results from sepsis. These injuries often have associated bowel lacerations. Accordingly, optimum initial treatment may now include stabilization of the ring with an external fixator followed by a laparotomy to perform a diverting colostomy. The open wounds can be debrided and kept packed open. By using a split mattress, a patient can be turned 360° for treatment of posterior pelvic wounds, if necessary. The pelvic frame permits full patient mobilization so that serial surgical debridements are possible without disrupting the healing pelvic ring tissues. We have treated four patients with major open pelvic injuries using this approach without any fatalities to date.

II Complex Open Fractures

The Hoffmann system is sufficiently versatile to stabilize complex fractures.
Injuries involving multiple fractures to a long bone can be simplified in
the following way. A standard transfixion pin group can be placed proximally
and distally to the fractured segment. If fractures extend too close to a
joint to permit the usual coronal pin group orientation, the pin group can
be oriented transversely or parallel with the joint surface (Fig. 1c). A
half pin group consisting of one, two or three pins, depending on the size
of the fragment, is then used to control each fracture segment or major fragment. These half pin groupings are either attached to rods on the basic
frame or they can be connected to each other with additional adjustable rods
(Edwards and Browner, 1981). The orthopedist can then compress or distract
each major fracture gap depending on the characteristics of that particular
fracture.

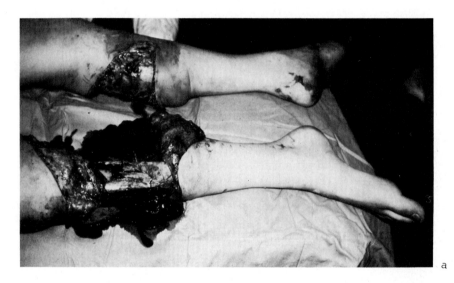

a

Fig. 1. "Floating knee" injuries treated with Hoffmann external
fixation and Ender nailing. a) Right: open femoral and tibial
fractures with bone, muscle, and popliteal skin loss; Left: open
tibial and hindfoot fractures and a closed femoral fracture.
b) and c) The right leg is treated with a "long-leg Hoffmann"
consisting of tibial and femoral frames joined by rods to stabilize injured soft tissues crossing the knee; the proximal tibial
3-pin group is placed horizontally due to the proximity of the
frame to the joint. The left leg is treated first with external
fixation of the tibia and foot. The fixator is then attached to
the fracture table footpiece (arrow). Traction can be applied
via the fixator to facilitate closed Ender nailing of the closed
femoral fracture. d) Subsequent reconstruction of the proximal
right tibial skin, muscle and bone defect using an iliac crest
composite graft. The graft is fixed with half pins before its
removal from the ileum; it is then attached to the tibial frame
before microvascular anastomosis.

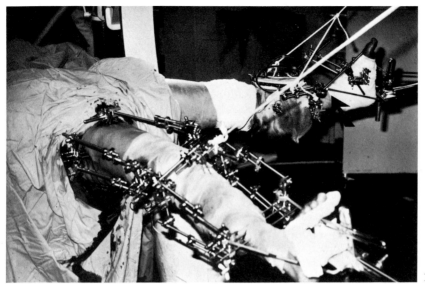

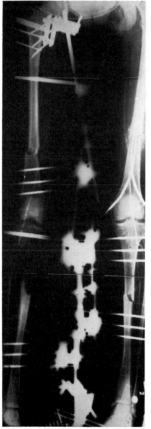

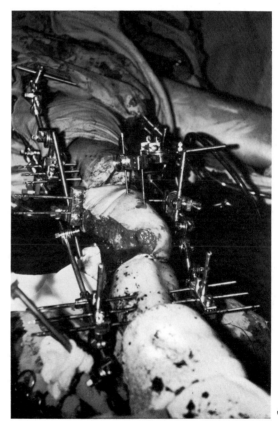

Fig. 1. (continued)

Hoffmann external fixation can easily be used combined with other fracture treatment systems in the same extremity. For example, an external fixation appliance for treatment of an open tibial fracture can be incorporated within a long leg traction cast used to treat a closed femoral fracture in a young patient (Browner et al, 1980; Edwards, 1979; 1980). Likewise, external fixation of open tibial and ankle injuries can simplify subsequent closed intramedullary nailing of the ipsilateral femur. The fixator can be clamped directly to the foot piece of the fracture table to facilitate leg positioning and traction for closed intramedullary nailing (Fig. 1a, b, c). Or, an external fixator can be used as a fracture reduction apparatus followed by definitive fixation incorporating the external fixation pins-in-plaster or with an internal fixation device.

Treatment of complex open fractures with a Hoffmann external fixator aids tissue reconstruction as well. One side of the standard quadrilateral or Vidal tibial frame can be removed for surgical access without compromising fracture stability. This facilitates serial wound debridements, split thickness skin grafting, and muscle flap tissue coverage procedures. Cross leg pedicle flaps, in particular, are simplified with the use of the Hoffmann fixator. A frame applied to the donor leg can be attached to the original frame on the injured extremity to comfortably fix the position of the two legs until the flap can be detached. This provides far more reliable fixation, comfort and better access to the flap than former bulky casting techniques (Edwards et al, 1979).

Another special indication for the Hoffmann fixator in reconstructing complex fractures is in the replacement of lost bone with an iliac composite graft. Full thickness iliac cortex can be transferred with surrounding muscle and overlying skin. A vascular supply can be maintained by anastomosing the feeding branch of the medial circumflex iliac artery to available vessels in the leg. The iliac bone can be fixed with a sagittally directed half pin group before its removal from the pelvis. This pin group can then be attached to the basic tibial Hoffmann frame to maintain the iliac composite graft in a stable position (Fig. 1c, d).

Hoffmann external fixation appears indicated for most open and/or severely comminuted humeral fractures. When fractures are associated with neurovascular injury, the Hoffmann fixator is particularly useful to stabilize the fracture and protect surgical repair of vessels or nerves. A humeral frame can be constructed lateral to the arm using two half pin groups connected by one or two adjustable rods (Edwards and Browner, 1981). We have had uniformly favorable results treating 20 open humeral fractures with this method (Browner et al, 1982).

External fixation may also be indicated in the treatment of closed humeral fractures in multiply-injured patients who must remain recumbent. Casting and splinting do not maintain reasonable fracture alignment in the recumbent patient. Olecranon traction techniques do not provide sufficient patient mobilization to permit necessary turning in bed. Additional experience is needed to determine if external fixation will become a better alternative for treatment of humeral shaft fractures in the recumbent patient.

III Evaluation of Amputation Candidates

It is possible to salvage a functional extremity if palm or sole innervation is present and if blood supply to the limb can be restored. Although legs requiring extensive bone and soft tissue reconstruction may be far from normal, a stiff but sensate limb may sometimes serve the patient better than a prosthesis. With external fixation, open wound treatment and advanced muscle and myocutaneous reconstructive techniques, there are few limbs which cannot be reconstructed or which require primary amputation. The decision whether to amputate or reconstruct a severely traumatized extremity is then based on the value of a particular reconstructed extremity weighed against the time, personal toil and cost required for each patient.

Primary external fixation of severely traumatized limbs which may have to be amputated permits careful assessment of the amputation question by both the physician and the patient. The physician may wish to proceed with one or more serial debridements, fluorescein dye injections or arteriography to fully assess the reconstruction potential of the limb. Even when amputation becomes the only reasonable alternative, patients appreciate the attempted limb salvage and the chance to participate in the amputation decision. We have found that patients allowed to participate in the decision are able to accept the amputation psychologically better than those patients who awaken from anesthesia to find that their unsalvageable limb has been amputated. Initial treatment with external fixation permits a full evaluation of both the limb and the patient's needs before definitive surgery.

IV Treatment Following Fasciotomy

Fasciotomy to treat a compartment syndrome generally converts a closed fracture to a grade III open fracture. This is because the compartment syndrome which necessitated fasciotomy has left the muscle ischemic and often with areas of focal necrosis. This ischemic muscle usually swells significantly creating a rather large soft tissue wound over the fracture.

Accordingly, we suggest applying an external fixator at the time of fasciotomy. In the case of a potentially stable fracture, without extensive comminution, a unilateral frame with half pin groups is generally sufficient. In order to avoid the fasciotomy wounds, the pins can be placed in the sagittal plane entering the tibia in an anterior to posterior direction (Fig. 2a, b). Extreme caution, however, must be exercised in passing the proximal tibial pin group through the posterior cortex of the tibia. It must be remembered that the tibial nerve and posterior tibial artery are in close approximation to the posterior tibial cortex. For this reason, dull tip half pins should be used and should be placed under image intensification control.

External fixation of the tibial fracture following fasciotomy permits good access for treatment of the exposed muscle and subsequent closure or split thickness skin grafting. It simplifies elevation in that the fixator can be tied to an overhead frame. Finally, it rigidly stabilizes the injured soft tissues decreasing their oxygen needs to achieve maximum soft tissue survival.

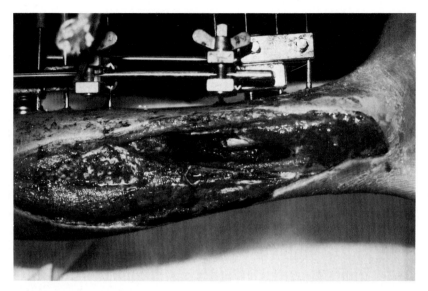

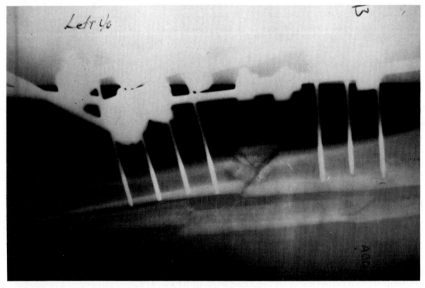

Fig. 2. a and b). Anterior tibial frame for stable
tibial fractures.
Following wide fasciotomies for a compartment syndrome,
half pins are inserted under image intensification control and an anterior double frame is assembled. This
frame configuration avoids muscle impalement, provides
good wound accessibility, and provides adequate fixation
for fractures without bone loss or extensive comminution.

V Definitive Treatment for Periarticular Comminution

External fixation can be indicated in the treatment of extensively comminuted articular or periarticular bone. Initial treatment consists of placing
pin groups on either side of the affected joint and then distracting between
these pin groups with adjustable rods. This neutralizes the compressive
forces from muscles which would normally act across the joint. The localized
traction can also pull fragments attached to surrounding soft tissues into
relative alignment - a concept known as "ligamentotaxis" (Vidal et al, 1979).

When the fractured articular surface includes two or more major fragments,
we recommend combining the neutralization frame with primary open reduction
and internal fixation of the major articular fragments. The internal fixation step can be delayed several days when treating contaminated wounds until
the wounds are clean. By using a small amount of metal (lag screws and
Kirschner wires) and avoiding large plates, we have had no cases of sepsis
or osteomyelitis associated with the use of this small amount of metal completely encased within bone. This principle is illustrated in the case of
a motorcycle rider who struck his left knee against a truck and suffered a
massive open fracture of the distal femur and proximal tibia (Fig. 3a).
Limited internal fixation with interfragmentary lag screws permitted accurate reestablishment of articular anatomy. The open metaphyseal fractures and
injured soft tissues were then immobilized by a Hoffmann apparatus which
initially extended from the proximal femur to the mid-tibia (Fig. 3b). Subsequent reconstruction includes repeated debridements until a clean and
viable base is achieved. A free microvascular latissimus dorsi flap can
also be used to restore soft tissue coverage. Following maturation of the
flap, a tibial bone graft is performed to replace missing bone and promote
fracture union.

In the case of a massive articular comminution, treatment is by ligamentotaxis alone. For the elbow, we connect a half pin group entering the lateral
or posterior distal humerus with a half pin group entering the proximal ulna.
For the ankle joint with extensive comminution of the distal tibia or talus,
one distracts between pin groups in the distal tibia and calcaneus; when
necessary, a half pin group is added into the first metatarsal to maintain
the forefoot in a neutral position (Edwards and Kenzora, 1981; Kenzora et
al, 1981). For the knee, the standard distal femoral transfixion pin group
is connected with a proximal tibial pin group. For the hip joint, a half
pin grouping is placed into each iliac crest and connected to the two pin
groups with a plain rod. Then, anterior and lateral half pin groups are
placed in the proximal femur also connected to each other with a rod. Finally, distraction is made between the pelvic and femoral frames with two
adjustable rods.

For example, a patient struck by an automobile suffered a chest contusion,
right femoral fracture, pelvic ring disruption and a highly comminuted left
central acetabular fracture (Fig. 4a). Optimum treatment for her lung contusion and associated injuries precluded skeletal traction. Initial orthopedic management included reduction and fixation of the pelvic dislocation
with a Slätis frame. A percutaneous trochanteric screw was inserted to reduce the acetabular fracture with lateral traction. Half pin groups placed

404

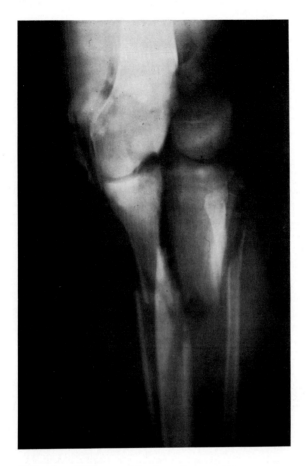

Fig. 3. Intra-articular fragments.
a) Open femoral and tibial fractures with
major displaced intra-articular fragments.

in the proximal femur were then attached to the pelvic frame with adjustable
rods. The trochanteric screw was removed and the femoral head was maintained
by traction under the roof of the acetabulum between the pelvic frame and
femoral pin groups (Fig. 4b). This "inboard traction" allowed good patient
mobilization as well. After three months, the fixator was removed. The
patient regained good hip range of motion and painless ambulation (Fig. 4c).

VI "Inboard Traction" for Multiple Fractures in an Extremity

Patients with severe injuries to multiple bones and/or joints in an extremity
have presented a major problem in management for the orthopedist. Placing an

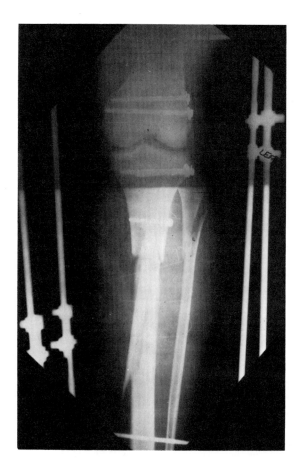

Fig. 3. (continued)
b) Initial treatment consists of application of external fixator to neutralize fractures and use of lag screws to restore articular congruity. During a subsequent debridement, additional pin groups and hinges can be applied to permit controlled knee motion.

extremity with multiple open injuries in balanced skeletal traction precludes essential patient mobilization and is, therefore, generally not appropriate for the multiple trauma victim. All the benefits of skeletal traction without its constraints can be achieved with Hoffmann external fixation. In the lower extremity, a standard femoral frame can be applied to span multiple femoral fractures and a quadrilateral tibial frame can be applied to span tibial fractures. A metatarsal and/or calcaneal pin group can be added to stabilize distal tibial and ankle disruptions. In cases of disruption of

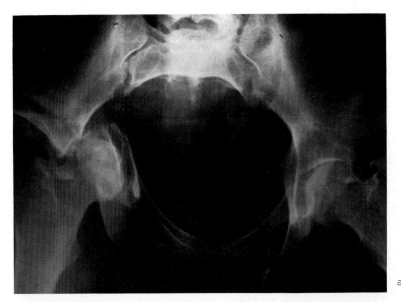

a

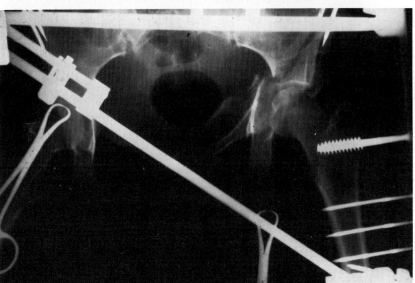

b

Fig. 4. Ligamentotaxis for treatment of hip joint comminution.
a) Comminuted central fracture dislocation of the hip, pelvic
ring disruption, and multiple injuries requiring patient mobilization. b) Initial treatment consisted of 1) application of
pelvic Hoffmann frame, 2) use of temporary lateral traction via
a trochanteric screw to reduce the hip, and 3) distraction between the pelvic frame and half pin groups in the proximal femur to maintain the position of the femoral head.

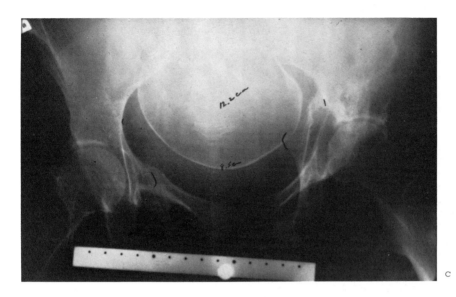

Fig. 4. (continued)
c) Preservation of a painless hip joint and a fully functional
pelvis 10 months postinjury (note fetal head).

the knee joint or periarticular fractures, the femoral and tibial frames can
be attached with additional rods. The various injured segments can then be
distracted to maintain length and relative alignment until definitive fixation can be accomplished.

Immediate inboard traction for multiple ipsilateral fractures offers several
advantages to the severely injured patient. It permits unrestricted patient
mobilization. It achieves rapid stabilization of the injured soft tissues
and fractures. It maintains length and alignment until wounds are clean and
the patient is sufficiently stable for delayed primary open reduction and
internal fixation and/or definitive external fixation.

The same principles and advantages apply to the upper extremity. For example,
a patient suffered open and contaminated fractures of the humerus, elbow
joint, and forearm resulting from a motorcycle accident (Fig. 5a). Initial
management consisted of debridement and irrigation followed by the application of a Hoffmann inboard-traction system for the upper extremity. A
standard lateral humeral half frame was applied first. Adjustable rods
were then used to connect the humeral frame with pins placed in the meta-
carpals. The rods were distracted to maintain length and relative alignment
of the comminuted elbow and forearm bone fractures (Fig. 5b). The arm was
elevated by tying the fixator to an overhead frame. The patient was then
taken back to the operating room twice for additional debridement. When the
wounds had a clean and viable base, open reduction and fixation of the elbow
fragments was performed using K wires and lag screws. Compression plates
were used to fix the forearm fractures. The distal extension of the fixator
was then removed. The proximal frame was left in place for definitive treatment of the open humeral fracture (Fig. 5c).

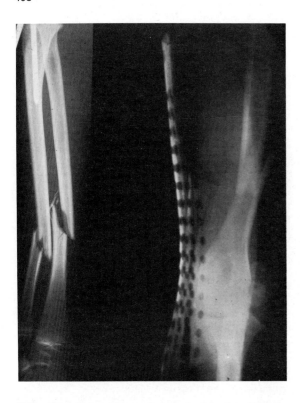

Fig. 5. Temporary "inboard-traction" for the upper extremity: a) Fractures of the forearm humerus and elbow complicated by contaminated wounds.

VII   Stabilization of Injured Soft Tissues Crossing Major Joints

One of our most gratifying uses for Hoffmann external fixation in the severely injured patient has been in the treatment of massive soft tissue injuries crossing major joints. Usually, these injuries are associated with open fractures. Due to the sparce amount of soft tissue overlying the joints, tissue grafting techniques are often necessary to obtain functional coverage. External fixation can simplify the treatment of these injuries. Adjacent fractures are stabilized with standard frames and then connected with plain rods and couplings to fix the position of the affected joint. This stabilizes the injured soft tissues to maximize their potential for recovery. It provides excellent access to the wounds for debridements, dressing changes and subsequent skin grafting or myocutaneous flap tissue reconstruction. In addition, fixing the joint in a functional position prevents unwanted contracture secondary to the pain flexion response or scar contracture.

Frame configurations for the treatment of soft tissue injuries crossing joints are essentially the same as for the definitive treatment of periarticular comminution. The main difference is that when the skeleton underlying the injured soft tissues is intact, unilateral frames and half pin groupings may be adequate.

The most common soft tissue injury affecting major joints is to the anterior muscle compartment of the tibia. High energy open fractures of the tibia are frequently accompanied by avulsion or major disruption of the anterior compartment tibial muscles. As a result, the patient loses active dorsiflexion of the ankle for at least several weeks following injury. Unless

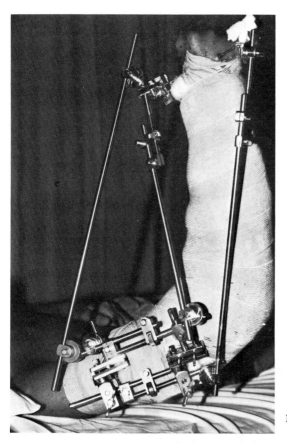

Fig. 5. (continued)
b) Use of adjustable rods between metacarpal pins and a
humeral frame to maintain traction across the elbow and forearm until wound condition permitted definitive internal fixation (c).

b

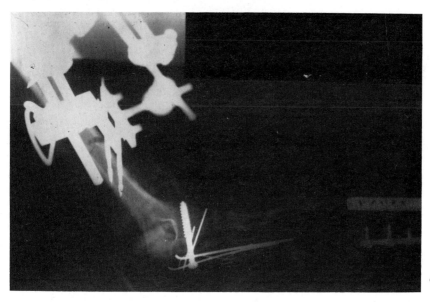

c

410

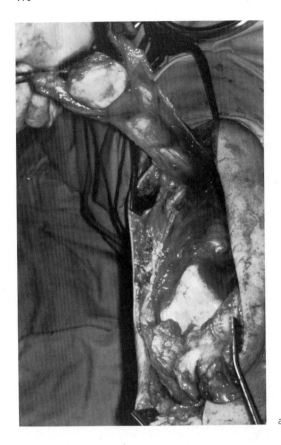
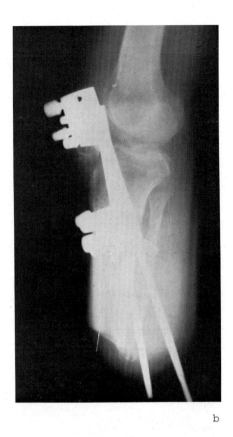

a

b

Fig. 6. Patellotibial fixation. a) Traumatic avulsion of the tibial tendon.
b) Protection of simple suture repair with a "Charnley" fixator. Single pins
pass through the patella and tibia in the coronal plane.

specific attention is directed towards maintaining the foot in a neutral
position, equinus deformity usually follows. In such cases, we suggest
attaching two half pins in the first metatarsals of the foot to the tibial
frame with a plain rod. This will hold the foot in neutral position and
encourage a functional tenodesis from scarring rather than an equinus contracture. The same basic tibiometatarsal frame can be used after avulsion
of skin or ligaments from the hindfoot and ankle. This provides excellent
tissue access and permits enough micromotion in the small joints of the foot
for articular cartilage survival (Edwards, 1979; 1980; Edwards and Kenzora,
1981).

Treatment of major soft tissue injuries crossing the knee is also simplified
with the use of Hoffmann fixation. For example, popliteal tissue avulsions
are almost always accompanied by adjacent open fractures. Treatment for
these complex injuries mandates fracture fixation, complete wound access and
soft tissue stability across the knee. Only a versatile external fixation
system can currently provide all these functions simultaneously (Fig. 1a, c).

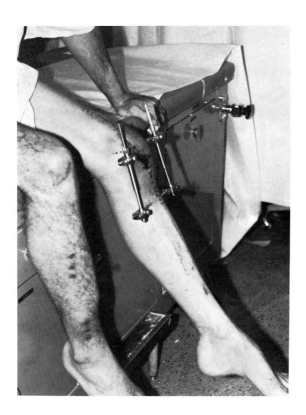

Fig. 6. (continued)
c) and d) Patellotibial fixation permits active knee motion.

c

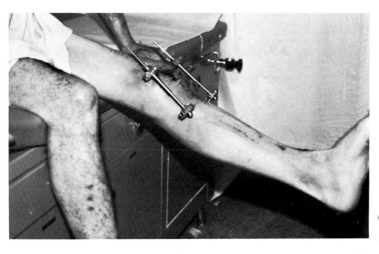

d

On the other hand, patellar tendon ruptures and avulsions can be treated by
a number of methods. These include direct suture, tendon graft weaves and
pullout suture techniques. We have used a simple external frame to protect
the tendon repair and speed subsequent rehabilitation (Edwards, 1979)(Fig.
6a). A threaded Steinmann or Bonnell pin is passed in the coronal plane
through the patella and another pin through the proximal tibia at the level

of the tibial tubercle (Fig. 6b). The two pins are then connected both medially and laterally by a simple external frame. When the Charnley frame is
used, the wing nut that tightens the frame to the pin should be removed to
allow rotation of the pin within the pin clamp.

The patellotibial frame concept offers several advantages. It can prevent
quadriceps contracture until an open wound has become clean enough for
patellar-tendon repair or reconstruction. It permits simple resorbable
suture repair of the patellar tendon since all tension forces are neutra-
lized by the external frame. It facilitates early active motion of the
knee to prevent adhesions and excessive quadriceps muscle atrophy (Fig. 6c,
d), and it allows the surgeon to load the healing tendon gradually by
lengthening the external frame.

External fixation across the hip or across the multiple joints of the foot
seems to provide enough micromotion for the articular cartilage and joint
structures to prevent significant loss of motion. Rigid fixation of the
knee or elbow, however, can lead to cartilage deterioration and the formation
of fibrous bands which will impair ultimate joint motion. Because some loss
of motion will inevitably follow rigid fixation of a joint for more than a
few weeks, we do not advise this technique for the treatment or protection
of closed ligamentous injuries to the knee or elbow. Even when external fixation is used to maintain a joint in one position for the treatment of open
dislocations or major soft tissue injuries, the surgeon must make provisions
to restore at least some motion to the joint as early as possible. Gradual
restoration of motion can be accomplished by first loosening the rods crossing the joints to passively move the joint through a small arc of motion each
day or by replacing the rods with hinges as soon as possible.

Summary

Experience at the University of Maryland and many other centers suggests that
the Hoffmann external fixation system can facilitate management of the severely injured patient. Because Hoffmann external fixation provides both the
immediate stability and late reconstructive requirements of injured segments
without interfering with patient mobility, it can be of great benefit to the
overall care and survival of multiply injured patients in particular. Yet,
application of external fixation is but one step in the reconstructive program. It accomplishes our treatment objectives for the initial management
of severe musculoskeletal injuries by providing versatile fracture fixation,
soft tissue stability, inboard traction and good tissue access. During the
reconstructive stage of treatment, however, it often must be combined with
bone and soft tissue grafting techniques and supplemental internal fixation
to achieve optimum results in severely injured patients.

References

1. Brown, S.A., Mayor, M.B. and Merrittik: Leukocyte migration inhibition
    test for metal sensitivity. Second conference on Materials for Use in
    Medicine and Biology. Brunel University, London, September 1976.

2. Browner, B.D., Edwards, C.C., Burgess, A., Hirtz, M.H. and Baugher, W.H.:
    Hoffmann external fixation in the treatment of complex humeral fractures.
    J. Bone & Jt. Surg. Transactions, 6, 1982.

3. Browner, B.D., Kenzora, J.E. and Edwards, C.C.: The use of modified
    Neufeld traction in the management of femoral fractures in polytrauma.
    J. Trauma, 1981.

4. Bucholz, R.W.: The pathologic anatomy of Malgaigne fracture - Dislocation
    of the pelvis. J. Bone Jt. Surg. 63A, 400, 1981.

5. Edwards, C.C.: New directions in Hoffmann external fixation. In, Vidal,
    J. (ed.), Proc. 7th Internat. Conf. on Hoffmann External Fixation.
    Diffinco SA, Geneva, 1979.

6. Edwards, C.C.: Management of multisegment injuries in the polytrauma
    patients. In, Johnston, R. (ed.), Advances in External Fixation.
    Yearbook Med. Publ., Miami, 1980.

7. Edwards, C.C. and Browner, B.D.: The Application of Hoffmann External
    Fixation, pp 30. Zimmer USA, Indiana, 1981.

8. Edwards, C.C., Jaworski, M.F., Solana, J., and Aronson, B.S.: Management
    of compound tibial fractures using external fixation. Amer. Surg. 45,
    190, 1979.

9. Edwards, C.C. and Kenzora, J.E.: External fixation about the foot and
    ankle. In, Uhthoff, H.K. (ed.), Current Concepts of External Fixation.
    Springer Verlag, New York, 1981.

10. Flint, L.M., Brown, A., Richardson, D., and Polk, H.C.: Definitive con-
    trol of bleeding from severe pelvis fractures. Ann. Surg. 189, 709,
    1979.

11. Kane, W.J.: Fracture of the pelvis. In, Rockwood, C.A. and Green, D.P.
    (eds.). Fractures, J.B. Lippincott Co., Philadelphia, 1975.

12. Karaharju, E.D., and Slätis, P.: External fixation of double vertical
    pelvic fractures with a trapezoid compression frame. Injury 10, 142,
    1978.

13. Kenzora, J.E., Edwards, C.C., Browner, B.D., DeSilva, J.B., and Gamble,
    J.G.: Acute management of trauma involving the foot and ankle with
    Hoffmann external fixator. Foot & Ankle 1, 348, 1981.

14. Mears, D.C. and Fu, F.: External fixation in pelvic fractures. Orthop.
    Clin. N. Amer. 11, 465, 1980.

15. Ring, E.J., Waltman, A.C., Athanasoukis, C., et al: Angiography in pel-
    vic trauma. Surg. Gynecol. Obstet. 139, 375, 1974.

16. Riska, E.B., Von Bonsdorff, H., Hakkinen, S., et al: External fixation
    of unstable pelvic fractures. Int. Orthop. 3, 183, 1979.

17. Schurman, D.J., Johnson, L.B., and Amstutz, H.C.: Knee joint infections:
    A study of the influence of antibiotics, metal debris, hemorrhage and
    steroids in a rabbit model. J. Bone Jt. Surg. (Proc) 56A, 850, 1974.

18. Vidal, J., Buscayret, C., and Lonnes, H.: Treatment of articular frac-
    tures by "ligamentotaxis" with external fixation. In, Brooker, A.F.
    and Edwards, C.C. (eds.), External Fixation: The Current State of the
    Art, Williams & Wilkins Company, Baltimore, 1979.

Shortcomings of External Fixation

J. J. Prieto and A. M. Pankovich

Applications and indications of external fixation have been considerably
extended and modified in recent years, and new fixation frames have been
designed, produced, and used. Certain shortcomings of external fixation
in the treatment of fractures have been recognized. A discussion of these
shortcomings should include fracture healing, external fixation frames,
complications, and the site in which external fixators are being used.

Healing of Fractures

It is important to recognize the three types of fracture healing: primary
healing, secondary healing, and healing by primary intention. It is also
important to understand contributions of the following three factors:

Blood supply. In diaphyseal cortical bone, it is derived almost entirely
from the nutrient intramedullary vessels. These vessels are disrupted at
the time the fracture occurs but are restored quite rapidly. Both intramedullary and periosteal vessels are present in the metaphyseal part of a
bone. It is quite obvious that good blood supply enhances healing and
that extensive injury of soft tissues around a bone, as in open fractures,
impairs blood supply and consequently delays healing. External fixation
generally tends to preserve and improve blood supply by avoiding dissection of soft tissues and by promoting revascularization by immobilization.

Stress and motion. These represent a dynamic factor which induces formation of external and internal callus. Significant increase in stress and
motion may lead to delay in healing and nonunion, usually the hypertrophic
type. On the other hand, absence of motion and stressing is characterized
by lack of external and internal callus.

Contact and compression. The two factors between fracture fragments may
or may not be significant. Thus, if the fracture fragments are separated
and no callus is formed, nonunion may develop, usually the atrophic type.

Primary healing (Fig. 1)

Recently described (Rahn et al, 1971; Rittmann and Perren, 1974), this mechanism of healing depends on contact and compression of fracture ends and
essentially no motion (less than 5-10 microns). These conditions allow for
formation of resorption cavities across the fracture line which then fill in
concentrically and centripetally with bone lamellae. Secondary osteons are
thus formed. When fixation is very rigid, essentially no external or internal callus is formed.

416

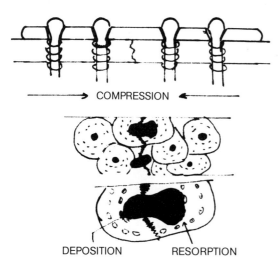

COMPRESSION

DEPOSITION   RESORPTION

Fig. 1. Primary bone healing (schematic representation). Top: Gross appearance of fracture line after application of compression to bone ends by a dynamic plate. Middle: Smaller magnification through the segment of fracture line showing a resorption in an osteon and in an interstitial area. Bottom: Larger magnification of the osteon shown in the middle, in which remodeling is occurring.

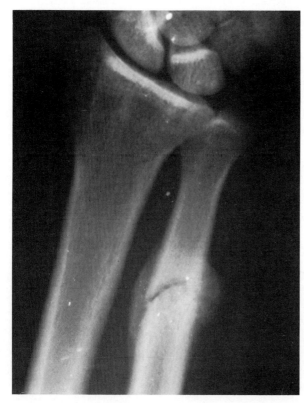

Fig. 2. Secondary (classic) healing by external and internal callus in the ulna is the result of motion at the fracture site. No immobilization was used in this case.

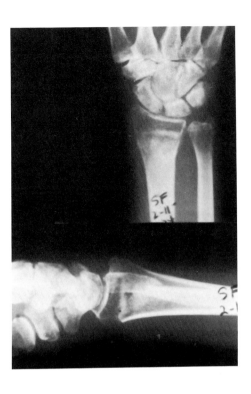

Fig. 3. Healing by primary intention. Healed Colles fracture, two months after the injury. Only endosteal callus is present.

Secondary healing (Fig. 2)

Formation of the osteocartilaginous external callus is the hallmark of this mechanism which depends on stress and motion of the fracture site. Some contact of fragments, usually cyclical, is desirable.

Healing by primary intention (Charnley et al, 1957; McLean, 1967).

This type of healing occurs typically in the femoral neck, where no periosteum exists, by endosteal fibrous callus which requires contact, compression, and rigid fixation for consolidation. This type of healing is found in the metaphyseal part of long bones where the tenuous periosteum may or may not form some external callus (Fig. 3).

Implications of various types of fracture healing become quite clear when considering the shortcomings of external fixation.

External Fixation Devices

In consideration of various external fixation frames, the following factors are important (Campbell and Kempson, 1981; Kempson and Campbell, 1981; Chao et al, 1979; Mears, 1979) (Table I):

Table I.

Device	Ease of Application	Versatility		Cost	Bulk	Rigidity
		Adjustment of Alignment	Adjustment of Rigidity			
AO old type double frame	demanding	slight lateral; none in AP and rotation	none	low	low	dependent on number of pins: high in lateral bending; low in AP bending
Hoffmann Vidal	relatively easy; requires use of a jig.	good in 3 planes	some with difficulty	high	high with double frame	varied with construction double vs. single frame
Denham (pin & cement single bar)	demanding	none	none	low	low	low
Kronner (ring-frame)	requires use of a jig	good in 3 planes	none	high	high	frame is rigid; long pins decrease rigidity
Day (Depuy)	relatively easy	good in 3 planes	none	moderate	moderate	intermediate
Fisher (Ace)	relatively easy; requires a jig	good in 3 planes	none	high	high	intermediate; allow for axial trading

Rigidity

The rigidity of an applied device, which includes the frames and the pins, can be increased by: a) increasing the diameter of the pins; b) increasing the number of pins; c) keeping the working length of the pins to a minimum; d) inserting pins in more than one plane; e) inserting anterior pins connected to a bar and even more so by connecting this single frame to side bars; f) using rectangular rather than circular bars; and, g) using double-sided frames (Chao et al, 1979).

Rigidity also depends on quality of bone and on security of engagement of bone by pins (Mears, 1979).

From Table I it is evident that various systems provide different rigidity at the fracture site, but none can be readily increased or decreased once applied. It would seemingly be advantageous if rigidity of a system could be decreased during treatment. In the beginning, more rigid construction would provide a favorable milieu for healing of soft tissues and revascularization. Later on, some motion of fracture fragments might induce formation of more abundant external and internal callus (Stone and Mears, 1981). Such a device is not yet available for general use.

Ease of application and realignment

These factors refer to the need for perfect reduction of fracture fragments and ability to realign fragments once the pins are inserted and the frame constructed. Insertion of the pins and reduction of the fracture must be perfect; yet, application of a double or single-sided frame is easy with an old AO system. On the other hand, insertion of pins and reduction of the fracture are not critical, but construction of a frame is demanding in the Hoffmann-Vidal system.

Bulk

Most external fixation devices are bulky, particularly the Kronner ring frame and the Hoffmann-Vidal double frame.

Cost

Cost is high for more versatile devices and therefore a significant shortcoming.

Complications

Pin tract infection.

The incidence of this complication in the current literature is estimated to be from 1 to 30% (Mears, 1981; Edwards, 1979). It can be minimized by avoiding skin tension and by making generous skin incisions around pins, and by cleaning skin-pin contact areas.

Pin Breakage

The risk of pin breakage can be reduced by inserting them parallel, by maintaining contact and compression at the fracture site, by keeping working
length of the pins to a minimum, by increasing the number of pins, and by
avoiding asymmetric compression (Chao et al, 1979).

Impalement of musculotendinous and
neurovascular structures

The impaling of musculotendinous structures by pins is more common and may
lead in some cases to joint stiffness.

Nonunion of fractures

Opponents of external fixation consider nonunion a direct consequence of the
method. Yet, it appears that lack or loss of contact and compression at
fracture site, bone loss, failure to graft early, infection, significant
soft tissue damage, and loss of vascularity are main causes in the development of nonunion (Lawyer and Lubber, 1980).

Refracture

This complication occurs after the device is removed, either through the
fracture site or through a pin hole, as a consequence of stress concentration and irregularities in the callus (Burny, 1979). Protection with a cast
following removal of a device, for four to six weeks, should decrease the
incidence of refracture.

Fracture Site

Upper extremity

Impalement of musculotendinous structures is a serious problem and may result
in loss of motion. Furthermore, multiplicity of neurovascular structures
make them an easy target for impalement by pins. Open exposure of bone before insertion of pins is mandatory (Mears, 1979).

Femur

The major shortcoming in the use of external fixation devices in femoral
fractures is impalement of the quadriceps muscle which commonly causes a
stiff knee. Another problem is the bulk of some devices, such as a triangular frame with Hoffmann apparatus, which is needed in extensive open fractures.

Tibia

Weight bearing is generally not allowed with external fixators in place.
Double frame and ring frame devices are bulky and cumbersome to wear and
weight bearing is difficult. Some authors permit weight bearing only in

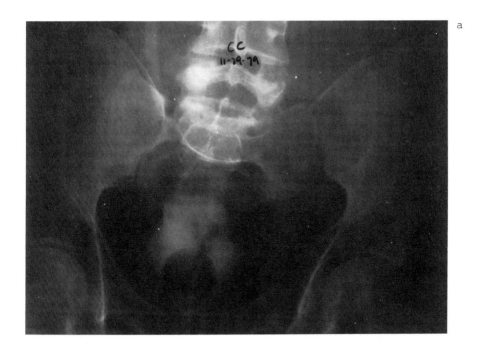

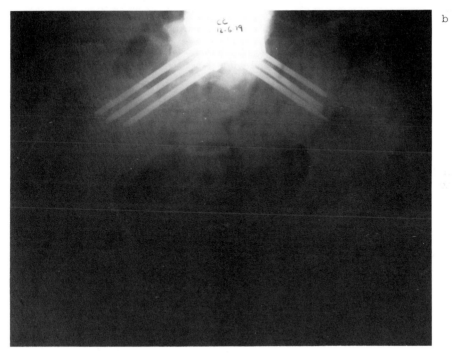

Fig. 4. Complete dislocation of the left sacroiliac joint.
a) Initial roentgenograms. b) One week after open reduction
and fixation with crossed Steinmann pins jointed by methylmethacrylate.

stable fractures, such as transverse and short oblique, but not on long oblique and spiral (Burny, 1979) and in very comminuted types. This is a major shortcoming of the method.

Pelvis

Fractures of the bony pelvis, particularly about the acetabulum, are commonly treated by open internal fixation. Sacroiliac dislocation, usually accompanied with a diastasis pubis, has been treated in pelvic sling traction, spica cast, and more recently with external fixation. In incomplete, open book dislocations (Johnson, 1979), in which the anterior sacroiliac ligaments rupture while the posterior are either intact or partially ruptured, reduction of the diastasis pubis is probably sufficient and can be conveniently accomplished by an anterior frame such as the Slätis design.

A complete sacroiliac dislocation, however, is difficult to reposition by closed reduction and difficult to keep reduced with the anterior frame. A hemihoop device (Mears, 1979) employs bilateral long iliac pins inserted through the iliac wings in an anteroposterior direction and connected with an anterior and a posterior frame. Though thus providing a stable immobilization of the sacroiliac joints, the method is demanding because of pin placement.

We have treated the unstable, displaced sacroiliac dislocation (Fig. 4a) by open reduction and found the procedure quite easy to perform. After reduction, three threaded Steinmann pins are inserted obliquely in both posterior iliac crests so that they cross each other in the midline. The pins are held in place by affixing one Hoffmann clamp at the end of each set of pins. The reduction is adjusted by sliding the clamps along the pins until an acceptable reduction is obtained. The clamps are then fixed in place with a bolus of methylmethacrylate (Fig. 4b). The patient can be turned in bed easily and allowed to sit in a chair within a week.

Shortcomings of external fixation of the pelvis are poor fixation of pins, difficulty in obtaining reduction, possibility of infection of intrapelvic hematoma, and insufficient stability of the unstable sacroiliac joint by anterior frames (Johnson 1979, Mears 1981).

References

1. Burny, F.L.: Elastic external fixation of tibial fractures. Study of 1421 cases. In, External Fixation, The Current State of the Art. The Williams and Wilkins Company, 1979.

2. Campbell, D., and Kemper, G.E.: Which external fixation device? Injury 12, 291, 1981.

3. Chao, E.Y.I., Briggs, B.T., and McCoy, M.T.: Theoretical and experimental analyses of Hoffmann-Vidal external fixation system. In, External Fixation, The Current State of the Art. Williams and Wilkins Co., 1979.

4. Charnley, B.J., and Purser, D.W.: The treatment of displaced fractures of the neck of the femur by compression. J.Bone Jt. Surg., 39B, 45, 1957.

5. Edwards, C.C.: Management of the polytrauma patient in a major U.S. center. In, External Fixation, The Current State of the Art. Williams and Wilkins, Co., 1979.

6. Johnson, R.: Stabilization of pelvic fractures with Hoffmann external fixation. In, Colorado Experience External Fixation, The Current State of the Art. Williams and Wilkins Co., 1979.

7. Kemper, G.E., and Campbell, D.: The comparative stiffness of external fixation frames. Injury, 12, 297, 1981.

8. Kronner, H.: The Kronner Circular Compression Frame. Richards Manufacturing Company, 1978.

9. Lawyer, R.B., and Lubber, L.M.: Use of Hoffmann apparatus in the treatment of unstable tibial fractures. J. Bone Jt. Surg., 62A, 1264, 1980.

10. Mears, D.C.: Materials and orthopaedic surgery. In, External Fixation, The Current State of the Art. Williams and Wilkins Co., 1979.

11. Mears, D.C.: The management of complex fractures. In, External Fixation, The Current State of the Art. Williams and Wilkins Co., 1979.

12. McLean, F.C.: Personal communication, 1967.

13. Rahn, B.A., Gallinaro, P., Baltensperger, A., and Perren, I.M.: Primary bone healing. An experimental study in the rabbit. J. Bone Jt. Surg., 53A, 783, 1971.

14. Rittmann, W.W., and Perren, I.M.: Cortical bone healing after internal fixation and infection. In, External Fixation, The Current State of the Art. Williams and Wilkins Co., 1979.

15. Stone, J.P., and Mears, D.C.: External fixation of open tibial fractures. Contemp.Orthop., 3, 310, 1981.

A New Bone Graft Substitute

V. Mooney and R. Holmes

The purpose of this presentation is to provide some information regarding the potentials for a material which appears to be as effective as autogenous graft in providing new bone formation at sites where bone deficits or delays in new bone formation exist. This material is made from sea coral by a system known as replamineform.

Weber and White (1973), at the Materials Research Laboratory of the Pennsylvania State University, recognized that the microstructure of certain scleractinian corals were similar to bone itself and might be used for the purpose of bone regeneration. The microstructural characteristics which were thought favorable to bone regeneration included: 1) channel diameters of adequate size; 2) a distribution of channel to channel interconnecting diameters nearly equal to the channel itself; 3) a high degree of permeability with a substantial void volume fraction. The coral microstructure is constructed by tiny animals (scleractinia) which secrete a calcium carbonate exoskeleton for porites. This channeled exoskeleton is about 230 micra in diameter, and the interconnecting fenestrations are about 190 micra in diameter. The void volume is approximately 65%. It seems to answer theoretic criteria.

It has been demonstrated with ceramics that bony ingrowth into porosities of over 100 micra is feasible, assuming the substrate is biocompatible, and that over 200 micra provides a more ideal environment (Hulbert, 1970). Most materials tested as a bone graft substitute in the form of a scaffolding do not have large interconnecting fenestrations; however, this is a natural event in these coral structures. Various types of hydroxyapatites and ceramics have been used but channeled void volume with interconnections is not the natural form of construction of these various materials. The structure of porites looks similar to cortical bone with the osteons removed except the interstitial bone lamellae (Fig. 1, 2). It is this similarity which presents the material as an ideal bone substitute.

The biocompatability of the limestone, however, was a limiting factor until a process named replamineform was discovered at the Pennsylvania State University. The coral calcium carbonate microstructure is converted hydrothermally to pure hydroxyapatite by a reaction with ammonium phosphate at a vapor pressure of water about 300°C (Roy and Linnehan, 1974). Preliminary studies by Chiroff (1975) demonstrated uniformly that new bone grew into the channels of the material when placed in the metaphysis of dogs. Experience at our center started with the work of Ralph Holmes (1978), chief of plastic surgery at the Dallas V.A. Hospital.

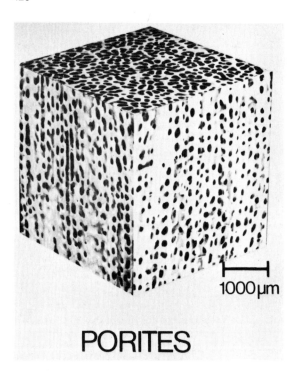

Fig. 1. Cube of porite coral. It demonstrates the interconnecting porosity and the linear alignment similar to cortical bone.

PORITES

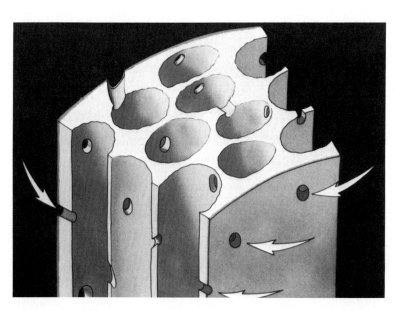

Fig. 2. Artist's representation of cortical bone with the osteons removed, thus demonstrating the interstitial bone. The similarity to porites is evident.

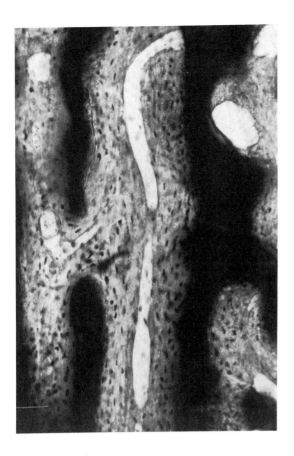

Fig. 3. Microscopic section of coral with new bone formation in the porosities. The black represents coral. The orientation of the osteons is evident with the interconnection vasculature also notable. No cartilage or fibrous tissue has ever been noted as a product of cellular activity within the coral.

The initial interest in this material was for the purpose of facial reconstruction, the first series of experimental studies being the replacement of dog mandible segments with coral. The host fragments were held in position by a metal bone tray, and the coral was placed in a 2 cm defect in the dog mandible. By six months, mature lamellar had regenerated across the 2 cm gap. One of the most significant aspects about the material, however, was that by 12 months 30% of the implant had undergone biodegradation and had been replaced by bone. Histologic examination of the soft tissue showed no evidence of inflammatory or foreign body reaction (Fig. 3, 4).

The toxicologic aspects of this material have been investigated at the Johnson and Johnson Research Center, where implants were placed in the ilium of dogs. Under these conditions, no abnormal reactions by the standard toxicologic tests could be identified.

Unfortunately, the material is more brittle than bone with an elastic modulus of $2\text{-}3 \times 10^{10}$ dyn.(cm^2) and, thus, cannot be used independent of other systems to take mechanical stress.

In an effort to evaluate the potentials for this material, several animal models have been developed. In all settings, the goal of the model was to

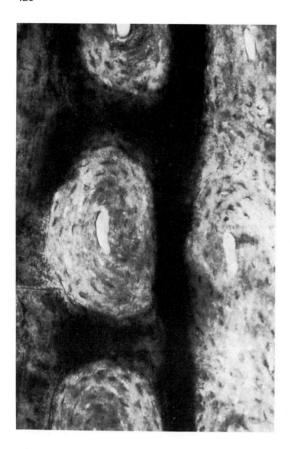

Fig. 4. Coral in cross section demonstrating the osteon-like orientation of the new bone formation. The black is the coral and, once again, cellular activity creates bone and not fibrous tissue.

compare the efficacy of the coral implant to autogenous bone graft. The models include a defect in the radius, a posterior spine fusion, and a tibial metaphyseal defect.

The experience with the radius defect has been excellent. Under these conditions in an ideal setting for new bone formation - a stable skeletal location - bone regeneration in the lattice work of the porites was extremely rapid. During the observation times of 2, 4, and 6 months, new bone was noted throughout. The defect of 2 cm, when compared to rate of new bone formation using autogenous graft, filled just as rapidly with new bone as the autogenous graft from the ilium (Fig. 5).

In the model of the posterior spine fusion, a standard lumbar facet fusion was used in the foxhound. One side was grafted with matchstick size autogenous grafts from the spinous processes of the segments operated on. The other side was filled with similar size grafts of coral. A facet fusion was accomplished in the standard manner on both sides. Findings from this study revealed that new bone formation was just as rapid in the autogenous side as on the coral side (Fig. 6). It was clear, however, that in those locations where motion was present, vascular invasion and regeneration of new bone needed for stability was initially achieved by a cartilaginous matrix filling

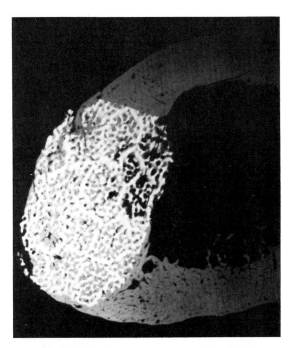

Fig. 5. Segment of dog radius which has had a coral implant. The white color is coral and the gray is bone growing into the coral in the orientation appropriate for the function of this diaphysis. (Note that no new bone formation is present in the intramedullary canal where apparently there is no biomechanical need.)

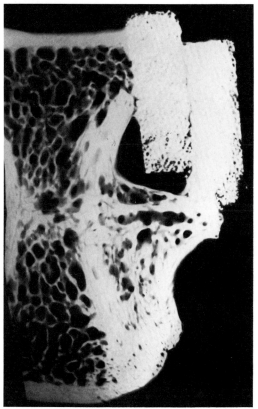

Fig. 6. Cross section of the dog spine fusion model. The autogenous bone is on the right, the coral replaced bone on the left. Again, infiltration of new bone in areas of need is noted.

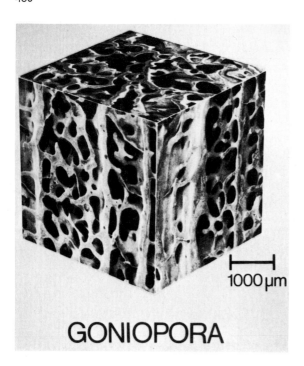

GONIOPORA

Fig. 7. Example of goniopora coral demonstrating a more cancellous-like orientation.

the space between graft and vascularized host bone. The size of this carti-laginous matrix gradually decreased until eventually solid bone traversed from host bone to graft bone. This model was an excellent demonstration of the negative effect of motion on new bone formation. Not until the system was fully stabilized by cartilaginous tissue did new bone formation develop. Thus, this is somewhat comparable to new bone formation at the epiphyseal plate.

Finally, one of the most interesting models was that of the metaphysis of a long bone - in this case the tibia of the foxhound. In this setting, a slightly different type of coral was used - one with greater porosity and void space - goniopora (Fig. 7). This coral has more of the appearance of cancellous bone and, thus, it was felt to be a more appropriate material in which cancellous bone might grow. Here again, when compared with autogenous graft filling of 1 cm defects in the metaphysis of the proximal tibia, new bone formation was avid and certainly as rapid as in the case of autogenous bone.

Consistently, at 6 months after the implant, osteoclastic activity was noted at the coral implant sites. The activity was most notable in settings where bone would not normally develop. At this point, we have no idea what signal causes the destruction of this ersatz skeletal tissue, or for that matter even what initiates new bone formation. Apparently it is stress related in that the ingrowth of bone routinely is seen in settings which provide a symmetrical distribution of forces.

One of the most remarkable aspects about this material is that because of its good biocompatibility and its now "native" structure of pure hydroxyapatite, it is not recognized as foreign. More important, as the need for the lattice changes, just as in the case of normal bone turnover, the material is removed. Thus, at points of time beginning at 6 months and well underway by 12 months, the coral hydroxyapatite is being removed in the normal manner by osteoclastic dissolution. The 2-year specimen shows nearly complete replacement of the implant material by new bone.

Thus, in summary, this material is biocompatible, has a lattice structure similar to cortical or cancellous bone, and provides an environment wherein new bone formation occurs as rapidly as in the case of autogenous grafts. New bone formation only occurs when total stability is available. Nonetheless, new bone formation will occur at depths greater than any other bone substitute material designed (2 cm in our most recent studies). Eventual use of this material, we hope, will be to provide opportunity for skeletal stability in settings wherein bone defects occurred either because of loss of tissue or due to crush of cancellous bone. Clinical trials for the material will begin later this year.

References

1. Chiroff, R.T.: Tissue ingrowth of replamineform. J. Biomed. Mat. Res. 9, 29, 1975

2. Holmes, R.E., and Salyer, K.E.: Bone regeneration in a coralline hydroxyapatite implant. Surg. Forum 24, 611, 1978.

3. Hulbert, S.F.: Potential of ceramic materials as permanently implantable skeletal prostheses. J. Biomed. Mat. Res. 4, 433, 1970.

4. Roy, D.M. and Linnehan, S.K.: Hydroxyapatite formed from coral skeletal carbonate by hydrothermal exchange. Nature 247, 220, 1974.

5. Weber, J.N., and White, E.W.: Carbonate minerals as precursors of new ceramic, metal and polymer material for biomedical applications. Min. Sc. Eng. 5, 151, 1973.

Subject Index

436

List of Contributors

BEHRENS, F.

Department of Orthopedic Surgery, St. Paul-Ramsey Medical Center, St. Paul, Minnesota, USA

BERNSTEIN, M.L.

Division of Orthopedic Surgery, University of California, Center for the Health Sciences, Los Angeles, CA 90024, USA

BISSERIÉ, M.

Hôpital de la Pitié, Paris, France

BOCK, J.J.

Department of Orthopedic and Hand Surgery, Ohio State University College of Medicine, 3545 Olentangy River Road, Suite 201, Columbus, Ohio, 43214, USA

BROWNER, B.D.

Division of Orthopedics, University of Maryland Hospital, 22 South Green Street, Baltimore, MD 21201 USA

BRUMPT, B.

Clinique Jouvenet, Paris, France

BUECHEL, R.L.

Wausau Hospital Centre, 524 Pine Ridge Boulevard, Wausau, WI 54401, USA

BURKE, D.L.

Department of Orthopedic Surgery, Montreal General Hospital, and Department of Surgery, McGill University, Montreal, Quebec, Canada

BURNY, F.

Department of Orthopaedics and Traumatology, Erasme University Hospital, Route de Lennik, 808, B-1070 Brussels, Belgium

BYRD, S.

University of Texas Health Science Center, Divisions of Orthopedic and Plastic Surgery, 5323 Harry Hines Boulevard, Dallas, Texas 75235, USA

CHERNOWITZ, A.

Berufsgenossenschaftliche Unfallklinik, Duisburg-Buchholz, West Germany

CIERNY, G., III

University of Texas Health Science Center, Divisions of Orthopedic and Plastic Surgery, 5323 Harry Hines Boulevard, Dallas, Texas 75235, USA

CLAUDI, B.	Orthopedic Trauma, Parkland Memorial Hospital, Dallas, Texas 75235, USA
DAY, B.	La Malmesbury Road, London, E18, England
DONKERWOLCKE, M.	Cliniques Universitaire de Bruxelles, Hopital Erasme. Centre Interdisciplinaire de Biomecanique Osseuse Route de Lennik, 808, 1070 Brussels, Belgium
EDWARDS, C.C.	Division of Orthopaedics, University of Maryland, Baltimore, MD 21201, USA
FERNANDEZ, D.L.	Department of Orthopedic Surgery, University of Berne, Switzerland. Klinik für Orthopädische Chirurgie, Inselspital, 3010 Bern, Switzerland
GIACHINO, A.	Division of Orthopedic Surgery, University of Ottawa, Ottawa, Canada.
GREEN, S.A.	Osteomyelitis Service, Rancho Los Amigos Hospital, Downey, CA; 389 Katella Avenus, Los Alantos, CA 90720, USA
HAX, P.-M.	Berufsgenossenschaftliche Unfallklinik, Duisburg-Buchholz, West Germany
HEDLEY, A.K.	Division of Orthopedic Surgery, University of California, Center for the Health Sciences, Los Angeles, CA 90024, USA
HELLINGER, J.	Orthopädische Klinik der Medizinischen Akademie "Carl Gustav Carus", Dresden, G.D.R.-8019 Dresden, Fetscherstrasse 74
HIERHOLZER, G.	Berufsgenossenschaftliche Unfallklinik, Duisburg-Buchholz, West Germany
HOLMES, R.	Division of Plastic Surgery, University of Texas Health Sciences Centre, and Dallas Veterans Administration Hospital, Dallas, Texas 75235, USA
JAKOB, R.P.	Department of Orthopaedic Surgery, University of Berne, Switzerland; Klinik für Orthopädische Chirurgie, Inselspital 3010, Berne, Switzerland
JONES, R.E.	University of Texas Health Science Center, Division of Orthopedic and Plastic Surgery, 5323 Harry Hines Boulevard, Dallas, Texas 75235, USA
JUDET, R.	Clinique Jouvenet, Paris, France
JUDET, Th.	Clinique Jouvenet, Hôpital de la Pitié, Paris, France

KAIRENTO, A.-L.   Division of Orthopaedic Surgery and Traumatology, Surgical Hospital, Kasarmikatu 11, 00130 Helsinki 13, Finland

KARAHARJU, E.O.   Division of Orthopaedic Surgery and Traumatology, Surgical Hospital, Kasarmikatu 11, 00130 Helsinki 13, Finland

KAUKONEN, J.-P.   Division of Orthopaedic Surgery and Traumatology, Surgical Hospital, Kasarmikatu 11, 00130 Helsinki 13, Finland

KING, J.   Department of Orthopedic Surgery, London Hospital Medical College, Whitechapel, England

KLEINING, R.   Berufsgenossenschaftliche Unfallklinik, Duisburg-Buchholz, West Germany

KLEMM, K.W.   Department of Post-traumatic Osteomyelitis, Berufsgenossenschaftliche Unfallklinik, Frankfurt am Main, Friedberger Landstrasse 430, D-600 Frankfurt am Main, West Germany

MAGERL, F.   Klinik für Orthopädische Chirurgie, Kantonsspital, 9007 St. Gallen, Switzerland

MAYER, G.   Orthopädische Klinik des Bezirkskrankenhauses Hoyerswerda, G.D.R.-7700 Hoyerswerda, Karl-Liebknecht-Strasse 1

MEARS, D.C.   University of Pittsburgh, 3601 Fifth Avenue, Pittsburgh, PA 15213, USA

MELKA, J.   Université de Montpellier (Montpellier, France) and Hôpital Saint Charles, Centre Hospitalier et Universitaire de Montpellier, France

MILLER, A.   4600 North Habana, Tampa, FLA 33614, USA

MOONEY, V.   Division of Orthopedic Surgery, University of Texas Southwestern Medical School, Dallas, Texas 65235, USA

MÜLLER, K.H.   Chirurgische Universitätsklinik "Bergmannsheil" Hundscheidtstr. 1, D-4630, Bochum, Germany

MURRAY, W.M.   Department of Orthopedic Surgery, Harrisburg Hospital, Front and Chestnut Streets, Harrisburg, PA 17101, USA

PANKOVICH, A.M.   Department of Orthopaedic Surgery, Northwestern University Medical School, Cook County Hospital, 1825 West Harrison Street, Chicago, ILL 60612, USA

PERREN, S.M.   Laboratory for Experimental Surgery, Davos,
                           Switzerland

PRIETO, J.J.   Department of Orthopaedic Surgery, Northwestern
                           University Medical School, Cook County Hospital,
                           1825 West Harrison Street, Chicago, Ill. 60612, USA

SARIC, O.   Cliniques Universitaire de Bruxelles, Hôpital
                           Erasme, Centre Interdisciplinaire de Biomecanique
                           Osseuse, Route de Lennik, 808; 1070 Brussels,
                           Belgium

SCHLÄPFER, F.   Laboratory for Experimental Surgery, Davos,
                           Switzerland

SEARLS, K.   Department of Orthopedic Surgery, St. Paul-Ramsay
                           Medical Centre, St. Paul, Minn, USA

SIGUIER, N.   Clinique Jouvenet, Paris, France

SLÄTIS, P.   Division of Orthopaedic Surgery and Traumatology
                           Surgical Hospital, Kasarmikatu 11, 00130 Helsinki 13,
                           Finland

SPIER, R.   Berufsgenossenschaftliche Unfallklinik,
                           6700 Ludwigshafen am Rhein, West Germany

STUHLER, Th.   Orthopaedic Clinic, König Ludwig Haus, University of
                           Würzburg, Würzburg, West German

VIDAL, J.   Université de Montpellier (France) and Hôpital
                           Saint-Charles, Centre Hospitalier et Universitaire
                           de Montpellier, France

WEISE, S.   Berufsgenossenschaftliche Unfallklinik, Tübingen,
                           West Germany

WELLER, S.   Berufsgenossenschaftliche Unfallklinik, Tübingen,
                           West Germany

WÖRSDÖRFER, O.   Laboratory for Experimental Surgery, Davos,
                           Switzerland

Current Concepts of Internal Fixation of Fractures

Editor: H.K. Uhthoff
Associate Editor: E. Stahl

1980. 287 figures, 51 tables. IX, 452 pages
ISBN 3-540-09846-1

Contents: Introduction. – Biomechanics of Internal Fixation. – Physical Properties and Choice of Biomaterials. – Biocompatibility of Implants. – Principles and Problems of Internal Fixation. – Screw Designs and Techniques of Insertion. – Rigid Internal Fixation: Experimental and Clinical Studies. – Less Rigid Internal Fixation: Experimental and Clinical Studies. – Intramedullary Fixation. – External Fixators.

The introduction of the compression technique for treating long bone fractures has led to numerous investigations into the mechanism of fracture healing and the factors influencing this process. Although most studies demonstrate the advantages of internal rigid fixation, heated arguments still abound as to the ideal mode of fracture fixation and fracture healing.
This book airs these arguments in a comprehensive review of the field. It contains contributions from researchers, surgeons, biomechanical engineers, traumatologists and metallurgists from all over the world. Among the reports are discussions of the advantages of rigid versus less rigid fixation. These presentations reflect the current state of applied research in internal fixation, providing researchers and clinicians with an invaluable reference source on the subject.

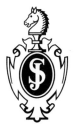

Springer-Verlag
Berlin
Heidelberg
New York

C.F. Brunner, B.G. Weber

Special Techniques in Internal Fixation

Translated by T.C. Telger
1981. 91 figures. X, 198 pages
ISBN 3-540-11056-9

J. Charnley

Low Friction Arthroplasty of the Hip

Theory and Practice
1979. 440 figures, 205 in color, 22 tables.
X, 376 pages
ISBN 3-540-08893-8

F. Freuler, U. Wiedmer, D. Bianchini

Cast Manual for Adults and Children

Forewords by A. Sarmiento, B.G. Weber
Translated from the German by P.A. Casey
1979. 121 figures in 352 separate illustrations,
2 tables. XII, 248 pages
ISBN 3-540-09590-X

U. Heim, K.M. Pfeiffer

Small Fragment Set Manual

Technique Recommended by the ASIF
Group
ASIF: Swiss Association for the Study of
Internal Fixation Translated from the
German by R.L. Batten, M.K. Pfeiffer
2nd edition. 1982. 215 figures in more than
500 separate illustration. Approx. 400 pages
ISBN 3-540-11143-3

R. Letourned, R. Judet

Fractures to the Acetabulum

Translated from the French and edited by
R.A. Elson
1980. 289 figures in 980 separate illustrations. XXI, 428 pages
ISBN 3-540-09875-5

Manual of Internal Fixation

Techniques Recommended by
the AO Group
By M.E. Müller, M. Allgöwer, R. Schneider,
H. Willenegger
In collaboration with W. Bandi, A. Boitzy,
R. Ganz, U. Heim, S.M. Perren, W.W. Rittmann, T. Rüedi, B.G. Weber, S. Weller
Translated from the German by J. Schatzker
2nd, expanded and revised edition 1979.
345 figures in color, 2 templates for Preoperative Planning. X, 409 pages
ISBN 3-540-09227-7

A. Sarmiento, L.L. Latta

Closed Functional Treatment of Fractures

1981. 545 figures, 85 tables. XII, 608 pages
ISBN 3-540-10384-8
Distribution rights for Japan:
Igaku Shoin Ltd, Tokyo

F. Séquin, R. Texhammar

AO/ASIF Instrumentation

Manual of Use and Care Introduction and
Scientific Aspects by H. Willenegger
Translated from the German by T.C. Telger
1981. Approx. 1300 figures. 17 separate
Checklists. XVI, 306 pages
ISBN 3-540-10337-6

Treatment of Fractures in Children and Adolescents

Editors: B.G. Weber, C. Brunner, F. Freuler
with contributions by numerous experts
1980. 462 figures, 27 tables. XII, 410 pages
ISBN 3-540-09313-3

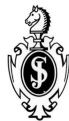

Springer-Verlag
Berlin
Heidelberg
New York